Lippincott's Illustrated Q&A Review of

Microbiology & Immunology

B. A. Buxton, PhD

Professor
Department of Pathology, Microbiology, Immunology,
and Forensic Medicine
Philadelphia College of Osteopathic Medicine-Georgia Campus
Suwanee, GA

Lauritz A. Jensen, DA

Professor and Chair,
Department of Microbiology and Immunology
Midwestern University
Glendale, AZ

Randal K. Gregg, PhD

Assistant Professor
Department of Pathology, Microbiology, Immunology,
and Forensic Medicine
Philadelphia College of Osteopathic Medicine-Georgia Campus
Suwanee, GA

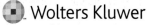 Wolters Kluwer | Lippincott Williams & Wilkins
Health

Philadelphia · Baltimore · New York · London
Buenos Aires · Hong Kong · Sydney · Tokyo

D0911481

Acquisitions Editor: Susan Rhyner
Managing Editor: Kelley A. Squazzo
Marketing Manager: Jennifer Kuklinski
Designer: Doug Smock
Compositor: Spi

First Edition

Library of Congress Cataloging-in-Publication Data

Buxton, B. A. (Bonnie A.)
  Lippincott's illustrated Q&A review of microbiology and immunology / B.A. Buxton, Lauritz A. Jensen, Randal K. Gregg. — 1st ed.
       p. ; cm.
  Includes bibliographical references and index.
  ISBN 978-1-58255-857-8 (alk. paper)
1. Microbiology—Outlines, syllabi, etc. 2. Microbiology—Examinations, questions, etc. 3. Immunology—Outlines, syllabi, etc. 4. Immunology—Examinations, questions, etc. I. Jensen, Lauritz A. II. Gregg, Randal K. III. Title. IV. Title: Illustrated Q&A review of microbiology and immunology. V. Title: Lipppincott's illustrated Q and A review of microbiology and immunology.
  [DNLM: 1. Microbiological Phenomena—Examination Questions. 2. Immune System Phenomena—Examination Questions. QW 18.2 B991L 2010]

  QR62.B89 2010
  616.9'041—dc22

                                                                    2009020547

DISCLAIMER

Care has been taken to confirm the accuracy of the information present and to describe generally accepted practices. However, the authors, editors, and publisher are not responsible for errors or omissions or for any consequences from application of the information in this book and make no warranty, expressed or implied, with respect to the currency, completeness, or accuracy of the contents of the publication. Application of this information in a particular situation remains the professional responsibility of the practitioner; the clinical treatments described and recommended may not be considered absolute and universal recommendations.

The authors, editors, and publisher have exerted every effort to ensure that drug selection and dosage set forth in this text are in accordance with the current recommendations and practice at the time of publication. However, in view of ongoing research, changes in government regulations, and the constant flow of information relating to drug therapy and drug reactions, the reader is urged to check the package insert for each drug for any change in indications and dosage and for added warnings and precautions. This is particularly important when the recommended agent is a new or infrequently employed drug.

Some drugs and medical devices presented in this publication have Food and Drug Administration (FDA) clearance for limited use in restricted research settings. It is the responsibility of the health-care provider to ascertain the FDA status of each drug or device planned for use in their clinical practice.

To purchase additional copies of this book, call our customer service department at (800) 638–3030 or fax orders to (301) 223–2320. International customers should call (301) 223–2300.

Visit Lippincott Williams & Wilkins on the Internet: http://www.lww.com. Lippincott Williams & Wilkins customer service representatives are available from 8:30 am to 6:00 pm, EST.

Dedication

This book is dedicated to our mentors who trained us, our students
who challenge us, and our families for their constant support.

Preface

Lippincott's Illustrated Q&A Review of Microbiology and Immunology presents essential concepts of medical microbiology and immunology for students preparing for Step 1 of the United States Medical Licensing Examination (USMLE) and the Comprehensive Osteopathic Medical Licensing Examination (COMLEX). Questions are written in the clinical vignette-style used on these examinations. Clinical vignette-style questions help develop problem-solving skills by requiring students to integrate a patient's clinical manifestations, history, and demographic information with physical exam findings and laboratory data to identify the disease and choose the correct management options. The questions also assess the student's ability to integrate basic and clinical science in order to solve problems. The questions are written at the level of competence expected of students who perform well on medical licensure examinations.

Many questions have accompanying photomicrographs. Complete explanations are provided for the answers, as well as each distracter. Questions are divided by chapter into the following categories: Bacteriology, Virology, Mycology, Parasitology, Infectious Diseases, Basic Immunology, and Clinical Immunology.

The review book is also designed to be used by medical students and allied health students as a companion to various microbiology and immunology textbooks. Use of this book will facilitate classroom learning and provide students with an opportunity for self-assessment in these two disciplines. Questions are also presented online. Students can work through the online questions in either "quiz" or "test" mode.

B.A. Buxton

Reviewers

Neal R. Chamberlain, PhD
Associate Professor
Department of Microbiology and Immunology
A.T. Still University of Health Sciences/KCOM
Kirksville, MO

Michael J. Parmely, PhD
Professor and Interim Chair
Microbiology, Molecular Genetics, and
Immunology
The University of Kansas
Lawrence, KS

Olivia Cronin
Medical Student
Loyola University Chicago-Stritch School
of Medicine
Chicago, IL

Sanjeet Patel
Medical Student
Baylor College of Medicine
Houston, TX

Pete Pelletier
Medical Student
University of Utah School of Medicine
Salt Lake City, UT

Niket Sonpal
Research Intern
Department of Gastroenterology
Brooklyn Queens Health Care
Brooklyn, NY

Garrick Tong
Resident
Department of Psychiatry
University of California, CA

Nathan Zilbert
Medical Student
New York University, NY

Contents

Preface v

Reviewers vii

Chapter 1 Bacteriology 1

Chapter 2 Virology 35

Chapter 3 Mycology 63

Chapter 4 Parasitology 79

Chapter 5 Infectious Diseases 109

Chapter 6 Basic Immunology 141

Chapter 7 Clinical Immunology 155

Figure Credits 176

Index 178

Chapter 1

Bacteriology

QUESTIONS

Select the best answer.
The next two questions are linked.

1 A 67-year-old diabetic woman is hospitalized with a 3-day history of fever, headache, diarrhea, dyspnea, and a cough productive of scant sputum. A chest radiograph reveals patchy, multilobar consolidation. No organisms are seen on sputum Gram stain; however, culture of sputum and blood on buffered charcoal yeast extract agar and blood agar are shown in the photograph. Bacteria from the colonies, stained with basic fuchsin, are also shown. Direct fluorescent antibody staining of cultured bacteria leads to a definitive diagnosis. With which organism is this woman infected?

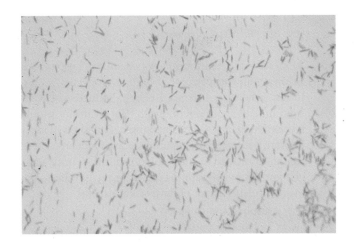

(A) *Actinomyces israelii*
(B) *Corynebacterium diphtheriae*
(C) *Haemophilus influenzae*
(D) *Legionella pneumophila*
(E) *Nocardia asteroides*

2 What is the source of infection for the patient in the above question?
(A) Aerosolized spores from soil
(B) Aerosols from contaminated water
(C) Colonization of the upper airways
(D) Inapparent carrier of the organism
(E) Person with the same disease

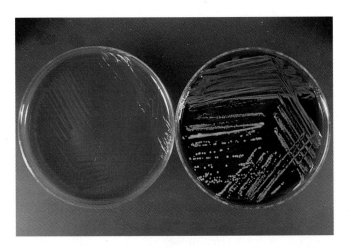

3 A 5-year-old child died from severe septic shock, disseminated intravascular coagulation, and cardiac insufficiency following a sudden onset of fever, severe headache, and vomiting. The causative agent, a Gram-negative diplococcus, was isolated from blood and cerebrospinal fluid (CSF) on Thayer–Martin agar and was also identified in CSF by latex agglutination. What is the most important virulence factor involved in disease production by the etiologic agent in this case?

1

(A) Exotoxin production
(B) Flagella
(C) Lipooligosaccharide
(D) Pili
(E) Polysaccharide capsule

4 Vaccination against which bacterial species has been most successful at reducing the number of cases of invasive diseases, including meningitis?
(A) *Escherichia coli* K1
(B) *Haemophilus influenzae* b
(C) *Listeria monocytogenes*
(D) *Neisseria meningitidis*
(E) *Streptococcus pneumoniae*

5 A 56-year-old renal transplant patient was hospitalized following an abrupt onset of high fever (39.6°C), confusion, headache, diarrhea, a cough productive of scant sputum, and shortness of breath. His chemistry profile revealed hyponatremia. A chest radiograph showed lobar infiltrates. Gram stain of sputum showed numerous neutrophils but failed to show any organisms. A urine antigen test was positive for the causative agent. What is the major virulence factor of the causative agent?
(A) Antiphagocytic capsule
(B) Cord factor
(C) Exotoxin production
(D) Intracellular growth
(E) Pyocyanin

6 A steer dies on a ranch in North Dakota and a veterinarian is consulted. Histological sections of the spleen from the deceased animal show evidence of a bacterial causative agent (shown in the photograph). The bacterium was also cultured aerobically on blood agar. Which of the following substances is associated with increased virulence of this isolate, and if detected, would alarm the state health officials and result in a more extensive investigation at the national level?

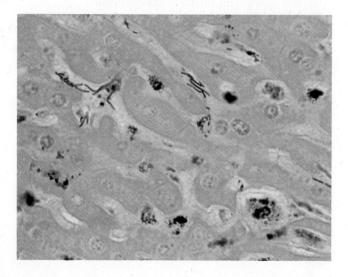

(A) Capsule
(B) H antigen
(C) Hemolysin
(D) Lipid A
(E) Lipoteichoic acid

The next two questions are linked.

7 Infected pressure sores were observed on the buttock of an elderly, bedridden patient recently treated for a malignancy of the rectum. Some of the lesions are conspicuously necrotic, exceptionally painful to the touch, and readily give off a musty sweet odor. Moreover, these lesions seem to have developed overnight. A Gram stain of the watery discharge from one of the lesions reveals an abundance of bacteria (shown in the photograph). What is the most likely diagnosis?

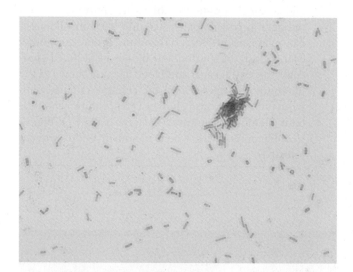

(A) Clostridial gas gangrene
(B) *Pseudomonas* ecthyma gangrenosum
(C) Staphylococcal cellulitis
(D) Staphylococcal pyomyositis
(E) Streptococcal necrotizing fasciitis

8 Which virulence factor is most important when considering the pathology of this case?
(A) α-Toxin (lecithinase)
(B) Enterotoxin
(C) Pyocyanin
(D) Pyrogenic exotoxin A
(E) Streptolysin S

9 While planting a tree, a man punctured his foot through his tennis shoe with the prongs of a rake. He was not initially concerned with the wound and washed it only superficially. At 4:00 AM, he awakened with excruciating pain in the foot and sought medical care at the emergency department. The lesion was cleaned and excised of devitalized tissue and an IV β-lactam antibiotic was administered, which subsequently cleared the infection. A Gram stain of an anaerobic culture taken from wound secretions is shown. Of the following microbial groups, which is most compatible with this case?

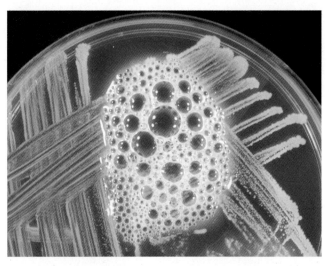

(A) β-lactamase
(B) Catalase
(C) Coagulase
(D) Staphylokinase
(E) Streptokinase

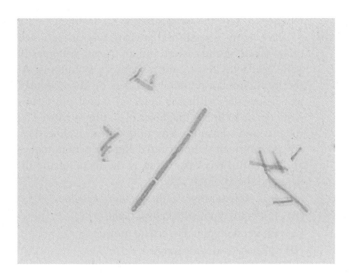

(A) Actinomycetes
(B) Clostridia
(C) Pseudomonads
(D) Staphylococci
(E) Streptococci

The next three questions are linked.

10 A patient injured herself at home in the garden, and after several days, the resulting skin lesion became infected and intensely painful and she sought medical help. Culture of the wound grew Gram-positive cocci that were β-hemolytic on blood agar. On nutrient agar, the organism produced effervescence when hydrogen peroxide was added to the colonies (shown in the photograph). What is the enzyme responsible for this bubbling?

11 Of the following organisms, what is the patient most likely infected with?
(A) *Clostridium* sp.
(B) *Enterococcus*
(C) Group A *Streptococcus*
(D) *Meningococcus*
(E) Methicillin-resistant *Staphylococcus aureus* (MRSA)

12 Based on these initial findings, what is the best antibiotic choice for the patient in the above case?
(A) Amoxicillin/clavulanate
(B) Cephalexin
(C) Dicloxacillin
(D) Polymyxin B
(E) Trimethoprim–sulfamethoxazole (TMP–SMZ)

13 A pediatric patient with a persistent cough is evaluated for sinopulmonary disease. History and physical examination determines that the child suffers from nasal polyps and, possibly, chronic airway obstruction. A sputum sample produces several bacterial species, including *Haemophilus influenzae* and a mucoid variety of *Pseudomonas aeruginosa*. Which of the following is the most likely diagnosis?
(A) Bronchiolitis
(B) Chronic obstructive pulmonary disease (COPD)
(C) Cystic fibrosis
(D) Interstitial pneumonia
(E) Sarcoidosis

14 During a medical mission to tropical Latin America, a woman presents with a chronic infection of her foot as seen in the accompanying photograph. Secretions from the lesions, upon Gram staining, clearly reveal the presence of filamentous Gram-positive cells. Which bacterial species is descriptive of the offending agent?

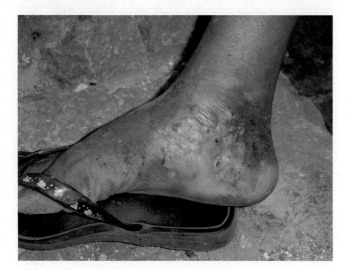

- (A) *Actinomyces israelii*
- (B) *Blastomyces dermatitidis*
- (C) *Clostridium perfringens*
- (D) *Mycobacterium leprae*
- (E) *Streptococcus pyogenes*

The next two questions are linked.

15 In early July, a middle-aged African-American male from rural southwestern Missouri is brought to regional urgent care facility. He has been vomiting most of the night and is currently febrile. Furthermore, he complains of "achy muscles" and a throbbing headache. Rales are detected on auscultation. Physical examination reveals a petechial rash on the forearms, and an engorged tick is removed from the groin area. Considering the particulars of this case, which of the following is the most crucial action that should be taken for successful management and a positive outcome?
- (A) Aggressive management of fluid intake to prevent rehydration
- (B) Chest radiographic study to rule out interstitial pneumonia
- (C) Gram stain clean-catch urine sample for evidence of a urinary tract infection (UTI)
- (D) Immediate initiation of doxycycline
- (E) Submit a blood sample for immunodiagnosis to the lab

16 With regard to the above case, which laboratory results would be most useful in confirming the clinical diagnosis?
- (A) Intracytoplasmic inclusions in McCoy tissue culture cells
- (B) Positive bacterial growth on selective and differential media
- (C) Twofold increase in a Weil–Felix Proteus OX-19 titer
- (D) Type-specific latex agglutination antibody titer of 1:64
- (E) Visualization of bacteria in the tissue by means of Gram stain

17 A Peace Corps agricultural advisor, who is stationed on an island in the eastern Indian Ocean, becomes ill with headache, fever, and respiratory symptoms. At the local clinic, a prominent eschar on the abdomen just below the beltline is detected. Local physicians easily make a clinical diagnosis of an illness carried by rodents and transmitted by mites. Doxycycline therapy is empirically administered and the patient makes an uneventful recovery. What is the name of the illness and the etiologic agent?
- (A) Brill–Zinsser disease/*Rickettsia rickettsiae*
- (B) Endemic typhus/*Rickettsia typhi*
- (C) Epidemic typhus/*Rickettsia prowazeki*
- (D) Q fever/*Coxiella burnetii*
- (E) Scrub typhus/*Orientia tsutsugamushi*

The next two questions are linked.

18 Physicians and state epidemiologists investigate a cluster of acute diarrheal cases in children who attend a preschool in a small Midwestern town. The children presented with fever, acute episodes of bloody diarrhea, and petechial rash or purpura. Two of the children have scanty urine output and are showing signs of renal failure. Fecal leukocytes and parasites are absent in microscopic smears, and no obvious pathogens are identified using standard microbiologic media. What is the most common infectious agent consistent with this clinical picture?
- (A) *Bacillus cereus*
- (B) Enterohemorrhagic *Escherichia coli* (EHEC)
- (C) *Salmonella typhi*
- (D) *Shigella flexneri*
- (E) *Yersinia enterocolitica*

19 The preschool in the above case only serves pasteurized milk and packaged cookies to the children and epidemiologists quickly rule out a food source as the risk factor. With this in mind, which of the following is the most plausible means by which the children were infected?

(A) Contagious transmission from an infected child

(B) Drinking water of the preschool is contaminated with the microbe

(C) Failure to wash hands after visiting a petting zoo

(D) Fecal–oral transmission, most likely from the restroom

(E) Visiting the elderly in an assisted-living or nursing home facility

The next three questions are linked.

20 Medical outreach physicians, working in a refugee camp in central Africa, are concerned with the number of young children presenting with high fever, bloody diarrhea, and dehydration. The crowded living conditions of the camp suggest person-to-person contact, but because of the remoteness of the site only limited laboratory studies are available. The suspected culprit is described as a nonmotile, Gram-negative bacillus that does not produce lactose-positive colonies on selective media. Based on these findings, which disease is more likely?

(A) Bacillary dysentery

(B) Campylobacteriosis

(C) Cholera (O:1 classic biotype)

(D) Nontyphoidal salmonellosis

(E) Staphylococcal food poisoning

21 A major virulence factor of the etiologic agent in the above question is a toxin. What is the role of this toxin in disease production?

(A) Acts as a superantigen thereby inducing inflammation

(B) Blocks protein synthesis causing intestinal cell death

(C) Increases cAMP concentration within intestinal cells

(D) Increases cGMP concentration within intestinal cells

(E) Suppresses cytokine secretion by immune cells

22 What is the proper course of action the physicians should take with regard to the management of the outbreak described in the above case?

(A) Advise patients to increase their vitamin intake due to the effects of diarrhea

(B) Avoid antibiotics and allow the symptoms to abate naturally

(C) Avoid contact with animal reservoirs to prevent reintroduction of the organism into the community

(D) Prescribe antimotility drugs to reduce transmission

(E) Treat affected patients with antibiotics

The next three questions are linked.

23 During the summer in western Massachusetts, a teenager complains of aching muscles and joints and mild fever. He notices a rash on the side of his upper leg (shown in the photograph), which prompts his mother to take him to the clinic. What is the most likely etiology and route of transmission?

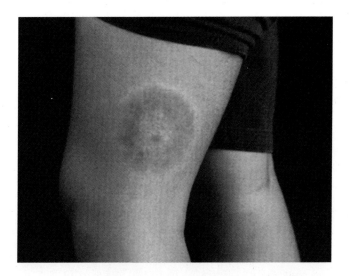

(A) *Borrelia burgdorferi*/tick bite

(B) *Ehrlichia chaffeensis*/tick bite

(C) *Francisella tularensis*/deer fly bite

(D) *Leptospira interrogans*/rodent bite

(E) Necrotic arachnidism/spider bite

24 How would the physician determine the diagnosis in the above case?

(A) CBC assessment and visualization of the microbe from the lesion by dark field microscopy

(B) History and clinical presentation of the patient plus elevated liver function tests

(C) History and clinical presentation of the patient alone

(D) Culture of the organism from blood and synovial fluid

(E) Serologic tests to detect antibodies in the patient serum against the organism

25 With regard to the above case, what is the drug of choice?

(A) Ceftriaxone

(B) Chloramphenicol

(C) Doxycycline

(D) Metronidazole

(E) Streptomycin

26 A 7-year-old female child is taken to an urgent care facility because of fever and periodic incontinence. The physician suspects a urinary tract infection. What is the most likely etiology of this child's infection?
(A) *Escherichia coli*
(B) *Proteus mirabilis*
(C) *Pseudomonas aeruginosa*
(D) *Staphylococcus saprophyticus*
(E) *Ureaplasma urealyticum*

The next two questions are linked.

27 During a gynecologic office visit, a positive leukocyte esterase test of the urine along with a voiding symptom prompts the physician to order a urine culture. The bacterium, which was isolated in clinically significant numbers, grows profusely on MacConkey agar, as shown in the accompanying photograph, and ferments lactose. Which of the following cellular attributes is most important in determining virulence and classifying this microbe as a uropathogen?

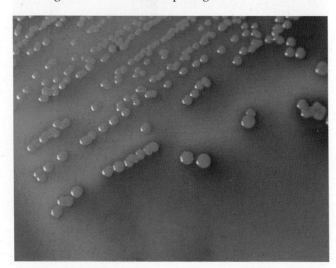

(A) β-lactamase
(B) Fimbriae
(C) Flagella
(D) Glycocalyx
(E) Urease

28 With reference to the above case, what is the most likely source and mode of transmission for this urinary bacterial isolate?
(A) Contamination with perianal and bowel flora
(B) Hematogenous spread from the kidneys
(C) Inadvertent inoculation with commensal organisms on skin
(D) Transmission from an uncircumcised sexual partner
(E) Waterborne spread

The next two questions are linked.

29 A 78-year-old hospitalized male with an indwelling catheter develops a new onset of fever. The urine sample has an alkaline pH. The bacterium isolated from the urine is a urease-producing, highly motile, Gram-negative bacillus. What is the most likely complication of this infection?
(A) Deposition of antigen–antibody complexes in the glomeruli
(B) Development of epididymitis
(C) Development of prostatitis
(D) Formation of struvite kidney stones
(E) Rapid dissemination throughout the body

30 What is the pathogen most likely involved in the above case?
(A) *Escherichia coli*
(B) *Proteus mirabilis*
(C) *Pseudomonas aeruginosa*
(D) *Staphylococcus saprophyticus*
(E) *Ureaplasma urealyticum*

The next two questions are linked.

31 An 85-year-old male nursing home patient with a history of alcoholism suddenly developed a flu-like illness. He complained of chills and fever and had frequent coughing spells productive of thick, bloody sputum. The attending physician diagnosed bronchopneumonia and prescribed antibiotics, but regrettably the patient died within a week. What is the most likely cause of the patient's pneumonia?
(A) *Haemophilus influenzae*
(B) *Klebsiella pneumoniae*
(C) *Legionella pneumophila*
(D) *Mycoplasma pneumoniae*
(E) *Streptococcus pneumoniae*

32 A bacterium, cultured on MacConkey agar (shown in the photograph), was isolated from sputum and blood of the patient in the above case. What is the primary function of the pathogenicity determinant depicted in this photo?

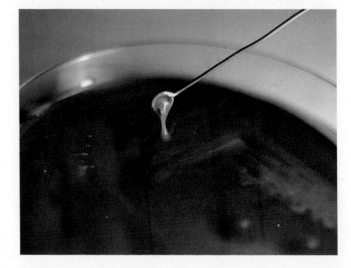

(A) Antiphagocytic, unless opsonization occurs

(B) Degrades secretory IgA on mucosal surfaces

(C) Inhibits the function of complement

(D) Lyses neutrophils and macrophages

(E) Protease activity and disrupts membranes

33 A bacterium was isolated from the central nervous system of a newborn that died of meningitis. The vagina of the mother was colonized with the same isolate as determined by the capsular antigen. The microbe grew well on standard blood and MacConkey agar at ambient atmospheric conditions. What is the most likely etiologic agent?

(A) *Escherichia coli* K1

(B) Group B *Streptococcus* type III capsule

(C) *Haemophilus influenzae* type b

(D) *Neisseria meningitidis* serogroup b

(E) *Streptococcus pneumoniae* (encapsulated variety)

34 An adult tourist visiting a remote area of Guatemala developed fever, prostration, malaise, dysentery, and dehydration. Based on current epidemiologic data of the region, a local physician reported that the causative agent was probably a diarrheogenic strain of *Escherichia coli* and did not prescribe antibiotic therapy. Presuming the Guatemalan doctor to be correct, which type of virulent *E. coli* is most consistent with this clinical picture?

(A) Enteroaggregative *E. coli* (EAEC)

(B) Enterohemorrhagic *E. coli* (EHEC)

(C) Enteroinvasive *E. coli* (EIEC)

(D) Enteropathogenic *E. coli* (EPEC)

(E) Enterotoxigenic *E. coli* (ETEC)

The next two questions are linked.

35 A 40-year-old man presented with a rubeola-like rash on the extremities, chills, fever, myalgia, and malaise 5 days after returning from a June fishing trip in Arkansas. A history of tick bites is noted and Rocky Mountain spotted fever (RMSF) is suspected. What is the etiologic agent of this disease?

(A) *Babesia microti*

(B) *Orientia tsutsugamushi*

(C) *Rickettsia prowazeki*

(D) *Rickettsia rickettsii*

(E) *Rickettsia typhi*

36 With reference to the above question, which antimicrobial agent should be employed?

(A) Chloramphenicol

(B) Ciprofloxacin

(C) Doxycycline

(D) Penicillin G

(E) TMP–SMZ

37 A previously healthy woman became nauseated and vomits 12 hours after eating home-pickled eggs. Within 24 hours, she developed a diffuse flaccid paralysis and respiratory impairment, necessitating hospitalization and mechanical ventilation. Other symptoms included diplopia and dysarthria. What is the most likely diagnosis?

(A) Botulism

(B) Brucellosis

(C) Gastrointestinal anthrax

(D) Legionellosis

(E) Meningococcal disease

The next three questions are linked.

38 A 52-year-old woman presented with indigestion and heartburn occurring shortly after meals which she treated with over-the-counter antacids. Physical examination revealed mild epigastric tenderness. A radiolabeled-urea breath test is positive. What is the most probable etiologic agent?

(A) *Campylobacter jejuni*

(B) *Clostridium difficile*

(C) *Helicobacter pylori*

(D) *Shigella dysenteriae*

(E) *Yersinia enterocolitica*

39 What cancer is the patient in the above case at risk for as a consequence of this infection?

(A) Pancreatic cancer

(B) Gastric adenocarcinoma

(C) Hepatoma

(D) Colon cancer

(E) Esophageal cancer

40 What virulence factor of the organism may be associated with induction of this cancer?

(A) cagA

(B) Heat shock protein B

(C) Mucinase

(D) Urease

(E) Vacuolating cytotoxin

41 Hemorrhagic colitis, hemolytic uremic syndrome, and thrombotic thrombocytopenic purpura are clinical manifestations of which bacterial species?

(A) *Campylobacter jejuni*

(B) *Escherichia coli* O157:H7

(C) *Shigella flexneri*

(D) *Vibrio cholerae*

(E) *Yersinia enterocolitica*

42 Over the course of a summer, several patients present to hospitals in the northwestern United States with complaints of fever, chills, headache, and other viral-like symptoms. Reportedly, with many of these patients, the fever subsides only to return with a vengeance later. Of significance is that spirochetes are observed in peripheral blood smears. Another common denominator is that all patients are outdoor enthusiasts and frequently engage in activities like camping, fishing, and hiking in mountainous areas. What is the most likely etiologic agent?

(A) *Borrelia hermsii*
(B) *Treponema pallidum*
(C) *Rickettsia rickettsiae*
(D) *Proteus vulgaris*
(E) *Vibrio vulnificus*

The next three questions are linked.

43 A 23-year-old male presents with ulcerated lesions on the penis as shown in the accompanying photograph as well as marked unilateral inguinal lymphadenopathy. The lymph node, however, is not particularly painful to the touch. The patient denies abnormal discharge and any discomfort during intercourse. He is presently afebrile. Consistent with the presentation, what is the probable causative etiology?

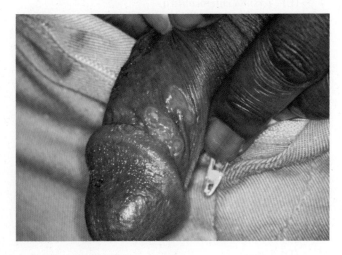

(A) *Chlamydia trachomatis*
(B) *Haemophilus ducreyi*
(C) *Neisseria gonorrhoeae*
(D) *Treponema pallidum*
(E) *Trichomonas vaginalis*

44 The 20-year-old pregnant partner of the above patient presented with a 2-week history of flu-like symptoms. Physical examination reveals a generalized nontender lymphadenopathy and numerous discrete cutaneous hyperpigmentations on the soles of the feet as shown in the accompanying photograph. Which of the following laboratory procedures would give you a definitive diagnosis?

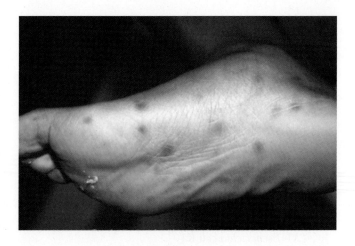

(A) Bacteriologic culture
(B) Giemsa-stained histological section
(C) Gram-stained smear
(D) Growth in cell culture
(E) Specific antibody test

45 Assuming that the patient in the above case has no drug allergies, which antibiotic would be the best choice for treatment?

(A) Ciprofloxacin
(B) Doxycycline
(C) Metronidazole
(D) Penicillin
(E) TMP–SMZ

46 A 5-day postoperative patient develops a high fever. An IV catheter is removed and culture of the tip reveals Gram-positive cocci believed to be *Staphylococcus aureus*. Which of the following laboratory test results would further support this belief?

(A) α-Hemolysis on blood agar
(B) Bacitracin sensitivity
(C) Coagulase positivity
(D) Lactose fermentation
(E) Urea hydrolysis

47 A high school student who was appropriately immunized with the diphtheria–tetanus–acellular pertussis (DTaP) series by kindergarten, but who had received no additional boosters since, stepped on a nail while walking barefoot. The nail was easily removed and the lesion freely bled. What should the student be given?

(A) Equine tetanus antitoxin
(B) Human tetanus immune globulin
(C) Prophylactic antibiotic treatment for *Clostridium tetani*
(D) No treatment
(E) Tetanus toxoid

The next two questions are linked.

48 The Gram-stained smear of urethral exudate from a male (shown in the photo) is diagnostic for which disease?

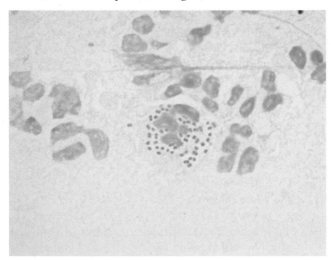

(A) Chancroid
(B) Gonorrhea
(C) Lymphogranuloma venereum
(D) Nongonococcal urethritis
(E) Primary syphilis

49 What is the appropriate therapy for the patient in the above case, assuming no further tests were conducted?
(A) Ceftriaxone
(B) Ceftriaxone plus azithromycin
(C) Ciprofloxacin
(D) Penicillin
(E) Tetracycline

50 A 24-year-old woman presents with a vagina discharge that is characterized by a thin milky appearance, a marked amine odor, and a pH of 4.5. A Gram-stain of the vaginal discharge is shown in the photograph. What is the most likely diagnosis?

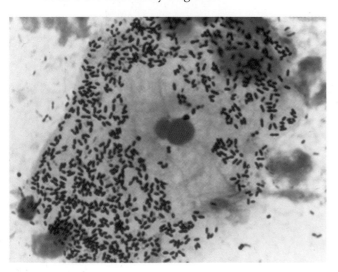

(A) Atrophic vaginitis
(B) Bacterial vaginosis
(C) Gonorrhea
(D) Group B strep colonization
(E) *Trichomonas vaginalis* infection

51 A tube dilution panel for a particular antibiotic gives results as illustrated in the accompanying photograph. With regard to the sensitivity of this particular bacterial isolate to the antibiotic tested, which statement is true?

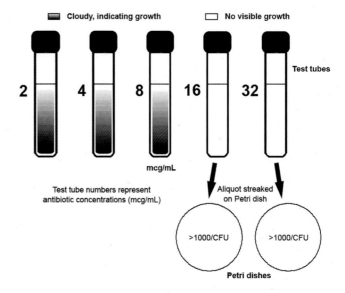

(A) Results reflect the bacteriostatic properties of the antibiotic
(B) The antibiotic is bactericidal at all tube dilution concentrations
(C) The minimum inhibitory concentration (MIC) is 8 mcg/mL
(D) The MIC is >32 mcg/mL
(E) The minimum bactericidal concentration (MBC) is 16 mcg/mL

52 A preschool-aged child from Georgia is hospitalized because of edema and hematuria. Of note is that the child was recently successfully treated for a pyoderma (see photo). Which microbe is likely associated with this child's condition?

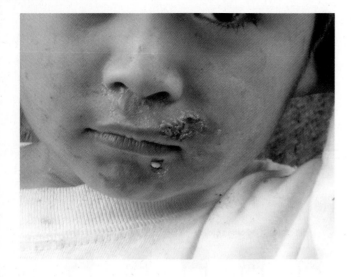

(A) Acid-fast *Nocardia asteroides* complex
(B) Coagulase-negative *Staphylococcus*
(C) *Escherichia coli* or related Gram-negative enteric
(D) Group A *Streptococcus*
(E) *Pseudomonas aeruginosa*

The next two questions are linked.

53 A 37-year-old man presented with a 2 day history of low grade fever, abdominal cramps diarrhea, nausea, and vomiting. One day prior to the onset of symptoms, six family members had eaten at an all-you-can-eat fried chicken buffet. Two other members of his family (his 82-year-old mother and a 14-month-old son) had similar symptoms. Examination of a fecal smear from the patient revealed abundant fecal leukocytes. Which of the following laboratory profiles is consistent with the most likely microbial cause of this man's condition?
(A) Aerobic, β-hemolytic, spore-forming Gram-positive rod
(B) Bacitracin-sensitive, Gram-negative cocci
(C) Coagulase-negative, Gram-positive cocci
(D) Nonlactose fermenting, Gram-negative bacilli
(E) Oxidase-positive, motile, curved, Gram-positive bacilli

54 Which of the following medications, if taken by the man in the above case, could have increased his susceptibility to the infection he developed?
(A) Acetaminophen
(B) Antacids
(C) β-Blockers
(D) Ibuprofen
(E) Statins

55 Which of the following bacterial agents has the lowest infective dose for producing gastrointestinal disease in the human host?
(A) Enteropathogenic *Escherichia coli*
(B) Enterotoxigenic *Escherichia coli*
(C) *Salmonella* (nontyphoid serotypes)
(D) *Shigella flexneri*
(E) *Vibrio cholerae*

56 Intestinal infection with which of the following organisms should not be treated with antibiotics?
(A) *Clostridium difficile*
(B) *Escherichia coli* O157:H7
(C) *Salmonella typhi*
(D) *Shigella sonnei*
(E) *Vibrio cholera*

57 Fimbriae-mediated adherence to intestinal epithelial cells, type III secretion system-mediated endocytosis and transport to the lamina propria to elicit a localized inflammatory response are descriptive of the infectivity and pathogenesis of which diarrheogenic agent?
(A) *Campylobacter jejuni*
(B) *Clostridium difficile*
(C) Enterotoxigenic *Escherichia coli*
(D) *Salmonella* sp.
(E) *Vibrio cholerae*

58 A critically ill patient, who has a Foley catheter, develops a serious UTI. The organism is identified as a motile, nonurease-producing, Gram-negative enteric bacillus with a high degree of antibiotic resistance that rarely causes disease in immune competent people. The agent formed pigments on nutrient agar cultivated at room temperature, as shown in the photograph. What is the etiology of this patient's UTI?

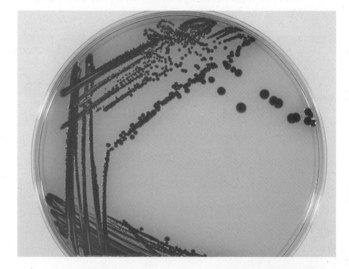

(A) *Escherichia coli*
(B) *Klebsiella pneumoniae*
(C) *Pseudomonas aeruginosa*
(D) *Proteus mirabilis*
(E) *Serratia marcescens*

59 A 3-year-old female child presented with a febrile headache, vomiting, and a swollen right knee that was exquisitely painful upon motion. Physical examination revealed a petechial rash on the skin. Gram stain of the synovial fluid revealed the presence of Gram-negative diplococci and culture suggested a strict aerobe that fermented glucose and maltose. Capsule antigens were also detected by serology. Which one of the following is most likely the causative agent of the disease?
(A) *Escherichia coli*
(B) *Neisseria meningitidis*
(C) *Neisseria gonorrhoeae*
(D) *Staphylococcus aureus*
(E) *Haemophilus influenzae* b

The next two questions are linked.

60 An 18-month-old male presents with fever, lethargy, malaise, productive coughing, and vomiting. Culture of cerebral spinal fluid samples with *Staphylococcus aureus* on blood agar reveals the presence of "satellite" colonies. Serology has indicated that the organism is polyribitol phosphate (PRP) positive. Gram stain of the colonies indicates the presence of a Gram-negative coccobacillus. Which one of the following organisms is most likely responsible for the disease?
(A) *Bordetella pertussis*
(B) *Campylobacter jejuni*
(C) *Escherichia coli*
(D) *Haemophilus influenzae* b
(E) *Pasteurella multocida*

61 How could the infection in the above case have been avoided?
(A) Improved community sanitation
(B) Avoidance of infants with similar symptoms
(C) Avoidance of day care facilities or other crowded situations
(D) Use of 10% bleach solution to clean toys shared with other infants
(E) Vaccination of the infant

62 A 78-year-old man developed endocarditis due to a vancomycin-resistant strain of *Enterococcus faecalis*. What is the molecular basis of resistance of this organism to vancomycin?

(A) A change in the terminal pentapeptide from D-ala-D-ala to D-ala-D-lac
(B) A mutation in the penicillin-binding protein
(C) A mutation in the porin protein
(D) The acquisition of an efflux pump
(E) The secretion of β-lactamase

63 A 47-year-old woman in India is becoming blind due to repeated infection with *Chlamydia trachomatis*. What is seen in the pus draining from her eyes and stained by immunofluorescence?
(A) Elementary bodies
(B) Inclusion bodies
(C) Negri bodies
(D) Gram-negative diplococci
(E) Gram-positive diplococci

64 A new rapid diagnostic test for strep throat was undergoing clinical trials. Among 500 culture-positive individuals with sore throat, 500 were positive by the test. Among 500 culture-negative individuals without sore throat, 200 were negative by the test. Describe the sensitivity and specificity of this test.
(A) High sensitivity; high specificity
(B) High sensitivity; low specificity
(C) Low sensitivity; high specificity
(D) Low sensitivity; low specificity

The next two questions are linked.

65 An 8-year-old girl presents to the urgent care facility with 1 day history of fever, sore throat, malaise, and headache. Physical examination reveals a temperature of 39 °C, cervical lymphadenopathy, and a whitish tonsillar exudate. A rapid diagnostic test is negative; however, culture of the exudate grew Gram-positive cocci in chains that caused β-hemolysis on blood agar. What complication is prevented by appropriate antibiotic therapy for this infection?
(A) Bacteremia
(B) Carditis
(C) Encephalitis
(D) Hepatitis
(E) Meningitis

66 What is the basis of serotyping of the pathogen in the above question?
(A) Capsular antigens
(B) Cell wall antigens
(C) Flagellar antigens
(D) O antigens
(E) M antigens

67 A resident in his first week of outpatient clinic work prescribes erythromycin for the treatment of a urinary tract infection, presumably a simple case of *Escherichia coli*. The attending physician countermands the resident's order and prescribes TMP–SMZ. Why is the therapeutic choice by the attending more appropriate?

(A) Bacterial glycocalyx impedes the absorption of erythromycin

(B) Erythromycin is likely to be inactivated by transpeptidases

(C) Macrolides are principally secreted in the feces

(D) Macrolides promote *Candida* overgrowth in women

(E) Oral macrolides are linked to Stevens–Johnson syndrome

The next two questions are linked.

68 A 10-month-old male child presents with episodes of repetitive coughing with intermittent large gasps of air as well as some vomiting. Parents indicate that the child has been suffering from this condition for about 1 week. Incidentally, the previous week he was reported to have a coldlike illness with a fever and sneezing. A white blood cell count shows 65% lymphocytes and 30% neutrophils. An oxidase-positive, Gram-negative coccobacillus is grown from a nasopharyngeal swab plated on Regan–Lowe charcoal agar. Which one of the following organisms is most likely responsible for this disease?

(A) *Bordetella pertussis*

(B) *Corynebacterium diphtheriae*

(C) *Haemophilus influenzae*

(D) *Mycoplasma pneumoniae*

(E) *Streptococcus pneumoniae*

69 What are the virulence factors of the organism in the above question that enable it to adhere to and kill ciliated respiratory epithelial cells?

(A) Capsular polysaccharide and diphtheria toxin

(B) M protein and pneumolysin

(C) Pertactin, filamentous hemagglutinin, and tracheal cytotoxin

(D) P-pili and lecithinase

(E) Polyribitol phosphate capsule and colonization factor

70 A 20-year-old male is brought to the emergency department with a 1-day history of delirium. He has had a sustained fever of up to 40 °C and a history of progressive headache, myalgia, and constipation which began 10 days previously as he was returning to the United States from a trip to visit relatives in India. Physical examination revealed hepatosplenomegaly, diffuse abdominal tenderness, and red spots on the chest and neck. Colonies of a Gram-negative bacillus that produced a characteristic "fish-eye" growth (lactose nonfermenter with sulfur reduction) are isolated on Hektoen agar from blood and stool samples as shown in the photograph. What is the most likely diagnosis?

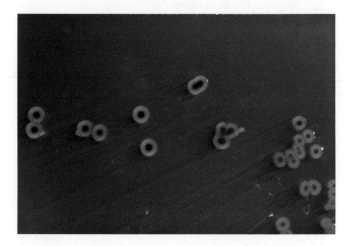

(A) Cholera

(B) Hemolytic uremic syndrome

(C) Shigellosis

(D) Tularemia

(E) Typhoid fever

71 A 35-year-old male became ill with watery diarrhea due to a bacterial infection while on a trip to South America. Which of the following is the key event that promotes the development of watery diarrhea?

(A) Decreased activity of adenylate cyclase

(B) Increase in the intestinal epithelial cell levels of cAMP

(C) Increase in the levels of intracellular chloride

(D) Movement of water from the intestinal lumen into the epithelial cells.

(E) Movement of ions such as potassium and sodium into the intestinal epithelial cells

72 A 47-year-old male is diagnosed with peptic ulcer disease. Treatment includes antibiotics for infection of the stomach with *Helicobacter pylori*. Which enzyme is secreted by this organism and enables it to survive in the acid environment of the stomach?

(A) Catalase
(B) Oxidase
(C) Protease
(D) Transpeptidase
(E) Urease

(A) *Enterobacter cloacae*
(B) *Klebsiella pneumoniae*
(C) *Proteus vulgaris*
(D) *Pseudomonas aeruginosa*
(E) *Serratia marcescens*

73 A 15-year-old boy presents with diarrhea, malaise, fever, and abdominal pain. The stools were positive for occult blood and fecal leukocytes. Microscopy of the stool also reveals the presence of curved bacilli that moved about on a slide in a darting motion. The etiologic agent, a Gram-negative, curved rod, grew on specialized medium in microaerophilic conditions. Which one of the following organisms is most likely responsible for the disease?
(A) *Campylobacter jejuni*
(B) Enterotoxigenic *Escherichia coli*
(C) *Salmonella* sp.
(D) *Shigella sonnei*
(E) *Vibrio cholerae*

74 A 3-year-old girl develops a wound infection on her hand following a cat bite. Culture of wound exudate on blood agar grew a Gram-negative coccobacillus that is a normal flora of the cat oropharynx. What is the most likely etiologic agent?
(A) *Bacteroides fragilis*
(B) β-Hemolytic *Streptococcus*
(C) *Capnocytophaga canimorsus*
(D) *Moraxella catarrhalis*
(E) *Pasteurella multocida*

75 A 27-year-old male was hospitalized suffering third-degree burns over 50% of his body from a house fire. After 6 days in the hospital, he becomes septic and the burn wounds show tissue necrosis in several areas. Blood and wound cultures grew an oxidase-positive, Gram-negative bacillus resistant to aminopenicillins, macrolides, and first-generation and second-generation cephalosporins. The organism growing on nutrient agar is shown in the photograph. What is the etiology of this man's burn infection?

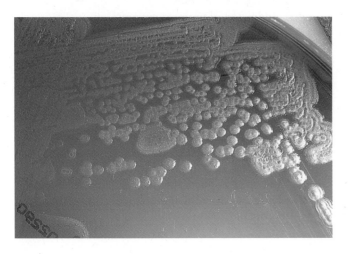

76 Five adults and seven children in a village in South Africa present over several days to a local clinic with voluminous watery diarrhea containing flecks of mucus. They show signs of severe dehydration and are treated with oral fluids and electrolytes. Stool cultures grew yellow colonies on thiosulfate citrate bile salt (TCBS) media. What is the etiology of this outbreak?
(A) Enteroinvasive *Escherichia coli*
(B) *Salmonella typhi*
(C) *Shigella dysenteriae*
(D) *Vibrio cholerae*
(E) *Yersinia enterocolitica*

77 An outbreak of pneumonic plague occurs in the Democratic Republic of the Congo killing over half of the affected individuals. How is this form of plague transmitted?
(A) Bite of infected flea
(B) Direct skin contact with bubos
(C) Ingestion of contaminated water
(D) Inhalation of aerosolized bacteria
(E) Introduction of bacteria into wounds while butchering infected animals

78 A 35-year-old man developed a flu-like illness that lasted 3 days and was followed by apparent recovery. Within days, he suffered a recurrence of illness with symptoms of meningitis and oliguria. He was hospitalized and diagnosed with Weil disease. Which of the following organisms is the cause?
(A) *Bartonella quintana*
(B) *Chlamydia psittaci*
(C) *Leptospira interrogans*
(D) *Mycobacterium leprae*
(E) *Ureaplasma urealyticum*

79 A 26-year-old man presents with a painless ulcer on the penis from which spiral-shaped bacteria could be visualized on dark-field microscopy. If left untreated, which of the following would be expected to occur within 6 weeks to 6 months?
(A) Ataxia
(B) Dementia
(C) Disseminated rash
(D) Kidney failure
(E) Meningitis

80 A 27-year-old woman presented with a 2-week history of low grade fever, chills, myalgia, headache, and non-productive cough. She was treated with an antibiotic that inhibits cell wall synthesis but did not improve because the causative agent lacks a cell wall. With which organism was she infected?
(A) *Chlamydophila pneumoniae*
(B) *Coxiella burnetii*
(C) *Ehrlichia chaffeensis*
(D) *Legionella pneumoniae*
(E) *Mycoplasma pneumoniae*

81 A 24-year-old woman was diagnosed with pelvic inflammatory disease. The infection was found to be polymicrobial and included a Gram-negative anaerobic rod. Identify the most likely anaerobe involved in the infection.
(A) *Actinomyces israelii*
(B) *Bacteroides fragilis*
(C) *Chlamydia trachomatis*
(D) *Neisseria gonorrhoeae*
(E) *Treponema pallidum*

82 A 12-year-old girl develops a low-grade fever, malaise, and tender lymphadenopathy in her right axial area. On her right hand are the scratches she received 10 days previously from her kitten. What is the most likely bacterial cause of this lymphadenopathy?
(A) *Actinomyces israelii*
(B) *Bartonella henselae*
(C) *Chlamydia psittaci*
(D) *Francisella tularensis*
(E) *Yersinia pestis*

83 A 25-year-male presented with fever, dry cough, and dyspnea. A sputum sample was induced but it failed to reveal organisms on Gram stain. The sputum also failed to grow organisms when cultured on a variety of agars; however, bacteria were isolated in cultured eukaryotic cells. What is the cause of this man's disease?
(A) *Chlamydophila pneumoniae*
(B) *Legionella pneumophila*
(C) *Mycobacterium intracellulare*
(D) *Mycobacterium tuberculosis*
(E) *Mycoplasma pneumoniae*

84 A 23-year-old female is treated for uncomplicated pyelonephritis with an antibiotic that inhibits bacterial DNA gyrase. Which antibiotic did she receive?
(A) Ampicillin
(B) Ceftriaxone
(C) Ciprofloxacin
(D) Gentamicin
(E) TMP–SMZ

85 A 61-year-old dialysis patient develops *Pseudomonas* septicemia for which she is given a β-lactam antibiotic with activity exclusively against aerobic, Gram-negative bacteria. Which antibiotic is she given?
(A) Aztreonam
(B) Ceftriaxone
(C) Cephalexin
(D) Gentamicin
(E) Imipenem

86 A 67-year-old moderately obese man presents with fever and an erythematous, swollen, tender, warm calf. He is diagnosed clinically with cellulitis and catalase-negative, β-hemolytic Gram-positive cocci are isolated from blood cultures. Which virulence factor of the causative organism enabled it to cause this invasive disease?
(A) An A-B exotoxin
(B) Lipopolysaccharide
(C) P fimbriae
(D) Streptokinase
(E) Yops proteins

87 A 22-year-old woman is admitted to the hospital with pelvic inflammatory disease. Her empiric antibiotic regimen requires coverage for anaerobes. Which antibiotic would provide appropriate anaerobic coverage?
(A) Azithromycin
(B) Ceftriaxone
(C) Gentamicin
(D) Linezolid
(E) Metronidazole

88 A 37-year-old male is seen at a sexually transmitted disease clinic for treatment of gonorrhea. Prior treatments for this disease have successfully eradicated the organism; however, the man has not changed his behavior and has been repeatedly reinfected. What is the most important strategy the organism employs which enables it to cause repeated infections?
(A) Antigenic variation
(B) Induction of immune suppression
(C) Intracellular growth in alveolar macrophages
(D) Polysaccharide capsule
(E) Secretion of IgG protease

89 A 76-year-old man receiving chemotherapy for cancer developed an abrupt onset of fever, chills, headache, nonproductive cough, and diarrhea. A chest radiograph suggested a diagnosis of pneumonia. The organism, isolated from sputum and blood culture, is an aquatic saprophyte that infects amoebas outside of the body and macrophages following infection. What is this organism?

(A) *Chlamydia pneumoniae*
(B) *Legionella pneumophila*
(C) *Mycobacterium tuberculosis*
(D) *Mycoplasma pneumoniae*
(E) *Streptococcus pneumoniae*

90 A 7-year-old child develops impetigo involving large areas of his body. He is given an antibiotic that inhibits cell wall synthesis. Which is the most likely antibiotic this child would have received?
(A) Ampicillin
(B) Cephalexin
(C) Ciprofloxacin
(D) Clindamycin
(E) Erythromycin

91 A 64-year-old woman is hospitalized with community-acquired pneumonia. Empiric antibiotic treatment consists of a drug that inhibits bacterial protein synthesis by binding to the 50S subunit of the bacterial ribosome and a β-lactam antibiotic. With which of the following should she be treated?
(A) Ampicillin plus gentamicin
(B) Azithromycin plus ceftriaxone
(C) Imipenem plus cilastatin
(D) Piperacillin plus tazobactam
(E) Trimethoprim plus sulfamethoxazole

92 A 34-year-old woman presents with fever, nausea, severe abdominal cramping, and bloody diarrhea that was fecal leukocyte-positive. A few days previously, she had eaten undercooked chicken. Of the following, which is the most likely etiologic agent?
(A) *Campylobacter jejuni*
(B) *Clostridium perfringens*
(C) *Salmonella typhi*
(D) *Shigella dysenteriae*
(E) *Yersinia enterocolitica*

The next two questions are linked.

93 A 48-year-old man has been hospitalized in intensive care for 3 weeks following an automobile accident. He develops a fever due to colonization of an intravenous line with Gram-positive cocci that are catalase-positive and coagulase-negative. What is the most likely cause of this man's fever?
(A) *Enterococcus faecalis*
(B) *Staphylococcus aureus*
(C) *Staphylococcus epidermidis*
(D) *Streptococcus mutans*
(E) *Streptococcus pyogenes*

94 What is the major virulence factor of the organism in the above case?
(A) Biofilm production
(B) Panton–Valentine leukocidin
(C) Pyrogenic exotoxin
(D) Streptokinase
(E) Vancomycin resistance

The next two questions are linked.

95 A 5-year-old girl from an orphanage in Ukraine was about to leave for the United States with her adoptive parents when she developed a fever, sore throat, cough, and malaise. A few days later, she was brought to the emergency room in respiratory distress. Physical examination revealed pronounced, bilateral cervical lymphadenopathy, inflamed pharyngeal area, and a thick, grayish, leathery exudate on the tonsils as shown in the photograph. Part of the exudate had become loose revealing bleeding of the underlying mucosal tissue. The etiologic agent was isolated on tellurite medium. What virulence factor accounts for the pathogenesis of this infection?

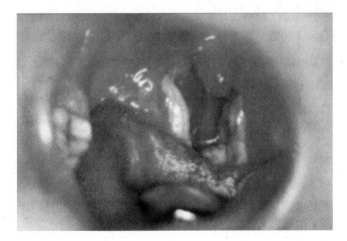

(A) Immune evasion following production of IgA protease
(B) Lipopolysaccharide-induced inflammation
(C) M protein-mediated resistance to phagocytosis
(D) Secretion of coagulase to facilitate invasion into mucosa
(E) Toxin-mediated inhibition of protein synthesis

96 Ten days after the onset of illness, the patient in the above case deteriorated and she subsequently died from a complication of her infection. What was the most likely cause of her death?
(A) Encephalitis
(B) Kidney failure
(C) Myocarditis
(D) Pneumonia
(E) Sepsis

97 Blood and urine cultures are taken from a 73-year-old man hospitalized with suspected *Escherichia coli* urosepsis. Which culture medium would allow selective growth of Gram-negative enterics while suppressing the growth of Gram-positive bacteria, *Haemophilus* and *Neisseria*?
(A) Blood agar
(B) Buffered charcoal-yeast extract agar
(C) Chocolate agar
(D) MacConkey agar
(E) Thayer–Martin agar

98 A 3-year-old boy developed bloody diarrhea after eating a poorly cooked hamburger. A few days later, he was hospitalized with oliguria and hypertension. With which organism is he most likely infected?
(A) *Clostridium perfringens*
(B) *Salmonella typhi*
(C) Enteroinvasive *E. coli*
(D) Shiga toxin-producing *E. coli*
(E) *Yersinia enterocolitica*

99 A surgery patient at risk for Gram-negative sepsis is part of a research project to prevent endotoxic shock using monoclonal antibodies to inhibit the endotoxin molecule. What is the active component of the endotoxin molecule against which the monoclonal antibody would most likely be directed?
(A) Core polysaccharide
(B) Lipid A
(C) N-acetylmuramic acid
(D) O side chain
(E) Teichoic acid

100 A 47-year-old man had a serious skin infection due to *Staphylococcus aureus*. He was unable to receive β-lactam antibiotics due to a history of penicillin-induced anaphylaxis. Which of the following antibiotics could he be given?
(A) Ampicillin
(B) Aztreoman
(C) Cefazolin
(D) Clindamycin
(E) Meropenem

The next three questions are linked.

101 A 22-year-old female college dorm resident presents with a sudden onset of fever of 104 °F and a severe headache. Nuchal rigidity and papilledema are seen on physical examination. Gram stain of the cerebral spinal fluid is shown in the accompanying photograph. What is the etiology of her infection?

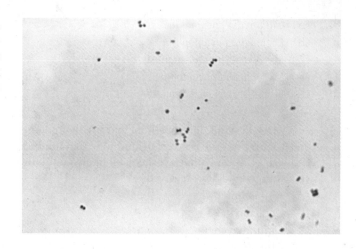

(A) Group B *Streptococcus*
(B) *Haemophilus influenzae* b
(C) *Listeria monocytogenes*
(D) *Neisseria meningitidis*
(E) *Streptococcus pneumoniae*

102 How could the infection in the above case have best been prevented?
(A) Improved sanitation within the dormitory
(B) Hand washing and use of hand sanitation gel
(C) Prophylactic γ-globulin
(D) Prophylactic ribavirin
(E) Vaccination

103 What is the drug of choice for treating the young woman in the above case?
(A) Azithromycin
(B) Aztreonam
(C) Cefazolin
(D) Imipenem
(E) Penicillin

104 An outbreak of watery diarrhea due to *Shigella* occurred in several day care centers in a Midwestern city. Which *Shigella* sp. is most likely involved?
(A) *S. boydii*
(B) *S. dysenteriae*
(C) *S. enterica*
(D) *S. flexneri*
(E) *S. sonnei*

The next two questions are linked.

105 While on vacation, a 68-year-old man develops fever, chills, night sweats, and malaise that began insidiously and progressed over several days. He sought care at an urgent care facility and was diagnosed clinically with the flu. He cuts his vacation short and returns home with the same symptoms plus weakness and dyspnea. He sees his primary care physician who hears a new onset of murmur on auscultation and admits the man to the hospital. Blood cultures grow the catalase-negative organism shown in the accompanying photographs. What is the cause of this man's infection?

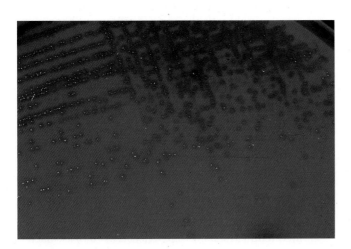

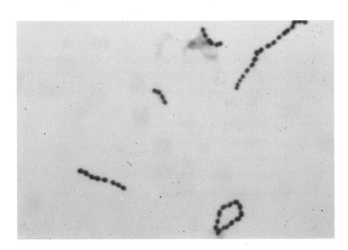

(A) Group A Streptococcus *pyogenes*
(B) Group B Streptococcus *agalactiae*
(C) *Staphylococcus aureus*
(D) *Staphylococcus epidermidis*
(E) Viridans group streptococci

106 Which of the following is an important virulence factor of the organisms in the above question?
(A) Dextran production
(B) Hyaluronidase
(C) Lipopolysaccharide
(D) Pyrogenic exotoxins
(E) Exfoliative toxins

107 A homeless man who is known to be HIV positive unexpectedly dies in a dormitory of a congregate nighttime shelter. A roommate states that during the night, he complained of periods of shaking chills and fever and appeared to be coughing up blood. An acid-fast stain slide of tissue from the lungs is shown in the photograph. Which statement best describes the disease process that is visible in the stained slide?

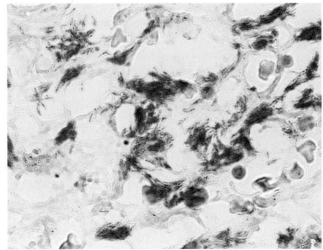

(A) Cytoplasmic inclusions associated with *Chlamydia*
(B) *Legionella* within alveoli indicating atypical pneumonia
(C) *Mycobacteria* overwhelming alveolar macrophages
(D) *Pseudomonas* microcolonies within lung parenchyma
(E) Signs of consolidation linked to typical pneumonia

The next two questions are linked.

108 A 6-year-old boy in Pakistan presents to a local hospital with involuntary limb movements. He also complains of pain and swelling in several joints including the wrists, elbows, knees, and ankles as well as weakness and shortness of breath. About 2 weeks earlier, he had been ill with fever and sore throat. A throat culture for group A *Streptococcus* was negative. What other test result would indicate a recent infection with this organism?

(A) Elevated C-reactive protein
(B) Elevated erythrocyte sedimentation rate
(C) Positive antistreptolysin O antibodies
(D) Positive Lancefield agglutination test
(E) Positive Rheumatoid factor test

109 With regard to the above question, what is the major virulence factor of this organism that plays a role in the pathogenesis of the boy's illness?
(A) Capsule
(B) M protein
(C) Phage-associated toxin
(D) Secretion of dextran
(E) Streptococcal superantigen

The next two questions are linked.

110 A 74-year-old woman is hospitalized with community-acquired pneumonia. Blood and sputum cultures grew the α-hemolytic catalase-negative, bile-soluble, optochin-sensitive organism shown in the photograph. It showed an intermediate degree of resistance to penicillin. What are the other important virulence factors of this organism?

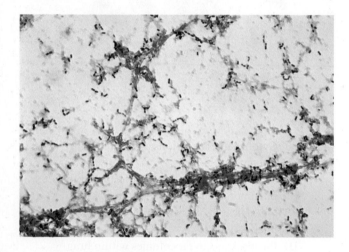

(A) Capsule and pneumolysin
(B) Filamentous hemagglutinin and superantigen
(C) Neuraminidase and hemagglutinin
(D) Pyocyanin and endotoxin
(E) Tracheal cytotoxin and pertactin

111 What is the molecular basis of resistance to penicillin shown by the organism in the above question?
(A) Altered penicillin-binding proteins
(B) Efflux pump
(C) Mutation of ribosomal binding site
(D) Mutated porin proteins
(E) Production of β-lactamase

112 Vaccination with Bacille Calmette-Guérin (BCG) has been shown to provide protection against tuberculosis by inducing cell-mediated immunity. What is the efficacy of this vaccine in preventing pulmonary infection?
(A) 10%
(B) 25%
(C) 50%
(D) 75%
(E) 90%

113 A 32-year-old woman presents to an urgent care facility with severe vomiting. She claims that several other people who ate at the church picnic 4 hours earlier are also sick with the same symptoms. She is clinically diagnosed with food poisoning. A health department investigation reveals that all affected individuals had eaten the ham salad. What is the bacterial agent responsible for the signs and symptoms?
(A) *Campylobacter jejuni*
(B) *Clostridium perfringens*
(C) *Bacillus cereus*
(D) *Salmonella* sp.
(E) *Staphylococcus aureus*

114 A 76-year-old hospitalized male being treated successfully with vancomycin for hospital-acquired methicillin-resistant *Staphylococcus aureus* bacteremia develops a new onset of fever. A urinary tract infection is suspected and a Gram stain of unspun urine reveals neutrophils and Gram-positive cocci. Antibiotic sensitivity results of the organism cultured from the urine reveal resistance to cephalosporins, TMP–SMZ, aminoglycosides, and vancomycin. Which bacteria is the most likely cause of his urinary tract infection?
(A) *Enterococcus faecalis*
(B) Group B *Streptococcus*
(C) *Peptostreptococcus*
(D) *Staphylococcus saprophyticus*
(E) *Streptococcus pyogenes*

115 A 4-year-old boy is being worked up for severe acute rhinosinusitis. Culture from material obtained from the maxillary sinus grew aerobic, oxidase-positive, and Gram-negative diplococci. How should this infection be treated?
(A) Ampicillin
(B) Amoxicillin–clavulanate
(C) Cephalexin
(D) Dicloxacillin
(E) Vancomycin

116 A 34-year-old woman in her third trimester of pregnancy delivers a stillborn infant. Her history is significant for a febrile illness with headache, back pain, and diarrhea prior to going into premature labor. A Gram-positive motile coccobacillus was isolated from blood and tissue samples of the mother and the infant cultured at 4°C. How did the mother acquire this infection?

(A) Acquisition of a respiratory pathogen that spread hematogenously

(B) Contamination of genital tract with normal intestinal flora

(C) Ingestion of contaminated food

(D) Overgrowth of normal vaginal flora

(E) Sexual transmission

117 A 54-year-old HIV-infected male with a CD4 cell count of 45/cmm presents with fever, shortness of breath, diarrhea, fatigue, night sweats, weight loss, and right upper quadrant abdominal pain of 2 weeks duration. He has refused antiretroviral therapy for the past 2 years due to debilitating side effects. Physical examination reveals a pale, ill appearing, cachectic male with hepatosplenomegaly. Lab tests reveal elevated transaminase and alkaline phosphatase levels. Blood cultures grew acid-fast bacilli. With which antibiotic regimen should this patient be treated?

(A) Clarithromycin plus ethambutol plus rifabutin

(B) Isoniazid plus rifampin

(C) Piperacillin plus tazobactam

(D) Trimathoprim plus sulfamethaxazole

(E) Vancomycin plus dalfopristin

118 A 7-year-old boy presents to the emergency department with fever, abdominal pain, and tenderness in the right lower quadrant. A white blood cell count reveals leukocytosis. Suspecting appendicitis, the child is taken to surgery; however, the removed appendix is grossly and histologically normal. The bacterial cause for the boy's symptoms was subsequently identified as a Gram-negative rod after cold enrichment of fecal cultures. What is the etiology of this infection?

(A) *Campylobacter jejuni*

(B) *Clostridium difficile*

(C) *Salmonella typhi*

(D) *Vibrio parahaemolyticus*

(E) *Yersinia enterocolitica*

119 A 60-year-old man with a history of chronic liver disease develops fever, cellulitis, and bullous skin lesions after spending 6 hours in flood waters following a hurricane that affected his residence along the Mississippi coast. Upon admission to the hospital, he is septic and hypotensive and dies the following day. Blood cultures grown on blood agar supplemented with 1% sodium chloride grew a curved, motile, Gram-negative rod. What is the etiology of this man's disease?

(A) *Clostridium perfringens*

(B) MRSA

(C) *Pseudomonas aeruginosa*

(D) *Streptococcus pyogenes*

(E) *Vibrio vulnificus*

ANSWERS

1   **The answer is D: *Legionella pneumophila.***   The clinical description is classic for this organism. The patient is elderly and has a chronic disease—diabetes. Those at risk for legionellosis are elderly, immune suppressed or those with diabetes or other chronic diseases. The disease often manifests extrapulmonary symptoms such as headache or GI symptoms. *Legionella* is a fastidious organism that does not grow on blood agar but requires specialized agar such as buffered charcoal yeast extract agar for growth. Although *Legionella* does not pick up the Gram stain, it can be stained with basic fuchsin. Direct immunofluorescent antibody staining can be used to make a definitive diagnosis either on sputum samples or, more likely, of cultured bacteria.

2   **The answer is B: Aerosols from contaminated water.**   This organism survives in aquatic environments and can be isolated from lakes and streams as well as air conditioning units, hot tubs, showers, and pipes bringing water into homes and hospitals. *Legionella* is not a spore-forming organism as are the endemic fungi that cause pneumonia. It does not colonize humans and has not been shown to be transmitted person to person.

3   **The answer is C: Lipooligosaccharide.**   The case describes a child with meningococcemia. Identification of *Neisseria meningitidis* as the etiologic agent is supported by the growth of Gram-negative diplococci on Thayer–Martin agar. *Neisseria* does not produce exotoxins or flagella. Although it has pili and *N. meningitidis* does produce a polysaccharide capsule, most of the disease manifestations are attributable to the endotoxin activity of lipooligosaccharide. This molecule is chemically distinct from lipopolysaccharide; however, its activities are similar.

4   **The answer is B: *Haemophilus influenzae* b.**   Very few cases of invasive diseases attributable to *H. influenzae* b occur in developed countries with high rates of vaccination. The incidence of invasive diseases due to *H. influenzae* b has decreased in the United States by 99% since the vaccine first became available in 1989. Although non-b serotypes of *H. influenzae* still cause disease, these strains are generally not involved in invasive diseases. Vaccines are also available for *S. pneumoniae* and *N. meningitidis*, and although the efficacy of these vaccines is still quite high, not all serotypes involved in disease are included in these two vaccines.

5   **The answer is D: Intracellular growth.**   The case describes an infection with *Legionella pneumophila*, an organism that grows within amoeba outside of the body and within alveolar macrophages following infection. Hallmarks of the infection include nonproductive cough, negative sputum Gram stain, and extrapulmonary signs (confusion, headache, and GI symptoms). The patient is immune compromised, an important risk factor for *Legionella* infection. Detection of *Legionella* antigens in urine is one way to make a definitive diagnosis. This test is specific for *L. pneumophila* serogroup 1, the major but not the only serogroup involved in causing this disease. Serogroup 6 can also be isolated from patients with Legionnaire disease in the United States.

6   **The answer is A: Capsule.**   Robust bacterial rods (bacilli) are clearly visible in the tissue section, and based on the shape of these bacterial cells and the overall clinical picture (death of the steer), a laboratory diagnosis of *Bacillus anthracis* seems plausible. *B. anthracis* is epizootic in certain areas of the United States and is described as a disease agent of cattle and sheep in the North Dakota region. The unwitting rancher exposed to the infected livestock could potentially develop cutaneous anthrax. Herbivores are believed to acquire the infection by ingesting endospores while grazing on the contaminated pastures. A foremost virulence determinant for *B. anthracis* is the polyglutamic acid capsule. If lacking, the potential for the microbe to be pathogenic and generate disease is effectively zero. As with other bacteria, this particular capsular type plays a role in protecting the bacterium against phagocytosis and bactericidal components of the immune system.

7   **The answer is A: Clostridial gas gangrene.**   See next question for discussion.

8   **The answer is A: α-Toxin (lecithinase).**   Several species of *Clostridium* have been linked to gas gangrene; however, *Clostridium perfringens* is the most common. Clostridia are anaerobes, emit strong odors—often described as fetid—and are gas producers in tissue or when grown in laboratory media. They produce endospores when challenged environmentally. The body reacts vigorously (sometimes to its detriment) to the huge array of exotoxins produced during an infection. These tissue-damaging toxins are virulence factors that allow the bacteria to "set up housekeeping" in the host. α-Toxin, a lecithinase that produces tissue necrosis, is of paramount importance in the pathogenesis of *C. perfringens*. Pyrogenic exotoxin A, an erythrogenic toxin of *Streptococcus pyogenes* (group A streptococci), is associated with scarlet fever; streptolysin S is linked to the β-hemolysis characteristically seen with group A streptococci on sheep blood agar; enterotoxin is responsible for eliciting the symptoms associated with food poisoning by *Staphylococcus aureus*; and pyocyanin is a bluish pigment and a primary virulence factor common to *Pseudomonas aeruginosa*.

9 The answer is B: Clostridia. Clostridial myonecrosis or gas gangrene is caused by a number of clostridial species, the most common being *Clostridium perfringens*. All are large, Gram-positive, anaerobic bacilli. When stressed, in the environment or possibly the laboratory, they will produce endospores. The soil contaminating the punctured wound was the vehicle for infection in this particular case. Infections often prove exquisitely painful. Gangrene is a fulminate condition, with severe illness and even mortalities possible within hours of the initial insult, especially if untreated. Clostridia are usually sensitive to penicillins and other β-lactam antibiotics.

10 The answer is B: Catalase. This enzyme catalyzes the conversion of hydrogen peroxide to water and oxygen gas, thereby creating the bubbles seen on the plate. It is produced by bacteria in defense against hydrogen peroxide production by neutrophils. β-lactamase is an enzyme that breaks the β-lactam ring of penicillin and related antibiotics. Coagulase is produced by *Staphylococcus aureus* and causes clot formation. Staphylokinase, also known as fibrinolysin, is produced by *S. aureus* and breaks down fibrin clots. Similarly, streptokinase, produced by *Streptococcus pyogenes*, dissolves fibrin clots.

11 The answer is E: Methicillin-resistant *staphyloccocus aureus* (MRSA). The organism fits the description of *S. aureus* (catalase-positive, Gram-positive coccus). The rapid onset and severity of symptoms fit the clinical picture of MRSA. Of the other organisms listed, only group A *Streptococcus* (GAS) and *Enterococcus* are Gram-positive cocci. While GAS is β-hemolytic, it is not catalase-positive. Enterococci are rarely β-hemolytic and are also catalase-negative.

12 The answer is E: (TMP–SMZ). This drug is commonly used for community-acquired MRSA infections. Amoxicillin/clavulanate, cephalexin, and dicloxacillin are β-lactam antibiotics used for β-lactamase-producing strains of *S. aureus*. The mechanism of β-lactam resistance in MRSA is due to the production of an altered penicillin-binding protein; thus, these are not appropriate antibiotics for this strain. Polymyxin B is an antifungal drug.

13 The answer is C: Cystic fibrosis. While chemical analysis of the chloride content of the sweat is the most reliable and preferred diagnostic tool for a cystic fibrosis (CF), isolation of a mucoid variant of *P. aeruginosa* is considered pathognomonic for the disease. *P. aeruginosa* is the pathogen most frequently isolated from the respiratory tracts of pediatric and adult patients with CF. *Burkholderia cepacia* is another opportunistic pseudomonad that can be isolated from CF patients, but its prevalence is significantly less. COPD needs time to develop and would not be expected in a child. The child does not present with typical signs of pneumonia. Sarcoidosis is a systemic disease that is often manifested by a granulomatous inflammation of the lungs. The etiology is unknown, and it is usually diagnosed in the adult patient. Bronchiolitis, a respiratory illness in children, is associated with the respiratory syncytial virus (RSV).

14 The answer is A: *Actinomyces israelii*. The actinomycetes, which include *A. israelii*, are a group of organisms characterized as Gram-positive rods commonly found in soil and decaying organic matter or as colonizers of body surfaces. They can infect humans causing cutaneous, pulmonary, or systemic disease. In culture and lesions, these organisms form filamentous or hyphae-like structures. The lesion shown is an actinomycetoma. In general, a mycetoma is described as a chronic granulomatous infection with subcutaneous tissue involvement. Eumycetoma, although a similar presentation, has a fungal origin. Mycetomas can form as a result of traumatic injury such as walking long distances on a jungle path in flip–flops as may have happened in this case. If treated early with a combination of antibiotics, a full recovery can be expected. None of the other organisms listed are causes of mycetomas.

15 The answer is D: Immediate initiation of doxycycline. Based on the fever, headache, a petechial rash, myalgia, GI and pulmonary issues, and a history of tick exposure in a prime endemic area in the United States, instigation of antibiotic therapy for Rocky Mountain spotted fever (RMSF) is probably warranted. In the United States, RMSF is the most commonly diagnosed rickettsial illness. *Rickettsia rickettsii*, the causative agent of RMSF, is an obligate intracellular microbe that exhibits tropism for endothelial cells of the small blood vessels. An intracellular parasitic niche seems to be advantageous for a bacterium because it can afford some degree of protection against the killing activities of white blood cells. Nevertheless, the endothelial cells are eventually damaged and vasculitides will develop in many sites in the body. For example, the characteristic cutaneous rash is directly linked to vasculitis. Even though this case reads like a textbook, a clinical diagnosis is often difficult to make with a high degree of certainty because it may be confused with other diseases like meningococcal meningitis, secondary syphilis, measles, etc. The rash, which first appears on the wrists and ankles within days of being infected, eventually spreads centripetally. The rash is often difficult to detect in darker pigmented patients. Furthermore, the disease is potentially more severe in African Americans, possibly because of a higher genetic likelihood of a glucose-6-phosphate dehydrogenase deficiency. The possibility for adverse complications, including a fatal outcome and the fact that seroconversion may not occur until well into the second week, justifies initiating antibiotic therapy (e.g., doxycycline or chloramphenicol) quickly. Delaying it would put this patient at risk for a more severe course.

16   The answer is D: Type-specific latex agglutination antibody titer of 1:64.   With regard to laboratory diagnosis, rickettsial organisms may be observed in a Giemsa-stain specimen; the Gram stain procedure is not optimal for visualizing rickettsiae. Also, rickettsial organisms are not cultured in the average clinical laboratory. The Weil–Felix reaction, which is based on a cross-reactivity or shared antigens with *Proteus vulgaris*, has a low sensitivity and specificity and, consequently, its use is limited. On the other hand, a positive serology, utilizing indirect immunofluorescence or latex agglutination procedures with a single diagnostic titer of 1:64 (or a fourfold increase), is invaluable and currently considered the preferred laboratory diagnostic measure. RMSF is a reportable disease.

17   The answer is E: Scrub typhus/*Orientia tsutsugamushi*. The geographic endemic area and the clinical presentation, especially the black eschar, are highly suggestive of scrub typhus. The causative agent, *O. tsutsugamushi*, is a rickettsial organism endemic to northern Australia and Southeastern Asian countries. Scrub typhus is acquired when an infected chigger, a trombiculid mite, bites the person. Avoiding contact with the mite limits the possibility of transmission. With regard to this case, paired sera giving a fourfold rise in antibody titer to the pathogen would have confirmed the diagnosis. Delaying treatment until a confirmation is available would only compound the illness. Although the other diseases listed cause some of the same symptoms (fever, headache, and rash), the vectors are different. Lice transmit *R. prowazeki*, fleas transmit *R. typhi*, and ticks transmit *C. burnetii* to cattle, sheep, and goats. Humans usually acquire Q fever through inhalation of the organism while handling infected animal tissues. Brill–Zinsser disease is a recurrence of *R. prowazeki* that persisted in the lymph nodes of a patient with epidemic typhus.

18   The answer is B: Enterohemorrhagic *E. coli* (EHEC).   This organism is associated with bloody diarrhea and hemolytic uremic syndrome (HUS), which is affecting two of the children. HUS is primarily a disease of infancy and early childhood caused by the production of a Shiga-like toxin that binds to and kills renal endothelial cells. HUS presents as a triad of microangiopathic hemolytic anemia and thrombocytopenia and can lead to acute renal failure. Diarrhea caused by *E. coli* O157:H7 is a precipitating factor and the use of antimotility drugs may increase the risk. The clinical picture of HUS can suggest a GI bleed because the stool may be grossly bloody. Urine output is reduced or absent with renal failure; petechiae, purpura, and fever are common findings. Schistocytes are markers of HUS. No *E. coli* was isolated from the blood because normal stool culturing does not reveal the organism (sorbitol–MacConkey medium is a screening that can give a preliminary identification). Antibiotics are not effective for EHEC. With the exception of *B. cereus*, which causes vomiting or watery diarrhea, all of the organisms listed can cause bloody diarrhea but none is associated with HUS. *Shigella dysenteriae* (not *S. flexneri*) can also cause HUS through the production of Shiga toxin.

19   The answer is C: Failure to wash hands after visiting a petting zoo.   Cattle are the reservoirs of *Escherichia coli* O157:H7; they show no signs of disease and shed the organism sporadically. Humans become infected when ingesting the organism in undercooked hamburger or foods contaminated with cattle fecal material. Children can also contract the organism by contaminating their hands through petting a cow. The organism is rarely isolated from chlorinated drinking water. *E. coli* O157:H7 can also be transmitted person-to-person in crowed settings such as day care centers; however, direct or indirect contact with cattle feces is a more likely route.

20   The answer is A: Bacillary dysentery.   Of the diseases listed, bacillary dysentery is the only one that fits the description. This disease is caused by *Shigella dysenteriae*, a nonmotile, Gram-negative rod that does not ferment lactose. *Shigella* species causing human disease include *S. dysenteriae*, *S. flexneri*, *S. boydii*, and *S. sonnei*. *S. dysenteriae* causes dysentery, a condition characterized by the passage of numerous small bloody stools containing mucus and pus. Humans are the only natural reservoir for *Shigella*. The organism is spread by ingestion of fecal-contaminated food or water. The infective dose is extremely low; as few as 200 bacteria can initiate the infection. Shigellosis occurs worldwide. *S. dysenteriae*,

S. flexneri, and *S. boydii* are found particularly in Asia, Africa, and Central and South America. They tend to occur whenever war, natural calamities (earthquakes, floods, etc.), or unhygienic living conditions result in overcrowding and poor sanitation. *Shigella sonnei* is the species found in developed countries such as the United States. It tends to cause watery diarrhea rather than bloody diarrhea.

21 **The answer is B: Blocks protein synthesis causing intestinal cell death.**   Shiga toxin is an AB toxin; the gene for which is carried on the chromosome of *Shigella dysenteriae*. The B portion of the toxin binds to the receptors on intestinal cells and the A subunit enters the cells and cleaves the 60 S subunit of the ribosome, preventing the binding of transfer RNA, thereby stopping protein synthesis. Intestinal cells die, leading to bloody diarrhea and facilitating the invasion of the organism into the lamina propria.

22 **The answer is E: Treat affected patients with antibiotics.** Antibiotic treatment decreases the duration of illness and reduces person-to-person spread. Suitable antibiotics include ampicillin and TMP–SMZ unless resistance is noted. If antibiotic susceptibility is unknown, parenteral ceftriaxone sodium, a fluoroquinolone, or azithromycin is the drug of choice. Improved community sanitation and personal hygiene should also be encouraged. Antimotility drugs are contraindicated for patients with bloody diarrhea as they may prolong the duration of fecal shedding of the organism and increase the risk of bacteremia. Humans are the only host for *Shigella*; the organisms have no animal reservoir.

23 **The answer is A: *Borrelia burgdorferi*/tick bite.**   The "bull's-eye" appearance of the skin lesion, the fever, muscle and joint pain, and the fact that the patient lives in an endemic area support a clinical diagnosis of tickborne Lyme disease caused by *B. burgdorferi*.

24 **The answer is C: History and clinical presentation of the patient alone.**   At this stage, the diagnosis is dependent primarily on the clinical picture of the patient. Erythema migrans, often a bull's-eye appearance, is highly suggestive of Lyme disease. Technically, however, it is not considered pathognomonic as similar lesions occur with insect bites and other tickborne agents. *Borrelia burgdorferi* cannot be readily visualized from lesions' samples. Culture is impractical due to the fastidious growth requirements of the bacterium. Liver function tests are not helpful in making a diagnosis of Lyme disease. The probability of a positive serology is low, as seroconversion usually takes

place several weeks following infection. When antibodies are present, diagnostic serology is based on a positive ELISA confirmed with a Western blot.

25 **The answer is C: Doxycycline.**   Most of the time, early Lyme disease responds well to the tetracyclines. The above patient is a teenager, with no pregnancy issues to contend with, and doxycycline is the appropriate choice. Misdiagnosed cases and failure to treat early in the course of the disease process could result in debilitating neurologic (e.g., meningitis, facial palsy) and cardiac complications (e.g., third-degree heart blocks, myocarditis, or pericarditis).

26 **The answer is A: *Escherichia coli*.**   *E. coli* is the most common cause of UTI in any age group. The other organisms can cause UTI but are much less common.

27 **The answer is B: Fimbriae.**   P-fimbriae and type-1 fimbriae are significant virulence determinants of uropathogenic strains of *Escherichia coli*, the most common cause of urinary tract infections. These fimbriae mediate attachment of uropathogenic strains to uroepithelial cells. *E. coli*, which grows on MacConkey agar and ferments lactose, accounts for 70% to 90% of all the uncomplicated UTIs.

28 **The answer is A: Contamination with perianal and bowel flora.**   Uropathogenic *E. coli* frequently colonizes the bowel and contamination of the female urethra is common. Sexual activity can promote ascension of uropathogenic *E. coli* to the bladder to cause a UTI. Circumcision reduces the risk of *E. coli* UTIs in boys.

29 **The answer is D: Formation of struvite kidney stones.**   Urease breaks down urea, releasing ammonia that, when converted to ammonium, raises the urine pH. This leads to the formation of struvite stones. Although the etiological organism (see next question) can be involved in epididymitis, prostatitis, immune complex deposition, and blood stream infections, it is more likely to cause the formation of struvite stones.

30 **The answer is B: *Proteus mirabilis*.**   This organism fits the description due to its involvement in struvite kidney stone production and because it is a highly motile, urease-producing, Gram-negative rod. Although *U. urealyticum* and *P. aeruginosa* have been reported to induce struvite stones, *Proteus* organisms are the most common cause.

31 **The answer is B: *Klebsiella pneumoniae*.**   All the organisms listed could have caused pneumonia in this patient. *M. pneumoniae* causes a mild illness. Sputum production is scant with *L. pneumophila*. Rust-colored sputum is typical for *S. pneumoniae*. Thick, bloody sputum, described as "currant jelly" sputum, is characteristic of pneumonia caused by *K. pneumoniae*. This organism is an opportunistic pathogen causing lung infections in middle-aged and older individuals with alcoholism and patients with diabetes or chronic bronchopulmonary disease. Growth of the organism in the lungs causes necrosis, inflammation, abscess formation, cavitation, empyema, pleural adhesions, and hemorrhage leading to prominent bloody sputum. It is a severe illness with rapid onset of high fever and chills, flu-like symptoms, and a cough productive of abundantly thick, tenacious, blood-tinged sputum. Mortality rate is over 50% despite early and appropriate antimicrobial treatment. Risk factors for infection include a compromised respiratory immune system, hospitalization, intubation, diabetes, and alcoholism.

32 **The answer is A: Antiphagocytic, unless opsonization occurs.** *Klebsiella* is a nonmotile, Gram-negative rod with a prominent polysaccharide capsule or K antigen. The capsule is the main determinant of pathogenicity, preventing phagocytosis of the organism unless it has been opsonized by complement or IgG. Other virulence factors include lipopolysaccharide or O antigen and siderophores involved in uptake of iron from the host.

33 **The answer is A: *Escherichia coli* K1.** All of the agents listed can cause meningitis. The most common causes of meningitis in infants less than 1 month of age are *E. coli* K1, Group B *Streptococcus*, and *Listeria monocytogenes*. The clue to the identification of *E. coli* as the etiologic agent is the fact that the organism grew on MacConkey agar—a selective medium for the growth of enteric, Gram-negative rods.

34 **The answer is C: Enteroinvasive *E.Coli* (EIEC).** The clinical picture described fits the description of enteroinvasive *E. coli* that causes a *Shigella*-like dysentery. ETEC is a cause of traveler's diarrhea. EPEC is a major cause of childhood diarrhea in developing countries. EIEC causes *Shigella*-like dysentery. EHEC causes hemorrhagic colitis; EAEC (30% of the traveler's diarrhea cases) is primarily associated with persistent diarrhea in children in developing countries.

35 **The answer is D: *Rickettsia rickettsii*.** This organism is the cause of RMSF. *B. microti* is transmitted by ticks and causes babesiosis; *O. tsutsugamushi* is transmitted by mites and causes scrub typhus. *R. prowazeki* is transmitted by lice and causes epidemic typhus. *R. typhi* is transmitted by fleas and causes endemic typhus.

36 **The answer is C: Doxycycline.** Tetracyclines are the drug of choice for rickettsial infections, and doxycycline is the preferred member of this group. Sulfonamides are contraindicated as they have been shown to worsen the symptoms.

37 **The answer is A: Botulism.** This case is a classic description of botulism. The disease, although rare, is associated with ingestion of home-canned food products. The symptoms of botulism are diffuse, flaccid paralysis, visual disturbances including diplopia (double vision), and speech difficulty (dysarthria). None of the other choices are associated with these disease manifestations.

38 **The answer is C: *Helicobacter pylori*.** While all of the organisms listed are associated with GI symptoms, this case is descriptive of peptic ulcer disease, which is associated with *H. pylori* infection. The other organisms cause diarrheal diseases.

39 **The answer is B: Gastric adenocarcinoma.**

40 **The answer is A: cagA.** All the items listed are virulence factors of *H. pylori*. Urease breaks down urea, releasing ammonia that neutralizes gastric acids, making a more favorable environment for the pathogen to survive. Heat shock protein B has been shown to enhance the activity of urease. Mucinase breaks down gastric mucus, allowing the organism to penetrate the thick mucus layer and adhere to the gastric epithelial cells. Vacuolating cytotoxin damages gastric epithelial cells and promotes inflammation, thereby playing an important role in ulcer formation. The role of cagA in carcinogenesis is supported by the fact that the protein is translocated into the host cells where it activates signal transduction molecules and induces morphological changes in the cells. In addition, cagA-negative strains of *H. pylori* are significantly less associated with gastric adenocarcinoma.

41 **The answer is *B: Escherichia coli* O157:H7.** All of the organisms listed are causes of diarrheal diseases; however, of the species listed, only *E. coli* O157:H7 is associated with this constellation of symptoms.

42 **The answer is A: *Borrelia hermsii*.** The case is descriptive of tickborne relapsing fever endemic to the western United States. Several spirochete species of the genus *Borrelia* are linked to this disease. *Borrelia recurrentis*, which causes another type of relapsing fever, is transmitted to humans by the Pediculus body louse and is found in certain areas of Africa and South America. Tickborne relapsing fever is usually successfully treated with antibiotics. Of the other organisms listed, only *T. pallidum*, the causative agent of syphilis, is a spirochete.

43 **The answer is D: *Treponema pallidum*.** No pain is reported with the ulcerated lesions (i.e., reports no discomfort during sexual activity) suggesting that this is a primary syphilic sore or chancre. The lymphadenopathy and lack of fever further supports the presumption of primary syphilis. The other agents listed are sexually transmitted agents. *H. ducreyi* causes a painful ulcer and tender, enlarged lymph nodes. *C. trachomatis*, *N. gonorrhoeae*, and *T. vaginalis* (a protozoan) cause a urethritis characterized by discharge.

44 **The answer is E: Specific antibody test.** Secondary syphilis commonly presents with macular brownish lesions on the soles of the feet and palms of the hands. Lesions may be diffusely distributed on the body but are often more visible on the soles and palms, especially in dark pigmented patients. Another clue that points to syphilis is the nontender lymphadenopathy. Although it is reported that these lesions are positive for treponemes and are often observed with darkfield microscopy, it is more practical in a busy clinic to employ a serological test. Nontreponemal tests such as the RPR and VDRL have general screening value but could mistakenly be interpreted as a positive result in a patient who is pregnant. Confirmation with the fluorescent treponemal antibody absorption (FTA-ABS) is a suitable test in this situation.

45 **The answer is D: Penicillin.** Although treponemes are sensitive to several different antibiotics, the patient is pregnant which makes penicillin the obvious choice. The other drugs listed are contraindicated in pregnant women.

46 **The answer is C: Coagulase positivity.** Catalase positivity separates staphylococci from streptococci. Coagulase positivity separates *S. aureus* from the so-called "coagulase-negative staph" including *S. epidermidis* and *S. saprophyticus*. *S. aureus* is β-hemolytic. Bacitracin sensitivity helps distinguish group A streptococci from other streptococcal species. Lactose fermentation is used to distinguish members of the Enterobacteriaceae group. Urea hydrolysis is a notable characteristic of *Proteus* sp. and *Helicobacter pylori*.

47 **The answer is E: Tetanus toxoid.** Assuming that the child has no deficiencies with humoral immunity, the standard of care is to provide a booster of tetanus toxoid to a patient with the above clinical picture. It is currently believed that the anamnestic response (i.e., memory cell activity) will produce ample antibody long before the tetanus bacillus is able to produce the damaging toxin. In other words, the patient is actively immunized.

48 **The answer is B: Gonorrhea.** Although the results are not very clear-cut in the female patient because of normal flora considerations, a Gram stain of urethral exudate from a male patient is a dependable diagnostic procedure. It is also very inexpensive to perform. In the male patient, the sensitivity is at least 90% and the specificity is 99%. Gram-negative diplococci within the neutrophils give little doubt that the patient has gonorrhea.

49 **The answer is B: Ceftriaxone plus azithromycin.** Due to the frequency of coinfection, the CDC recommends treating cases of *gonococcal* urethritis with additional antibiotics for *Chlamydia trachomatis* if the latter has not been ruled out. Suitable combinations include ceftriaxone for *N. gonorrhoeae* plus azithromycin or doxycycline for *C. trachomatis*. Resistance to penicillins, tetracyclines, fluoroquinolones, and azithromycin preclude the use of these antibiotics for the treatment of *Neisseria gonorrhoeae*.

50 **The answer is B: Bacterial vaginosis.** Usually a physician will make the diagnosis of bacterial vaginosis or BV from the clinical presentation of the woman and the identification of clue cells (epithelial cells with an overgrowth of bacteria on the surface) in a wet mount. The overgrowth will generally appear as a stippling over the surface of the cell. The photograph is a Gram stain showing adherent bacteria on a vaginal epithelial cell. Also of note is that the margins of the epithelial cell are somewhat ragged, which is further evidence of BV. *Gardnerella vaginalis* will often give a Gram-variable reaction (shown); however, it is important to recognize that there are other bacterial causes of BV, including *Lactobacillus*, *Mobiluncus*, *Bacteroides*, and *Mycoplasma hominis*. In fact, it is probably more proper to refer to the condition as a polymicrobial infection rather than attributing it to only *Gardnerella*. The discharge is described as milky in consistency, gray in color, and possibly with foul odor characteristic of anaerobic bacteria. It is treated with metronidazole; untreated cases have been linked to pelvic inflammatory disease and other gynecological conditions.

51 **The answer is A: Results reflect the bacteriostatic properties of the antibiotic.** The MIC is the concentration of antibiotic that results in no visible growth of bacteria in the tube. If the antibiotic is bacteriostatic (inhibiting the growth of bacteria), then when the aliquots of the tube showing the MIC are plated on agar, growth of the organism would result. This is what is seen in the above example. If the antibiotic was bacteriocidal, no organisms would have grown when aliquots of the tube showing the MIC were plated on agar. Many antibiotics are bactericidal for some species of bacteria but bacteriostatic for others. This may be a relevant piece of information, especially if the patient is critically ill. Tube dilution MICs and MBCs on agar plates will provide this information.

52 **The answer is D: Group A *Streptococcus*.** The child was diagnosed with impetigo contagiosa, a pyoderma. The two most common agents are coagulase-positive staph (*Staphylococcus aureus*) and group A strep (*Streptococcus pyogenes*). Mixed infections of both organisms regularly occur, but this fact has little relevance with the current status of the child. What is relevant, however, and what distinguishes this case, is the probable glomerulonephritis as noted by the clinical presentation. Described as a rare immune-mediated disease, glomerulonephritis is precipitated by certain strains of strep A pyoderma. Glomerulonephritis can occur even if the impetigo was successfully treated.

53 **The answer is D: Nonlactose fermenting, Gram-negative bacilli.** The two most common bacterial causes of foodborne illness in the United States are *Campylobacter* and *Salmonella*. Both are associated with undercooked poultry and cause invasive (inflammatory) GI disease with the induction of fecal leukocytes. *Salmonella* are Gram-negative rods that are unable to ferment lactose. *Campylobacters* are motile, curved, Gram-negative rods that are isolated under microaerophilic conditions (5% oxygen, 5% to 10% carbon dioxide) on selective media such as Skirrow agar.

54 **The answer is B: Antacids.** Decreased gastric acid increases susceptibility to GI disease caused by *Salmonella* and *Vibrio*. The elderly and young children are also at an increased risk of infection.

55 **The answer is D: *Shigella flexneri*.** Both of the virulent *E. coli* varieties, *V. cholerae* and the nontyphoid *Salmonella* serotypes, have an infective dose (ID) of around 10^6. Actually, the ID of many nontyphoid salmonellae vary and may be as high as 10^9 (1 billion). Host factors that influence a person's predisposition to infection include immunologic deficiencies, inflammatory bowel disease, disruption of GI flora due to broad-spectrum antibiotic use, and the use of stomach acid reducing agents (e.g., antacid, proton pump inhibitors, H_2 blockers, etc.). Of the choices given in the question, clearly *Shigella* has the lowest ID, sometimes as low as 10 organisms. Two other foodborne-fecal agents (not part of the question) that have low infective dose (ca. 10^2) are *Salmonella typhi* and *Campylobacter jejuni*.

56 **The answer is B: *E. coli* O175:H7.** Infection with this strain of *E. coli* is associated with hemolytic uremic syndrome. This complication may be more likely to occur if the patient is treated with antibiotics. Cholera, typhoid fever, pseudomembraneous colitis, and shigellosis respond favorably to antibiotic treatment.

57 **The answer is D: *Salmonella* sp.** After ingestion, the bacterium adheres via fimbriae to M cells, a type of intestinal epithelial cell. The organisms then insert, via a type III secretion system, proteins that induce actin reorganization leading to M cell membrane riffling and engulfment of *Salmonella*. The organisms replicate with phagosomes, leading to M cell death and allowing further spread of the pathogen to neighboring epithelial cells and macrophages. Hence, *Salmonella* is correctly referred to as a facultative intracellular pathogen able to elude specific immune defenses and disseminate deeper into the organ or body. Other bacterial microbes that subjugate the macrophages include *Legionella*, *Yersinia*, *Francisella*, and *Mycobacterium*.

58 **The answer is E: *Serratia marcescens*.** *Serratia* is a motile, Gram-negative bacillus of the family Enterobacteriaceae (includes *E. coli*, *K. pneumoniae*, *Shigellae dysenteriae*, etc.). The species is commonly found in the environment. It can also produce urinary infections in debilitated patients. Unfortunately, this organism has a notorious history of antibiotic resistance, especially to the aminoglycosides and many of the β-lactam antibiotics. The red pigment or prodigiosin is actually an antibiotic produced by certain strains which gives the microbe a competitive advantage against other nearby environmental bacteria. Prodigiosin is most pronounced in cultures grown at room temperature; only a small percentage of the isolates produce this pigment. None of the other organisms listed fit the description provided in the case. The only organism other than *Serratia* that produces pigment, causes disease in immune compromised individuals, and has a high degree of antibiotic resistance is *P. aeruginosa*; however, it does not belong to the family of Gram-negative, enteric bacteria, the Enterobacteriaceae. *E. coli* is a frequent cause of disease in immune competent individuals, *P. mirabilis* produces urease and *K. pneumoniae* is nonmotile.

59 **The answer is B: *Neisseria meningitidis*.** The case describes a toddler with septic arthritis. Many bacteria cause septic arthritis in pediatric patients. The most common cause is *S. aureus*; however, the organism found on Gram stain of the synovial fluid was a Gram-negative diplococcus. Of the organisms listed, only *Neisseria* are Gram-negative diplococci, and both species cause septic arthritis. The fact that the infant had a petechial rash strongly suggests *N. meningitidis*. Other information that supports this organism as the cause is the fact that it ferments glucose and maltose (*N. gonorrhoeae* only ferments glucose) as well as the finding of capsular antigens by serology (*N. gonorrhoeae* lacks a capsule).

60 **The answer is D: *Haemophilus influenzae* b.** The child in the case has meningitis. Organisms that cause meningitis in a child of this age include *Streptococcus pneumoniae*, *Neisseria meningitides*, and *H. influenzae* b. No other organism shares the culture characteristics of *Haemophilus*. This group of organisms is nutritionally fastidious and able to grow on chocolate agar (which supplies necessary nutrients from lysed red blood cells) or as satellite colonies surrounding β-hemolytic colonies of *S. aureus* on blood agar.

61 **The answer is E: Vaccination of the infant.** The *Haemophilus influenzae* b (Hib) vaccine has had remarkable success in reducing the numbers of serious, life-threatening infections due to *H. influenzae* b. Infants are routinely vaccinated with Hib starting at 1 month of age. *H. influenzae* b is transmitted through respiratory droplets and causes a variety of diseases in people of various ages. Thus, avoidance of infants with meningitis would not have protected this infant from infection. Improved community sanitation (treatment and disposal of human waste, clean water, etc.) is not an issue in the transmission of this pathogen. The use of 10% bleach solution to clean toys shared with other infants is recommended to reduce infections and avoidance of day care facilities or other crowded situations could decrease exposure of the infant to infection with this agent. Neither of these options can replace vaccination as a way to prevent infection with *H. influenzae* b.

62 **The answer is A: A change in the terminal pentapeptide from D-ala-D-ala to D-ala-D-lac.** The other mechanisms listed account for resistance to various antibiotics in other bacterial species.

63 **The answer is A: Elementary bodies.** There are two forms of the bacterium *C. trachomatis*, the infectious but nonmetabolically active elementary bodies and the metabolically active but noninfectious reticulate bodies. The Chlamydiaceae is the only family of bacteria which have morphologically distinct phases of their replication cycle. These organisms, similar to viruses, are obligate intracellular pathogens. They can be isolated only in cells and are unable to grow in standard bacteriologic medium. Elementary bodies are found in discharges from the sites of infection (pus from the eye, vaginal or urethral discharges in genital infections, etc.). Contact with these discharges transmits the organism from person to person. Receptors for elementary bodies are found on mucosal epithelial cells and facilitate the uptake of the organism by the cell. Upon entrance into the cytoplasm of the cell, elementary bodies transform into reticulate bodies, replicating within endosomes and forming an inclusion body that can be seen by electron microscopy

or histopathology. Prior to exiting the cell, reticulate bodies transform back into elementary bodies that are able to infect additional cells or be shed from the body. Negri bodies are inclusion bodies formed by rabies virus. Although *Chlamydia* are Gram-negative in the cell wall makeup, they are not cocci.

64 **The answer is B: High sensitivity; low specificity.** Sensitivity and specificity are important criteria for diagnostic tests. The sensitivity is calculated as (true positives/true positives + false negatives) × 100. In this case, the sensitivity is 100%, i.e., (500/500 + 0) × 100 = 100%. The specificity is calculated as (true negatives/false positives + true negatives) × 100. The specificity of this test is (200/300 + 200) × 100 = 40%.

65 **The answer is B: Carditis.** The infection described is strep throat caused by *Streptococcus pyogenes*, also referred to as group A *Streptococcus*. A potential complication of some strains is rheumatic fever, the manifestations of which include carditis, arthritis, and Sydenham chorea. Antibiotic treatment is recommended to prevent this complication. *S. pyogenes* is also associated with skin infections and necrotizing fasciitis. Strep throat very rarely leads to bacteremia. The organism is not associated with encephalitis, hepatitis, or meningitis.

66 **The answer is E: M antigens.** There are over 100 serotypes of *Streptococcus pyogenes* which vary in their pathogenic potential. Certain strains are more invasive than others, and rheumatogenic strains are associated with acute rheumatic fever. Serotypes are based on antigenic differences in the M protein, a coiled, dimeric protein that functions as an important virulence factor. It is coded for by the bacterial *emm* family of genes. The N terminus of the M protein dimer extends above the cell wall and is highly variable while the carboxyl terminus, anchored in the cytoplasmic membrane, is highly conserved between strains. The M protein functions in adhesion and has antiphagocytic properties. Some strains of *S. pyogenes* have a capsule. Capsular antigens distinguish virulent strains of *S. pneumoniae* from less virulent strains; however, strains are not distinguished from one another by variation in capsular antigens. Cell wall antigens are the basis of Lancefield classification of streptococcal species. This organism lacks flagella as well as O antigens, which are part of the structure of lipopolysacccharide, a component of Gram-negative cell walls.

67 **The answer is C: Macrolides are principally secreted in the feces.** The macrolide group (e.g., erythromycin, clarithromycin, and azithromycin) is concentrated in the liver and biliary excretion is the reason why the drug does not give good coverage for urinary tract infections (UTIs) caused by enteric and staphylococcal organisms. Only minute quantities of macrolides are secreted in the urine. Stevens–Johnson syndrome, a rare hypersensitivity reaction, may be drug related but is not the reason for the change in the choice of antibiotic. TMP–SMZ is appropriate but the attending physician could have also ordered a fluoroquinolone or an aminopenicillin. All are concentrated in the urine and have good activity against most bacterial UTI agents. The glycocalyx, transpeptases (β-lactamases), and candidiasis are not significant factors in the decision to change antibiotics.

68 **The answer is A: *Bordetella pertussis*.** The case fits the description of whooping cough or pertussis. This disease is characterized by repetitive bouts of unrelenting coughing punctuated by gasps of air and often end in vomiting. A whooping sound is often made when patients gasp for air. Lymphocytosis, at times as high as 70% of the peripheral white blood cell count, is typical for this disease. The causative agent is *Bordetella pertussis*, a fastidious organism that can be cultured on Regan–Lowe charcoal agar. While the other organisms listed cause respiratory disease, they are not associated with the disease described or microbiologic characteristics of the organism causing this case.

69 **The answer is C: Pertactin, filamentous hemagglutinin, and tracheal cytotoxin.** Both pertactin and filamentous hemagglutinin mediate binding to the ciliated epithelial cells while tracheal cytotoxin, a peptidoglycan like molecule, specifically kills ciliated respiratory epithelial cells. M protein is an adhesive structure found on group A streptococci; pneumolysin is a virulence factor of *Streptococcus pneumoniae* which may kill ciliated epithelial cells; P-pili are adhesive structures of uropathogenic *E. coli*; and lecithinase is secreted by *Clostridium perfringens*. While capsular polysaccharide can promote adhesion, *B. pertussis* is not encapsulated. Polyribitol phosphate capsule is characteristic of *Haemophilus influenzae* and colonization factor is a virulence factor of *Vibrio cholerae*.

70 **The answer is E: Typhoid fever.** The case described is typical for typhoid fever caused by *Salmonella typhi*. This multiorgan system disease is due to the dissemination of the microbe within macrophages. *S. typhi* enters the intestine, infects local macrophages, and is transported around the body, replicating in macrophages in the lymph nodes, spleen, liver, and bone marrow. The infection is accompanied by high fever and evidence of toxemia. Replication of the organism in Peyer patches leads to inflammation of the bowel

wall and subsequent constipation. Bacterial emboli to the skin cause the rose spots seen on the patient's chest and neck. *S. typhi* is isolated on specialized media such as Hektoen agar on which the production of hydrogen sulfide by *Salmonella* is demonstrated as a black center within the colony. None of the other bacterial diseases cause the symptoms or have the microbiological characteristics described in the case. Cholera, caused by the Gram-negative, curved rod *Vibrio cholerae*, is characterized by watery diarrhea. Hemolytic uremic syndrome, caused most commonly by *E. coli* O157:H7, is characterized by bloody diarrhea, kidney failure, and thrombocytopenia. Shigellosis is generally associated with bloody diarrhea. While *Shigella* and *Salmonella* are both grown on Hektoen agar, *Shigella* produces greenish-blue colonies without black centers. Tularemia can manifest in different ways, including ulcers with regional lymphadenopathy, eye infections, pneumonia, and a typhoidal form characterized by fever, malaise, myalgias, and weight loss.

71 **The answer is B: Increase in the intestinal epithelial cell levels of cAMP.** Bacterial causes of watery diarrhea include *Vibrio cholerae* and enterotoxigenic *Escherichia coli*. Both of these organisms produce a toxin (cholera toxin and labile toxin, respectively) whose active portion acts to increase intracellular levels of cyclic AMP (cAMP). cAMP prevents sodium absorption into the intestinal cells and increases chloride secretion from the cells. Water moves from the cells into the lumen of the intestine in response to the movement of ions, thereby leading to watery diarrhea.

72 **The answer is E: Urease.** This enzyme neutralizes gastric acids. The organism also secretes catalase and superoxide dismutase which provide resistance to killing by neutrophils and mucinase that breaks down the mucus, allowing the organism to contact gastric epithelial cells. Another important virulence factor of this organism is vacuolating cytotoxin that leads to epithelial cell injury and neutrophil infiltration.

73 **The answer is A: *Campylobacter jejuni*.** All the organisms listed cause diarrhea; however, only *C. jejuni* and *Salmonella* sp. typically cause bloody diarrhea. *Shigella flexneri* causes bloody diarrhea whereas *S. sonnei* typically causes a watery diarrhea. Of the organisms listed, only *C. jejuni* is a microaerophilic (requiring reduced oxygen in the environment to grow), Gram-negative, curved rod that demonstrates darting motility when viewed under a microscope.

74 **The answer is E: *Pasteurella multocida*.** While animal bite wounds are typically polymicrobial, *Pasteurella multocida* is the most common organism isolated from cat bite wounds. It is a Gram-negative coccobacillus and a commensal organism found in the oropharynx of cats.

75 **The answer is D: *Pseudomonas aeruginosa*.** All of the organisms listed are Gram-negative rods; however, only *P. aeruginosa* fits the microbiologic description. It is oxidase-positive, a test often used to distinguish this species from other Gram-negative bacteria such as the other organisms listed. The photograph demonstrates the characteristic pigment production by *P. aeruginosa*. This organism produces two pigments, pyocyanin and pyoverdin, which are important virulence factors. *P. aeruginosa* is an important nosocomial pathogen resistant to many antibiotics. In the hospital, it is an important cause of burn wound infections as well as urinary tract infections, pneumonia, and bacteremia.

76 **The answer is D: *Vibrio cholerae*.** The case describes an outbreak of cholera characterized by abundant "rice water" stools and rapidly leading to dehydration. Control of the outbreak is essential and, where possible, definitive diagnosis of the etiologic agent is recommended and the organism is cultured on TCBS media. The other organisms listed typically cause bloody diarrhea.

77 **The answer is D: Inhalation of aerosolized bacteria.** Plague is a zoonotic infection of rodents caused by *Yersinia pestis*. It is transmitted among rodents and rarely to people by fleas. Human infection resulting from the bite of an infected flea results in bubonic plague characterized by high fever and painful, enlarged lymph nodes or bubos. Bubonic plague is not transmitted person-to-person. Bacteremia can occur in untreated individuals with bubonic plague, leading to lung infection or pneumonic plague. This form of plague is transmissible person-to-person through respiratory aerosols.

78 **The answer is C: *Leptospira interrogans*.** This organism is the cause of Weil disease. *Bartonella quintana* causes trench fever, an emerging disease among urban homeless individuals in developed nations. *Chlamydia psittaci* is an avian pathogen that can cause fever and respiratory illness in persons with pet birds. *M. leprae* is the cause of leprosy. *U. urealyticum* is a bacterium that colonizes the urogenital tract and can occasionally cause nongonococcal urethritis.

79 **The answer is C: Disseminated rash.** The case describes a man with a primary syphilis chancre (painless ulcer on the genitalia). The chancre will spontaneously heal even without treatment, allowing individuals to believe their infection to be cured. Secondary syphilis, which develops in untreated patients, typically presents as a disseminated rash occurring weeks to months following resolution of the chancre. This stage is also highly infectious. Tertiary syphilis occurs years after infection and can present as dementia, ataxia, and numerous other ways depending on the organ system involved.

80 **The answer is E: *Mycoplasma pneumoniae*.** *Mycoplasma* is one of the few bacterial groups that lack a cell wall. *M. pneumoniae* is an important cause of community-acquired pneumonia.

81 **The answer is B: *Bacteroides fragilis*.** Of the organism listed, *Bacteroides fragilis* is the only one that fits the description. It is a Gram-negative, anaerobic rod involved in intra-abdominal infections such as pelvic inflammatory disease (PID). *C. trachomatis* and *N. gonorrhoeae* are the leading causes of PID and would be the most likely additional organisms involved in this woman's PID; however, they are not anaerobic, Gram-negative rods. *C. trachomatis* is an obligate intracellular pathogen which does not pick up a Gram stain and *Neisseria gonorrhoeae* is a Gram-negative diplococcus. *A. israelii* is an anaerobic, nonspore forming Gram-positive rod. *T. pallidum* is the spiral-shaped bacterial cause of syphilis.

82 **The answer is B: *Bartonella henselae*.** The case is descriptive of cat scratch fever caused by *Bartonella henselae*. This organism colonizes cats, particularly kittens, and is transmitted to humans through bites and scratches. A chronic regional lymphadenopathy develops about 10 days after being scratched or bitten. Infection with the other organisms listed is not linked to cat scratches.

83 **The answer is A: *Chlamydophila pneumoniae*.** All of the organisms listed cause pneumonia and none of them are detected on Gram stain of the sputum. *Chlamydophila pneumoniae* is the only organism listed that requires growth in cultured eukaryotic cells rather than agar or broth.

84 **The answer is C: Ciprofloxacin.** This antibiotic is a fluoroquinolone that acts by inhibiting bacterial topoisomerases (including DNA gyrase), which regulate bacterial DNA supercoiling. While the other antibiotics listed are used for urinary tract infections, they do not have this mechanism of action. Ampicillin is an aminopenicillin and ceftriaxone is a third-generation cephalosporin. Both are β-lactam antibiotics which inhibit cell wall synthesis. Gentamicin is an aminoglycoside that blocks protein synthesis by binding to the 30 S ribosome. TMP–SMZ is an antimetabolite that interferes with folic acid metabolism.

85 The answer is A: Aztreonam. This agent is a monobactam with activity only against aerobic, Gram-negative bacteria including many strains of *Pseudomonas aeruginosa*. It is a good drug to choose for this particular case as it has virtually no renal toxicity. Ceftriaxone is a third-generation cephalosporin which, as a group, has limited activity against *Pseudomonas*. The third-generation cephalosporin ceftazidime is an exception in that it does have activity against this organism. Cephalexin is a first-generation cephalosporin which, as a group, has limited activity against Gram-negative bacteria. Gentamicin has excellent activity against aerobic, Gram-negative bacteria; however, it is an aminoglycoside, not a β-lactam. Gentamicin is also useful against some aerobic, Gram-positive organisms when used synergistically with a β-lactam that enhances uptake of the aminoglycoside through the disrupted cell wall.

86 The answer is D: Streptokinase. This is cellulitis caused by group A *Streptococcus*, or *Streptococcus pyogenes*. Streptokinase lyses clots, enabling the bacteria to spread in the tissues. None of the other virulence factors listed are associated with *S. pyogenes*. A-B exotoxins are made by a variety of toxigenic bacteria such as *Clostridium botulinum* or *Corynebacterium diphtheriae*. Lipopolysaccharide is a component of the outer membrane of Gram-negative bacteria. Uropathogenic strains of *E. coli* express P fimbriae. Yops proteins are virulence factors of *Yersinia pestis*.

87 The answer is E: Metronidazole. Of the listed antibiotics, only metronidazole is useful for anaerobic infections. This drug was first used for treatment of certain protozoal infections such as *Trichomonas vaginalis*, *Entamoeba histolytica*, and *Giardia lamblia*. It is useful against most anaerobic infections.

88 The answer is A: Antigenic variation. *Neisseria gonorrhoeae* spontaneously changes the composition of its pilin proteins by switching between the expression of several different pilin-encoding genes. Antigenic variation also occurs with the opa proteins through changes in the number of nucleotide repeats at the 5′ end of the gene. These changes occur during DNA replication and result in changes in the amino acid sequence of the opa proteins expressed in the cell membrane. *Neisseria gonorrhoeae* does not induce immune suppression or grow in alveolar macrophages. It is not encapsulated and while it secretes an IgA protease, it does not secrete an IgG protease.

89 The answer is B: *Legionella pneumophila*. The case is descriptive of legionellosis. This disease typically occurs in immune compromised patients and presents with pulmonary and nonpulmonary symptoms (headache and diarrhea in this case). *L. pneumophila* lives outside the human host in aquatic environments by infecting free-living amebas. Within the human host, it replicates in alveolar macrophages. Although they all cause pneumonia, none of the other bacteria listed have this combination of characteristics.

90 The answer is B: Cephalexin. Impetigo can be caused by either *Streptococcus pyogenes* or *Staphylococcus aureus*; thus, antibiotics that cover these two organisms must be chosen. Cephalexin, a first-generation cephalosporin, is a β-lactam antibiotic that inhibits cell wall synthesis. It is a drug of choice for treating impetigo involving large areas of the body. Ampicillin is useful against *S. pyogenes*; however, many strains of *S. aureus* secrete β-lactamases that break down this antibiotic. The R1 side chains of first-generation cephalosporins such as cephalexin render the molecules resistant to staphylococcal β-lactamases. Ciprofloxacin is a fluoroquinolone that inhibits topoisomerases involved in bacterial DNA replication. Although they have activity against *S. pyogenes* and some strains of *S. aureus*, and can be used to treat impetigo, fluoroquinolones are generally contra-indicated in young children. Erythromycin and clindamycin are also used for systemic treatment of wide-spread impetigo; however, they do not inhibit cell wall synthesis. They both act to inhibit protein synthesis by binding to the 50S ribosome. Clindamycin is useful for treating skin infections caused by community-acquired methicillin resistant *S. aureus*.

91 The answer is B: Azithromycin plus ceftriaxone. This combination is recommended as an empiric therapy for inpatient treatment of community-acquired pneumonia in adults as it covers both typical and atypical pathogens. Azithromycin is a macrolide antibiotic that binds to the 50S ribosome and inhibits bacterial protein synthesis. It has good activity against the atypical organisms *Chlamydia*, *Mycoplasma*, and *Legionella* as well as against some strains of *Streptococcus pneumoniae* and *Haemophilus influenzae*. Ceftriaxone is a third-generation cephalosporin, a β-lactam antibiotic. It has activity against *H. influenzae* and most strains of *S. pneumoniae*. None of the other antibiotic combinations fit the described mechanisms of action. Ampicillin plus gentamicin is a combination used to treat many severe infections but is not a combination recommended for empiric therapy of community-acquired pneumonia in adults. In addition, while ampicillin is a β-lactam and gentamicin inhibits protein synthesis, it does so by binding to the 30S ribosome. Imipenem is a β-lactam antibiotic in the carbapenem group. Cilastatin is added to this antibiotic to inhibit its rapid metabolism by the renal enzyme dehydropeptidase I. While this combination is useful against *S. pneumoniae* and *H. influenzae*, carbapenems are not useful against the atypical pneumonia pathogens. The combination of piperacillin (an extended-spectrum penicillin) plus tazobactam (a β-lactamase inhibitor) is useful against many Gram-positive and Gram-negative organisms including *Pseudomonas aeruginosa*. Despite its broad spectrum of activity, it is not useful against atypical bacteria. The combination of trimethoprim plus sulfamethoxazole acts by interfering with folate metabolism. This inexpensive drug has activity against a broad range of aerobic bacteria but is not effective against atypical pneumonia pathogens.

92 **The answer is A: *Campylobacter jejuni*.** This organism and nontyphoid strains of *Salmonella* are associated with ingestion of undercooked chicken or raw eggs. Both are common causes of foodborne infections in the United States and both cause a bloody diarrhea that is fecal leukocyte-positive. *C. perfringens* food poisoning is associated with ingestion of contaminated meat products including poultry. This organism causes an intoxication characterized by abdominal cramps and watery diarrhea occurring 8 to 24h after ingestion. *S. typhi* and *S. dysenteriae* are strict human pathogens and are not associated with ingestion of undercooked chicken. Both are uncommon in the United States. *Y. enterocolitica* infection, also uncommon in the United States, is generally associated with ingestion of contaminated dairy products.

93 **The answer is C: *Staphylococcus epidermidis*.** All the organisms listed are Gram-positive cocci. Staphylococci are distinguished from Streptococci and Enterococci by catalase production. Thus, the organism is a species of *Staphylococcus*. Coagulase production distinguishes *S. aureus* from the other staphylococcal species, which are often referred to as coagulase-negative staphylococci. Thus, the etiological agent in this case is *S. epidermidis*.

94 **The answer is A: Biofilm production.** *Staphylococcus epidermidis* produces a polysaccharide, referred to as a slime layer or biofilm, that surrounds the growing colony of organisms. The polysaccharide enables the bacteria to attach firmly to medical devises such as catheters as well as prosthetic joints or heart valves. The biofilm also protects the organisms from opsonins and phagocytes and slows the penetration of antibiotics. Panton–Valentine leukocidin is a cytotoxin found in some strains of *Staphylococcus aureus*, particularly community-acquired MRSA. Pyrogenic exotoxin and streptokinase are important virulence factors of group A streptococci. Some strains of enterococci are noted for vancomycin resistance.

95 **The answer is E: Toxin-mediated inhibition of protein synthesis.** The case is descriptive of diphtheria caused by *Corynebacterium diphtheriae*. This bacterium produces a toxin that inhibits protein synthesis by inactivating elongation factor-2. It does not express any of the other virulence factors listed. It is not known to secrete an IgA protease as does *Neisseria*. As a Gram-positive organism, *C. diphtheriae* lacks lipopolysaccharide. *Streptococcus pyogenes* produces M protein as an important virulence factor. *C. diphtheriae* is not known to produce coagulase as does *Staphylococcus aureus*.

96 **The answer is C: Myocarditis.** Myocarditis can occur about 1–2 weeks following the onset of diphtheria. The diphtheria toxin interacts with receptors on myocardial cells resulting in the inhibition of protein synthesis. The heart is particularly susceptible to the effects of the toxin as myocytes express high levels of the toxin receptor and the toxin's effect is manifested as severe impairment of contractility. Myocarditis is seen in up to 60% of the patients. Death due to diphtheria is usually because of blockage of air passages by the pseudomembrane or myocarditis.

97 **The answer is D: MacConkey agar.** This is one of the most commonly used solid media, enabling differentiation of lactose-fermenting and nonfermenting enteric Gram-negative bacteria and inhibiting the growth of Gram-positive organisms and nonenteric Gram-negative organisms such as *Neisseria*. Blood agar allows for the nonselective growth of a broad range of nonfastidious bacteria. Buffered charcoal yeast extract agar is used to isolate *Legionella*. Chocolate agar is made with lysed sheep red blood cells and is used to isolate fastidious organisms like *Neisseria* and *Haemophilus*. Thayer–Martin agar is used to isolate *Neisseria gonorrhoeae* in specimens collected from nonsterile sites. This agar allows for the growth of *N. gonorrhoeae* while suppressing the growth of other bacterial contaminants in the specimens.

98 **The answer is D: Shiga toxin-producing *E. coli*.** The case is descriptive of hemolytic uremic syndrome associated with infection with *E. coli* O157:H7. This strain of *E. coli* produces phage-associated Shiga toxins (Stx-1 and/or Stx-2) that are functionally and antigenically similar to that produced by *Shigella dysenteriae*. None of the other organisms listed are associated with hemolytic uremic syndrome, although some do cause a bloody diarrhea. *C. perfringens* is associated with ingestion of contaminated meats but it causes watery diarrhea. *S. typhi*, rare in the United States, causes typhoid fever. Enteroinvasive *E. coli* strains are uncommon causes of diarrhea. *Y. enterocolitica*, also rare in the United States, causes a bloody diarrhea.

99 **The answer is B: Lipid A.** Endotoxin is another name for lipopolysaccharide (LPS). This molecule is found projecting from the outer membrane of Gram-negative bacteria. It is composed of a glycolipid called lipid A which is anchored in the outer membrane. Attached to the lipid A is a group of sugars that make up the core polysaccharide and O side chain regions of the molecule. The toxic activity of LPS is attributed to lipid A, which is able to activate immune cells through the stimulation of Toll-like receptor 4 (TLR-4). Activation of cells through TLR-4 leads to NF-κ B-dependent transcription of proinflammatory cytokines such as tumor necrosis factor and interleukin-1. When endotoxin is present in large amounts in the blood, the massive release of these vasoactive cytokines increases vascular permeability leading to hypotension, or endotoxic shock. N-acetylmuramic acid is a component of peptidoglycan which makes up the bacterial cell wall. Teichoic acid is a polymer of ribose and glycerol and is found in the cell wall of Gram-positive bacteria.

100 **The answer is D: Clindamycin.** Clindamycin is a lincosamide antibiotic that is active against aerobic, Gram-positive bacteria such as S. aureus, including community-acquired methicillin resistant strains. It is also used for anaerobic bacterial infections. It is the only antibiotic listed that does not contain a β-lactam ring. People with a history of serious allergic reactions to penicillin should not be given any of the β-lactam antibiotics.

101 **The answer is D: Neisseria meningitidis.** The case is descriptive of meningitis. All the organisms listed can cause meningitis; however, only N. meningitidis is a Gram-negative diplococcus. It is an important cause of meningitis in children and young adults whose spread is facilitated by crowded, confined living situations such as dormitories.

102 **The answer is E: Vaccination.** Many colleges require proof of immunization against this organism of its students. Prophylactic therapy with rifampin or ciprofloxacin is recommended for close contacts of infected individuals. This organism is spread by respiratory aerosols. Hand washing and improved sanitation would not protect against infection. There are no γ-globulin products for protection against this infection. Ribavirin is an antiviral medication and, thus, would provide no protection against this bacterial disease.

103 **The answer is E: Penicillin.** Neisseria meningitidis shows little antibiotic resistance and intravenous penicillin or ceftriaxone is recommended for treatment.

104 **The answer is E: S. sonnei.** There are four species of Shigella: S. dysenteriae, S. flexneri, S. sonnei, and S. boydii. Shigella sonnei is the most common in developed countries and generally causes a watery diarrhea. Shigella flexneri, the most common species in developing countries, also causes some outbreaks in the United States, but it is more likely to cause bloody diarrhea. Shigella dysenteriae causes dysentery characterized by tenesmus and the production of scant, bloody stools.

105 **The answer is E: Viridans group streptococci.** This case is descriptive of subacute endocarditis. The Gram stain shows Gram-positive cocci in chains and the culture shows α-hemolysis. This information, along with the fact that the organism is catalase-negative, suggests that the organism is a viridans group Streptococcus. This group comprises several species. They are important causes of dental plaque and can be introduced into the blood stream where they cause subacute endocarditis. Both group A and group B streptococci are β-hemolytic. Staphylococcal species are catalase-positive.

106 **The answer is A: Dextran production.** The secretion of dextran, a sticky polysaccharide, enables the organisms to adhere to surfaces such as tooth enamel or heart valves. Hyaluronidase is produced by invasive organisms. Viridans group streptococci are not characterized as invasive. Lipopolysaccharide is a component of the outer membrane of Gram-negative bacteria. Pyrogenic exotoxins are produced by certain strains of group A Streptococci associated with scarlet fever. Exfoliative toxins are produced by certain strains of Staphylococcus aureus and are responsible for scalded skin syndrome.

107 **The answer is C: Mycobacteria overwhelming alveolar macrophages.** The case suggests that the man was suffering from progressive primary tuberculosis or a fulminant pulmonary infection. The TB bacillus is described as an intracellular parasite that, in this case, has successfully multiplied to exponential numbers within the phagosomes of macrophages. A virulence determinant of Mycobacterium tuberculosis prevents phagosome–lysosome fusion and, in so doing, escapes the killing effects of the lysosomal enzymes. A major clue with this question is the fact that the organisms here are acid-fast bacilli. This would immediately eliminate all the other choices. In addition, there is no evidence in the visual of consolidation or intracellular inclusions. Although patients with AIDS are at risk for Legionella pneumophila, the clinical findings in this case are not reflective of legionellosis. Lastly, Pseudomonas aeruginosa certainly produces isolated areas of limited growth, especially in burn patients, but huge numbers of bacilli present in the tissue section are beyond the microcolony level.

108 **The answer is C: Positive antistreptolysin O antibodies.** This case is descriptive of acute rheumatic fever. This complication of pharyngeal infection with group A *Streptococci* presents usually 2 to 3 weeks after recovery from sore throat, manifests as a combination of symptoms including polyarthritis, carditis, and chorea, and is uncommon in developed countries where antibiotic treatment of strep throat prevents the occurrence of rheumatic fever. Repeat episodes of rheumatic fever lead to chronic rheumatic heart disease, one of the leading causes of childhood heart diease in the developing world. Because it occurs weeks after pharyngeal infection, throat cultures are seldom positive. Detection of antibodies to streptolysin O, a pore-forming cytolysin released from group A streptococci, is used to document recent infection with this organism. Elevated C-reactive protein and elevated erythroyte sedimentation rate are indicative of an acute phase response. They are two of the "minor criteria" for the diagnosis of acute rheumatic fever using the Jones criteria. They are a nonspecific indicator of a systemic inflammatory response. Lancefield agglutination tests enable laboratory classification of a streptococcal isolate into the various Lancefield groups. This test is not used to make a diagnosis of recent streptococcal infection. The rheumatoid factor test is used as an aid in the diagnosis of rheumatoid arthritis, an autoimmune disease.

109 **The answer is B: M protein.** The M protein is a dimeric, helical protein anchored in the cytoplasmic membrane and extending through the cell wall and capsule of group A streptococci (GAS). It is highly antigenically variable and is the basis for distinguishing the 90+ serotypes of GAS. The M protein of those strains associated with acute rheumatic fever (rheumatogenic strains) is antigenically similar to components of heart valves and connective tissue in joints. Thus, an immune response directed against the M proteins of rheumatogenic strains cross reacts with similar epitopes on heart valves or joint connective tissue leading to acute rheumatic fever. The capsule is an important virulence factor for GAS but does not incite the autoimmune attack that is at the heart of the pathogenesis of acute rheumatic fever. The other virulence factors listed do not play a role in this disease.

110 **The answer is A: Capsule and pneumolysin.** The organism described in this case is *Streptococcus pneumoniae*. It is an important cause of community-acquired pneumonia and strains range in sensitivity to penicillin from fully susceptible to intermediately susceptible to highly resistant. Virulent strains of *S. pneumoniae*, also called pneumococcus, produce a thick, polysaccharide capsule that provides protection against complement activation and phagocytosis. Pneumolysin is a unique cytotoxin elaborated by pneumococci. It induces pores in host cell plasma membranes following binding to cholesterol

residues, thereby damaging ciliated respiratory epithelial cells and neutrophils. The organism does not elaborate any of the other virulence factors listed. Filamentous hemagglutinin, tracheal cytotoxin, and pertactin are virulence factors of *Bordetella pertussis*. Neuraminidase and hemagglutinin are envelope glycoproteins of influenza virus. Pyocyanin and endotoxin are two of the multiple virulence factors of *Pseudomonas aeruginosa*.

111 **The answer is A: Altered penicillin-binding proteins.** An increasing number of pneumococcal strains make penicillin-binding proteins that are not optimally recognized by penicillins and aminopenicillins. Pneumococci do not make β-lactamase. Growing resistance to macrolides, tetracycline, and sulfa drugs is also occurring in strains of this organism, possibly by some of the mechanisms listed.

112 **The answer is C: 50%.** The BCG vaccine is reported to reduce the risk of pulmonary TB by 50%. It provides a significantly higher level of protection in children against miliary tuberculosis and TB meningitis and is the main reason for its use in countries with high prevalence of TB.

113 **The answer is E: *Staphylococcus aureus*.** This organism, a frequent skin colonizer, can contaminate food during preparation. The food is then left at room temperature for several hours during which time the bacteria replicate and secrete heat-stable enterotoxins. The toxins enter the blood and affect the vomiting control center of the brain, inducing vomiting 1 to 6 hours following ingestion of contaminated foods. Settings at risk for outbreak of staphylococcal food poisoning include group picnics, restaurants, and school cafeterias or other situations in which large numbers of people eat food made in batches by food handlers, colonized with the bacteria, who do not use precautions to prevent contamination. Foods that are most frequently implicated are those that are high in salt or sugar, such as salted meats, ham, potato or macaroni salad, and cream-filled pastries or pies. *C. jejuni* causes a diarrheal illness and is associated with the consumption of undercooked chicken. *C. perfringens* also causes a diarrheal illness with an incubation period of 8 to 14 hours following ingestion of contaminated food. *B. cereus* causes vomiting and is most frequently associated with the consumption of fried rice. *Salmonella* food poisoning causes a bloody diarrhea 16 hours to 2 days after ingestion of undercooked chicken, eggs, or other contaminated foods.

114 **The answer is A: *Enterococcus faecalis*.** Enterococci are important causes of nosocomial urinary tract infections (UTIs). They are found as normal intestinal flora and cause disease when introduced into the body. UTI is the most common disease manifestation of this group. Enterococci are innately resistant to cephalosporins as this group of antibiotics cannot bind to enterococcal penicillin-binding proteins. Enterococci are able to utilize folic acid in their environment and are thus insensitive to TMP–SMZ. Although ampicillin plus an aminoglycoside is often used to treat enterococcal UTIs, these organisms show intrinsic resistance to aminoglycosides alone. Vancomycin resistance is the most alarming form of resistance among strains of enterococci as it is feared that the gene for this resistance could be shared among other species of bacteria, most notably, methicillin-resistant *Staphylococcus aureus*. Of the other organisms listed, only *S. saprophyticus* is a common uropathogen; however, it is usually associated with community rather than hospital-acquired UTIs and it is not noted for significant antibiotic resistance.

115 **The answer is B: Amoxicillin–clavulanate.** The organism described is *Moraxella catarrhalis*—a Gram-negative diplococci associated with sinusitis, otitis media, and community-acquired pneumonia. Most strains of *M. catarrhalis* produce β-lactamases, making them resistant to penicillins like ampicillin and first-generation cephalosporins like cephalexin. The addition of the β-lactamase inhibitor clavulanate to amoxicillin makes this a suitable drug for the treatment of this agent. Dicloxacillin is an antistaphylococcal penicillin resistant to β-lactamases produced by this group of organisms. Vancomycin is used for methacillin resistant *Staphylococcus aureus* and other antibiotic resistant Gram-positive organisms.

116 **The answer is C: Ingestion of contaminated food.** The case describes the outcome of an infection with *Listeria monocytogenes* in a pregnant woman. *L. monocytogenes* is a motile, Gram-positive coccobacillus that can grow at refrigerated temperatures, a characteristic exploited for laboratory diagnosis of this pathogen. Infections with *L. monocytogenes* are linked with contamination of food with fecal material from cattle or other animals whose intestines are colonized by this organism. Infection of young, healthy adults is often asymptomatic or leads to a flu-like illness or diarrhea. Immune compromised individuals, pregnant women, and the elderly can expierence life-threatening bacteremia or meningitis. Fetal infection can lead to fetal death or early onset of neonatal disease characterized by widespread abscesses and granulomas in many organs. Transient intestinal colonization with *L. monocytogenes* can occur in humans; however, colonization

does not lead to disease. The organism is not transmitted person-to-person.

117 **The answer is A: Clarithromycin plus ethambutol plus rifabutin.** The patient in the case has disseminated *Mycobacterium avium* complex. This organism is an acid-fast bacillus that causes multiorgan system disease in AIDS patients with CD4 counts of less than 50/cmm. With the advent of highly active antiretroviral therapy, the incidence of the disease among AIDS patients has markedly declined. The above triple drug regimen is recommended for treatment of this disease in AIDS patients as well as pulmonary disease in immune competent individuals. AIDS patients with CD4 counts of less than 50/cmm should receive prophylactic clarithromycin or azithromycin to prevent infection with this organism.

118 **The answer is E: *Yersinia enterocolitica*.** This Gram-negative rod usually causes a diarrheal illness but can also cause infections that mimic appendicitis. *Y. enterocolitica* is part of the normal intestinal flora of cattle and other farm animals. Human infection occurs by ingestion of food or water contaminated with animal feces. The organism is able to grow at refrigerated temperatures while other organisms present in the same fecal sample cannot. This isolation technique is known as cold enrichment. *S. typhi* and *C. jejuni* have been isolated from diseased appendices; however, these organisms are isolated at 37°C. *C. difficile* is an anaerobic, Gram-positive rod causing antibiotic-associated diarrhea and pseudomembranous colitis. *Vibrio parahaemolyticus*, a curved, Gram-negative rod, causes a diarrheal illness following ingestion of inadequately cooked seafood.

119 **The answer is E: *Vibrio vulnificus*.** This organism is a cause of severe wound infections associated with prolonged contact with salt water. The organism is found in the waters of the Gulf Coast of the United States as well as other warm waters around the world. Infections follow ingestion of contaminated seafood or water or exposure of the skin to organisms in seawater. An increase in infections during coastal hurricanes has been reported. People with renal or liver disease or immune suppression are at an increased risk of bullous skin lesions and septic shock following infection with this organism. The other organisms listed also cause serious skin and wound infections. Of these, only *P. aeruginosa* is a Gram-negative rod; however, it is most commonly associated with wound infections caused by burns rather than exposure to seawater.

Chapter 2

Virology

QUESTIONS

Select the single best answer.

1 An outbreak of Calicivirus occurs in a home for disabled adults. What is an important characteristic of this virus group that influences the occurrence of disease outbreaks and their control and prevention?
   (A) Long-term immunity after infection or vaccination
   (B) Low infectious dose required for infection
   (C) Susceptibility of the virus to chlorine cleaning agents
   (D) Susceptibility of the virus to desiccation
   (E) Transmission by inhalation of aerosolized virus particles

2 A new antiviral agent is found to prevent uncoating in a number of different viruses. At which part in the generalized virus replication cycle does uncoating occur?
   (A) Attachment, Penetration, Replication, Assembly, Release, Uncoating
   (B) Attachment, Penetration, Replication, Assembly, Uncoating, Release
   (C) Attachment, Penetration, Uncoating, Replication, Assembly, Release
   (D) Attachment, Uncoating, Penetration, Assembly, Replication, Release
   (E) Uncoating, Attachment, Penetration, Replication, Assembly, Release

3 A new immune modulator is developed which enhances early immunologic responses to viral infection. Which of the following is the earliest immunological event that could be the target of this new drug?
   (A) Activation of natural killer cells
   (B) Activation of naïve viral-specific B cells
   (C) Activation of naïve viral-specific T cells
   (D) Antigen presentation by dendritic cells
   (E) Production of IFN-γ by antiviral cytotoxic T cells

4 A 60-year-old female presents with symptoms of encephalitis and an RNA viral agent is suspected to be responsible for the symptoms. Which one of the following gene probe techniques is most appropriate for identification of an RNA virus in a sample of cerebrospinal fluid?
   (A) Dot blot
   (B) Fluorescent in situ hybridization (FISH)
   (C) Northern blot
   (D) Southern blot
   (E) Western blot

The next two questions are linked.

5 The 27-year-old pregnant mother of a child diagnosed with erythema infectiosum is concerned for the health of her fetus. What would be the most likely outcome of fetal infection with the virus causing her child's disease?
   (A) Hydrocephalus
   (B) Hydrops fetalis
   (C) Mental retardation
   (D) Microcephaly
   (E) Patent ductus arteriosus

6 The effect on the fetus in the above question was caused by virus replication in which fetal cells or tissues?
   (A) Cells of the aortic arch
   (B) Endothelial cells of the central nervous system
   (C) Meninges
   (D) Neurons of the developing nervous system
   (E) Pre-erythrocytes

7 A newly diagnosed HIV-infected male is being evaluated prior to being placed on antiretroviral therapy. What technique is used to determine the number of CD4⁺ cells in his peripheral blood?
   (A) Direct fluorescent antibody test
   (B) Enzyme-linked immunoassay
   (C) Flow cytometry
   (D) Immunoprecipitation
   (E) Quantitative polymerase chain reaction

35

8 Amantadine is a drug used to reduce the ill effects of an influenza virus A infection; however, increasing levels of resistance have limited its usefulness. Resistant strains of influenza A contain single amino acid substitutions in the M_2 protein. With which aspect of the virus replication cycle is this protein involved?

(A) Attachment
(B) Genome replication
(C) Penetration
(D) Release
(E) Uncoating

The next two questions are linked.

9 A 66-year-old man was bitten on the right index finger by a bat while in his bed. He washed the wound but did not seek medical care for the bite. Five weeks later, he went to the emergency room complaining of headache, malaise, drowsiness, pain, and weakness in his right hand. From his history of the bat bite, he was immediately treated with rabies prophylaxis. What was he given?

(A) Interferon-α plus rabies immune globulin
(B) Rabies immune globulin
(C) Rabies immune globulin plus rabies vaccine
(D) Rabies vaccine plus interferon-α
(E) Ribavirin plus interferon-α

10 Why was the man in the above question given rabies prophylaxis?

(A) Interferon enhances the efficacy of rabies vaccine
(B) Prophylaxis with antiviral drugs and interferon blocks viral replication
(C) Rabies prophylaxis reduces the person-to-person spread of rabies
(D) The immune globulin provides immediate but short-lived protection and the vaccine generates long-lasting neutralizing antibodies
(E) The vaccine generates antibody directed against host viral receptors preventing migration of rabies virus into the CNS

11 HIV can infect any cell expressing the appropriate co-receptors but a productive infection occurs only in activated cells. What is the most likely reason for this observation?

(A) Activated cells decrease their cell surface expression of the coreceptors, so budding virions can easily escape to infect new host cells
(B) Activated cells do not have the capacity to induce the antiviral state
(C) Resting cells have sensitive TLR molecules which bind HIV RNA molecules and activate the antiviral state, resulting in degradation of the integrated HIV DNA
(D) Activated cells express transcription factors and polymerases required for transcription of HIV genes
(E) Resting cells are resistant to HIV attachment and penetration due to low expression of the HIV coreceptors

12 A patient seeks treatment for the recurrent lesion seen in the accompanying photograph. Which antiviral would he be given?

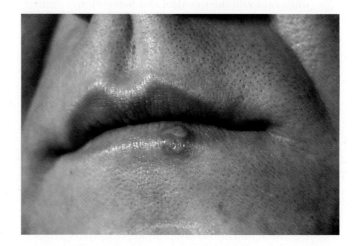

(A) Azidothymidine
(B) Foscarnet
(C) Ganciclovir
(D) Penciclovir
(E) Ribavirin

13 A prophylactic drug is being developed to prevent infection of cells by M-tropic HIV strains following exposure at mucosal sites (vagina, colon). M-tropic HIV strains primarily infect which of the following cell types?

(A) Colonic mucosal cells
(B) Intestinal M cells
(C) Macrophages
(D) Mast cells
(E) Vaginal mucosal cells

14 The CTL response to HIV infection is quite robust; however, these activated CD8$^+$ T cells have little impact on viral clearance or inhibition of AIDS progression. Which one of the following offers an explanation for this observation?
(A) HIV can directly infect CTL causing their lysis upon viral replication
(B) HIV infection of CTL results in insertion of viral DNA into areas of the host genome critical for cell function, thus, infected CTL are functionally impaired
(C) HIV peptides generated in infected cells do not fit into the grooves of the host cell class II MHC molecules, thereby, inhibiting CTL recognition and killing
(D) HIV peptides have alterations which do not permit efficient CTL TCR interactions
(E) HIV reverse transcriptase is highly efficient (not error prone) and thus protein mutation is a rare event

The next two questions are linked.

15 In January, a 66-year-old woman presents a fever of 102°F, chills, back pain, headache, and marked fatigue. Her physician prescribes oseltamivir and she rapidly recovers. With which etiologic agent was she infected?
(A) Coronavirus
(B) Influenza virus
(C) Parainfluenza virus
(D) Respiratory syncytial virus
(E) Varicella-zoster virus

16 What is the mechanism of action of oseltamivir?
(A) Directly prevents replication of the viral genome
(B) Prevents the release of mature virions from the infected host cell
(C) Inhibits the uncoating of the virus
(D) Inhibits the translocation of the viral genome to the nucleus
(E) Binds directly to the virus RNA polymerase active site

17 Type I interferon is used in the treatment of certain viral infections. Which one of the following best describes the mode of action of this antiviral?

(A) Decreases class I MHC expression of infected host cells
(B) Increases degradation of mRNA of infected host cells
(C) Decreases expression of viral receptors on the surface of host cells
(D) Directly lyses free virions in the blood
(E) Attaches to free virus and provides a binding site for opsonizing antibodies

The next two questions are linked.

18 A 55-year-old male develops a rash along the T6 dermatome on the right side of his body as seen in the accompanying photograph. His history is significant for immunosuppressive drug therapy for a transplantation surgery. Which virus is the most likely etiologic agent of this man's condition?

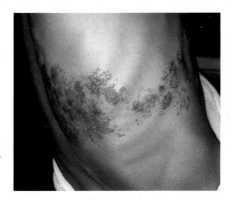

(A) Herpes simplex virus
(B) Measles virus
(C) Molluscum contagiosum virus
(D) Rubella virus
(E) Varicella-zoster virus

19 The man in the above case was placed on which medication to reduce the severity of which possible complication of this infection?
(A) Acyclovir/postherpetic neuralgia
(B) Corticosteroids/scarring from lesions
(C) Ganciclovir/re-establishment of latency
(D) Valacyclovir/prevent cutaneous spread of the lesions
(E) Varicella-zoster immune globulin/prevent spread of the virus into the central nervous system (CNS)

20 Active HIV infection requires susceptible host cells to be in an activated state; however, once they are infected, these host cells rarely undergo mitosis. Which one of the following is most likely an explanation for this observation?

(A) The infected host cell is rapidly lysed by exiting HIV virion

(B) HIV Rev prevents first stages of mitotic division

(C) HIV Nef promotes Bax expression and host cell apoptosis

(D) Infected host cell detects inserted HIV DNA and stops cell cycling to activate DNA polymerase in order to remove the viral genome

(E) HIV Vpr stops cell cycling in G2

21   A number of antivirals are termed nucleoside analogs. Which one of the following best describes the mode of action of nucleoside analogs?

(A) Insert within the helix of DNA to prevent viral replication

(B) Bind to ribosomes and prevent anticodon–codon interactions thereby inhibiting protein synthesis

(C) Substitute for nucleosides resulting in replication termination (chain termination).

(D) Bind directly to DNA polymerase binding sites on viral genome to prevent viral replication

(E) Bind directly to RNA polymerase binding sites on viral genome to prevent expression of viral gene products

The next three questions are linked.

22   A 56-year-old Southeast Asian immigrant is diagnosed with chronic hepatitis B virus infection. Considering the epidemiology of this infection in endemic countries, what is the most likely way that this man became infected?

(A) Heterosexual sex

(B) Homosexual sex

(C) Intravenous drug abuse

(D) Needlestick injury

(E) Perinatally

23   The patient in the above question is treated with a regimen that included pegylated interferon-α. Shortly after initiating therapy, the patient's serum liver enzymes increase, indicating liver cell death. What mechanism of action of α-interferon could account for this transient spike in serum liver enzymes?

(A) Down-regulation of expression of viral proteins on infected cells

(B) Increased expression of MHC-I on infected cells

(C) Interference with reverse transcriptase activity

(D) Interference with DNA-dependent DNA polymerase activity

(E) Interference with viral assembly

24   The other medication the patient was given acts by inhibiting reverse transcriptase. Which antiviral medication, used for chronic HBV infections, works by inhibiting this enzyme?

(A) Acyclovir

(B) Amprenavir

(C) Fomivirsen

(D) Ganciclovir

(E) Lamivudine

25   A 6-month-old female infant presents with a history of sudden fever of 103.4°F followed by the appearance of an erythematous maculopapular rash on the trunk and extremities. She is diagnosed with roseola. What is the cause of her condition?

(A) Coxsackievirus

(B) Human herpes virus type 6

(C) Measles virus

(D) Parvovirus

(E) Rubella virus

The next three questions are linked.

26   A 23-year-old woman presented with an insidious onset of fever, fatigue, joint pain, nausea, anorexia, and abdominal pain. Physical exam revealed hepatomegaly. A hepatitis panel revealed:

HBsAg-positive

Anti-HBsAg-negative

Anti-HBcAg IgM-positive

HBeAg-positive

Anti-HAV IgG-positive

What is a correct interpretation of the hepatitis panel?

(A) Acute infection with HBV

(B) Chronic infection with HAV

(C) Coinfection with HAV and HBV

(D) Past infection with HBV

(E) Vaccinated against HBV

27   Considering the epidemiology of this disease in the United States, what would the history of the above patient most likely include?

(A) Alcoholism

(B) Cocaine addiction

(C) Intravenous drug abuse

(D) Recent transfusion

(E) Unprotected sex with multiple partners

28 The patient in the above question is seen 2 years later for treatment of gonorrhea. Liver function tests reveal elevated alanine transferase levels. A follow-up hepatitis panel revealed:

HBsAg-positive
Anti-HBsAg-negative
Anti-HBcAg IgM-negative
Total anti-HBcAg-positive
HBeAg-positive
Anti-HBeAg-negative
Anti-HAV IgG-positive

What is a correct interpretation of the hepatitis panel?
(A) Acute infection with HBV
(B) Chronic infection with HBV
(C) Coinfection with HBV and HAV
(D) Recovery from HBV infection
(E) Vaccination against HBV and HAV

29 A 28-year-old man was clinically diagnosed with the flu after presenting to his physician with a fever of 102 °F, severe myalgia, fatigue, and rhinorrhea of 12 h duration. The physician had read local health department reports that said both AH1N1 and B viruses were circulating in the area. Which medication did she most likely prescribe?
(A) Amantadine
(B) Foscarnet
(C) Ribavirin
(D) Ritonavir
(E) Zanamivir

The next two questions are linked.

30 A 37-year-old man presents to your office in a panic, stating that he tested positive for HIV based on the results from a saliva-based rapid test offered at a health fair. The man reports no risk factors for HIV. Which of the following tests should be ordered right away?
(A) CBC and differential
(B) Lipid profile
(C) Serologies for hepatitis viruses
(D) Viral load and resistance testing
(E) Western blot for HIV

31 If the prevalence of HIV infection is 0.5% in the area where the man in the above case lives, and the sensitivity and specificity of the rapid test used at the health fair is 100% and 99.5% respectively, what is the positive predictive value of the test?

(A) 10%
(B) 25%
(C) 50%
(D) 75%
(E) 100%

32 A 2-year-old girl was brought to the emergency department by frantic parents with a 3-day history of coldlike illness and a 1-day history of difficulty breathing and an unusual, barklike cough. Physical exam revealed a fever of 38 °C, tachypnea, and tachycardia and stridor. A chest radiograph revealed narrowing of the upper airways (a steeple sign); however, lungs were free of infiltrates. A rapid antigen detection test on respiratory secretions was positive for parainfluenza virus. What is the clinical diagnosis?
(A) Bronchitis
(B) Bronchiolitis
(C) Croup
(D) Epiglottitis
(E) Pneumonia

33 A 21-year-old college student contracted mumps infection as did several other students at the college. He had received a single dose of the measles, mumps, rubella (MMR) vaccine at 15 months of age. What is the most likely reason that he became infected despite having been vaccinated?
(A) Early vaccines only contained one of the four strains of mumps virus
(B) Early versions of the mumps vaccine were heat inactivated and induced immune suppression in some recipients
(C) Fifteen months of age is too early to receive the MMR vaccine
(D) Mumps virus rapidly undergoes antigenic variation
(E) Some individuals who receive a single dose of mumps vaccine do not respond adequately

The next two questions are linked.

34 A 16-year-old boy presented with a 1-week history of sore throat, fever, and profound fatigue. Physical exam revealed a fever of 39.5 °C, cervical lymphadenopathy, exudative pharyngitis, and mild hepatosplenomegaly. His white blood cell count was 12,500/µL with 20% neutrophils, 24% monocytes, 42% lymphocytes, and 12% atypical lymphocytes. A rapid serologic test performed at the physician's office revealed the presence of heterophil antibodies. What is the cause of this boy's illness?

(A) Adenovirus

(B) Cytomegalovirus

(C) Enterovirus

(D) Epstein–Barr virus

(E) Human immunodeficiency virus

35 Which cells infected by the virus in the above question allow full virus replication and which may become transformed by the virus?

(A) Lymph node dendritic cells and T cells, respectively

(B) Monocytes and cells of the oropharynx, respectively

(C) Monocytes and hepatocytes, respectively

(D) Nasopharyngeal epithelial cells and B cells, respectively

(E) T cells and splenic macrophages, respectively

36 Five patients aged 45 to 67 were admitted to an urban hospital between February and March with severe pneumonia. Clinical manifestations included high fever, nonproductive cough, and dense lower lobe infiltrates. All five had underlying lung disease or were smokers. Gram stain of induced sputum showed no pathogens. None of the patients responded to empiric antibiotics pending bacterial and fungal cultures, which were subsequently reported as negative A DNA virus was isolated in cell cultures. Which virus is the most likely cause?

(A) Adenovirus

(B) Hantavirus

(C) Influenza virus

(D) Parainfluenza virus

(E) Respiratory syncytial virus

37 A 43-year-old man, recently infected with hepatitis C virus, donates blood during the window period of the infection. The blood is screened for antibodies to HCV and other bloodborne agents. What is the clinical significance of the time period during which the screening was performed?

(A) Anti-HCV antibodies would not be demonstrable

(B) His blood would be rejected for donation based on the antibody test results

(C) He would be negative for antibodies to HCV by ELISA, but positive by western blot

(D) The results of the screening test would be reported to the health department

(E) Viral RNA tests would be negative

The next two questions are linked.

38 A 3-year-old child presents with a 3-day history of cough, a profusely runny nose, and conjunctivitis, and a 1-day history of 40°C fever, and a blotchy, erythematous, maculopapular rash that began on his face and is now appearing on his chest. The child is toxic appearing. His history is significant for a lack of most childhood vaccines due to family religious beliefs. Which is the most likely diagnosis?

(A) Echovirus summer rash

(B) Measles

(C) Mumps

(D) Rubella

(E) Varicella

39 The child in the above case recovered uneventfully, was re-exposed to the same agent a year later, but did not become ill. What prevented the child from becoming infected on subsequent encounter with the agent?

(A) Activated macrophages

(B) Interferon-α

(C) Naïve cytotoxic T cells specific for the agent

(D) Neutralizing IgG antibodies specific for the agent

(E) NK cells

40 A 9-month-old child is hospitalized with viral pneumonia. Which virus is the most likely cause?

(A) Adenovirus

(B) Influenza virus

(C) Parainfluenza virus

(D) Respiratory syncytial virus

(E) Varicella-zoster virus

41 A 15-year-old boy presents to his family physician in a small Georgia town with an acute onset of nausea, vomiting, and abdominal pain. Hepatomegaly and icteric sclera are noted on physical exam. Alanine transferase and aspartate transferase levels are markedly elevated. Over the next 3 days, 10 more people in the town seek medical attention with similar complaints. How is the most likely cause of this outbreak definitively diagnosed?

(A) Antigen detection in the stool

(B) Culture of organism on MacConkey agar

(C) Demonstration of IgM antibodies against the agent

(D) Ova and parasite exam

(E) Virus isolation from the blood

42 An HIV-infected man with a CD4 cell count of 400/cmm develops a painful, vesicular rash as seen in the accompanying photograph. What does this skin rash indicate about his immune system?

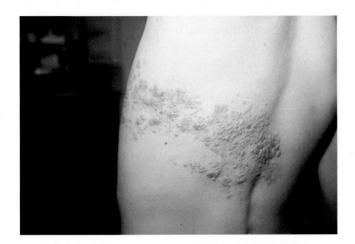

(A) He can no longer produce anti-HIV antibodies
(B) His B cells can no longer control the agent causing the skin infection
(C) His CD4 cells cannot activate CD8 cells
(D) His CD4 to CD8 ratio is increased
(E) His complement C5 to C9 is depleted

43 A 58-year-old AIDS patient has failed several antiretroviral regimens due to viral drug resistance. Which of the following drugs blocks the entry of HIV into cells and is used in combination therapy after other regimens have failed?
(A) Efavirenz
(B) Enfuvirtide
(C) Fosamprenavir
(D) Lamivudine
(E) Ritonavir

The next three questions are linked.

44 A 40-year-old woman in apparent good health is found to have slightly elevated serum liver enzymes during an insurance physical. Follow-up investigations revealed antibodies to hepatitis C virus. What test could be done to distinguish between current infection and previous infection with full recovery?
(A) ELISA
(B) Indirect fluorescent antibody
(C) Reverse transcriptase polymerase chain reaction
(D) Western blot
(E) Viral culture

45 As part of the initial workup of this patient, the genotype of HCV was determined. What is the clinical significance of genome testing?
(A) Predicts response to therapy
(B) Predicts risk of cirrhosis
(C) Predicts risk of extrahepatic manifestations of disease
(D) Predicts risk of hepatoma
(E) Predicts viral load

46 Three years following diagnosis with hepatitis C virus, liver biopsy from the above patient reveals sufficient damage to consider antiviral therapy. With which drug combination should she be treated?
(A) Adefovir plus lamivudine
(B) Amoxicillin plus sulbactam
(C) Lamivudine plus zidovudine
(D) Pegylated interferon and ribavirin
(E) Trimethoprim plus sulfamethoxazole

The next two questions are linked.

47 An infant is born prematurely in February. Concerned about the risk of serious infection with respiratory syncytial virus, he is treated with the monoclonal antibody palivizumab before being released from the hospital. What is the viral target of this monoclonal antibody?
(A) Capsid protein
(B) Fusion protein
(C) Hemagglutinin protein
(D) Neuraminidase protein
(E) Matrix protein

48 A fourth year medical student sustains a needlestick from a patient being evaluated for jaundice. A hepatitis panel is ordered on the student the same day and finds:
HBsAg-negative
Anti-HBsAg-positive
Anti-HBcAg IgM-negative
Anti-HBcAg total negative
Anti-HAV IgG-positive
Anti-HCV-negative

What is a correct interpretation of the hepatitis panel?
(A) Acute infection with HAV
(B) Acute infection with HBV
(C) Chronic infection with HBV
(D) Past infection with HBV
(E) Vaccinated against HBV and HAV

49 A 4-month-old child develops a viral infection with fever and vesicular lesions in the anterior portion of the mouth, as well as around the mouth. This infection occurred 2 weeks after her mother had a cold sore. The lesions lasted for about 3 weeks during which time the child was not eating or drinking normally due to the discomfort. Which of the following will be the most likely consequence of this infection in the child?

(A) Acute infection with complete recovery
(B) Encephalitis
(C) Esophagitis
(D) Keratitis
(E) Latency with periodic recurrences

50 An 8-year-old boy attending 4-week summer camp presented in August with a 3-day history of fever, sore throat and conjunctivitis. Seven other children and two camp counselors developed similar symptoms over the next few days. All described a gritty feeling in their eyes. A similar outbreak had occurred at the camp in July. The cause of the outbreak of fever, sore throat, and conjunctivitis was found to be a virus traced to the camp's underchlorinated, turbid swimming pool. Which virus is the cause of this outbreak?

(A) Adenovirus
(B) Influenza virus
(C) Parainfluenza virus
(D) Respiratory syncytial virus
(E) Rotavirus

The next three questions are linked.

51 A 17-year-old girl presents with fever, stiff neck, malaise, inguinal lymphadenopathy, vaginal discharge, and vesicular lesions on her external genitalia. A direct fluorescent antibody stain of the genital lesions showed nuclear fluorescence. She admits to being sexually active but has never had symptoms like these before. What is the recommended treatment for this infection?

(A) Acyclovir
(B) Imiquimod
(C) Ketoconazole
(D) Lamivudine
(E) Zanamivir

52 Upon administration, the antiviral medication in the above question is in an inactive form. Upon uptake by virally infected cells, the drug is activated by the action of a viral-specific kinase. Which one of the following best describes why the viral kinase would activate this antiviral?

(A) Resting cells express higher levels of viral receptors on their cell surface due to the action of the viral kinases
(B) Resting cells have unphosphorylated nucleosides which are phosphorylated by the viral kinases in order to be usable for viral replication by viral DNA polymerase
(C) Viruses infecting resting cells do not permit viral access to the nucleus without the action of viral kinases on the nuclear pore complex
(D) Viruses infecting resting cells require the action of viral kinases to promote associations of the small and large subunits of the host ribosomes for viral protein synthesis
(E) Viral kinases induce activation of resting cells resulting in increased host cell membrane permeability

53 How are recurrences of the infection in the above question best prevented?

(A) Antiviral medication
(B) A strong antiviral cell mediated immune response
(C) High levels of α-interferon
(D) High titers of antiviral IgG
(E) Highly active natural killer cells

54 A previously healthy 56-year-old woman in Florida dies of eastern equine encephalitis virus. Viral activity had been detected at that time by the local health department in which reservoir and vector species, respectively?

(A) Birds; mosquitoes
(B) Cattle; soft bodied ticks
(C) Foxes; hard bodies ticks
(D) Horses; mosquitoes
(E) Rats; fleas

55 A researcher wanted to induce the replication of HIV in a cell culture line because it was easier than culturing human T cells. What molecule, in addition to CD4, would she have to transfect into the cultured cell line in order to make the cells susceptible to HIV infection?

(A) CD3
(B) CD25 (γ chain of IL-2 receptor)
(C) CD80/81
(D) CXCR4 or CCR5
(E) DC-SIGN

The next two questions are linked.

56 A 35-year-old male is diagnosed with acute hepatitis due to hepatitis C virus. Based on the epidemiology of this infection in the United States, how did this man most likely become infected?

(A) Intravenous drug abuse
(B) Needlestick injury
(C) Recent transfusion
(D) Unprotected heterosexual sex
(E) Unprotected homosexual sex

57 The patient in the above question ultimately requires treatment for chronic hepatitis C and is given pegylated interferon and ribavirin. What is the mechanism of action of ribavirin?
(A) Enhances cell-mediated immunity to kill viral-infected cells
(B) Inhibits fusion of the virus with host cell membrane
(C) Inhibits insertion of viral genetic material into the host chromosome
(D) Inhibits synthesis of guanosine triphosphate (GTP)
(E) Inhibits viral DNA polymerase

The next two questions are linked.

58 A 29-year-old pregnant nurse presents with a mononucleosislike syndrome. She states that she had infectious mononucleosis as a teenager, and is concerned that she may have contracted cytomegalovirus from her 18-month-old son who attends day care. Her concern is for her unborn child. What is the incidence of congenital cytomegalovirus infection in the United States?
(A) 1/100,000 live births
(B) 1/10,000 live births
(C) 1/1,000 spontaneous abortions
(D) 1/100 live births
(E) 1/10 spontaneous abortions

59 What neurological sequelae are most likely if the fetus in the above question is born with symptoms of in utero infection with cytomegalovirus?
(A) Aneurisms of blood vessels in the brain
(B) Intracranial hemorrhages
(C) Mental retardation and deafness
(D) Recurrent episodes of meningitis
(E) Seizures

The next five questions are linked.

60 You are a physician working for a public health agency charged with reducing the incidence of HIV infection. To understand the impact of the disease, you ask many questions about the epidemiology of the disease in the United States and around the world. According to recent statistics, approximately how many new infections with HIV occur yearly around the world?

(A) 2,500
(B) 25,000
(C) 40,000
(D) 400,000
(E) 2.5 million

61 Approximately how many new infections with HIV occur yearly in the United States?
(A) 2,500
(B) 25,000
(C) 40,000
(D) 400,000
(E) 2.5 million

62 Which area in the world has the highest prevalence of HIV/AIDS?
(A) Indian subcontinent
(B) Southeast Asia
(C) States of the former Soviet Union
(D) Sub-Saharan Africa
(E) The United States

63 What is the most common route of transmission of HIV around the world?
(A) Heterosexual sex
(B) Homosexual sex
(C) IV drug use
(D) Perinatal
(E) Transfusion

64 Persons in which transmission category in the United States currently have the highest number of newly diagnosed cases of HIV/AIDS?
(A) High risk heterosexual contact
(B) Intravenous drug use
(C) Medically related
(D) Male-to-male sexual contact
(E) Perinatal

65 A 23-year-old heterosexual male was diagnosed with acute retroviral syndrome. His CD4 count and viral load at the time of diagnosis were 450/µL (normal 500 to 1,500) and 80,000 copies, respectively. He returns in 6 weeks, and is asymptomatic. What changes in the CD4 count and viral load are typically expected at this time in the infection?
(A) Decrease in CD4 cells, decrease in viral load
(B) Decrease in CD4 cells, increase in viral load
(C) Increase in CD4 cells, decrease in viral load
(D) Increase in CD4 cells, increase in viral load
(E) No significant change would be expected

66 A 43-year-old woman has been infected with human immunodeficiency virus for the past 12 years. Which of the following, if it occurs, will indicate that the woman's disease has progressed to fit the case definition of AIDS?
(A) Herpes zoster
(B) Invasive cervical cancer
(C) Pelvic inflammatory disease
(D) Recurrent fever, night sweats, and generalized lymphadenopathy
(E) Recurrent, severe vaginal yeast infections

67 A 21-year-old man infected with herpes simplex virus-type 2 is given an antiviral drug that interferes with the production of viral early proteins. What is the function of the early proteins in the replication of herpes viruses?
(A) Assembly
(B) Capsid formation
(C) Penetration into the nucleus
(D) Replication of viral DNA
(E) Translation of viral mRNA

68 An individual is infected with a virus that replicates causing clinical manifestations. The manifestations later subside; however, virus is not cleared from the body. Viral replication occurs continuously throughout life. Which term describes this type of infection?
(A) Acute
(B) Chronic
(C) Latent
(D) Localized
(E) Slow

69 A 43-year-old man is hospitalized after presenting to the emergency department with fever, chest pain, and shortness of breath after mild exertion. Physical exam reveals tachycardia out of proportion with his fever. He reports a flulike illness 2 weeks previously. A biopsy, taken after the patient began to show signs of heart failure, reveals mononuclear infiltration in the myocardial tissue. Reverse transcriptase PCR identified a viral cause. What is the most likely etiological agent causing this man's condition?
(A) Adenovirus type 7
(B) Coxsackievirus B
(C) Influenza virus
(D) Measles virus
(E) Parvovirus B19

70 A patient with HIV is shown to have neutralizing antibodies against HIV gp120. Which aspect of the virus's replication cycle is directly blocked by these antibodies?

(A) Adsorption
(B) Assembly
(C) Genome replication
(D) Reverse transcription
(E) Uncoating

The next two questions are linked.

71 A 57-year-old AIDS patient with a CD4 cell count of 75/cmm develops vision problems in the right eye. Fundoscopic examination of the eye reveals widespread necrosis and hemorrhage as shown in the accompanying photograph. A viral cause for these findings is suspected. What is the most likely etiology of this man's visual loss?

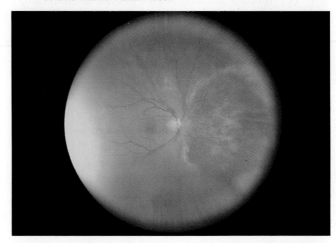

(A) Adenovirus
(B) Cytomegalovirus
(C) Human herpes virus type 8
(D) Lymphocytic choriomeningitis virus
(E) Metapneumovirus

72 The patient in the above question could be treated with an intraocular implant of which antiviral drug?
(A) Acyclovir
(B) Famciclovir
(C) Ganciclovir
(D) Valacyclovir
(E) Zanamivir

73 A 16-year-old boy who competes on the high school wrestling team presents with several firm, flesh-colored, 3 to 4 mm diameter, umbilicated papules on the chest, arms, and groin area. He is diagnosed clinically with molluscum contagiosum. What is the viral etiology of this condition?
(A) Adenovirus
(B) Herpesvirus
(C) Papillomavirus
(D) Polyomavirus
(E) Poxvirus

74 A 56-year-old AIDS patient fails his third regimen of antiretroviral drugs despite being very compliant about taking his medications properly. His failure reflects the development of resistance in his population of viruses to various antiretroviral drugs. The protein product of which gene of HIV is responsible for the rapid production of mutations that leads to antiretroviral drug resistance?

(A) *env*
(B) *nef*
(C) *pol*
(D) *tat*
(E) *vpu*

The next two questions are linked.

75 A 45-year-old homeless Caucasian male presents with multiple 3 to 5 cm erythematous macular lesions on his back, arms, chest, and face. His history is significant for homosexuality and IV drug use. Physical exam reveals an afebrile male in no acute distress with no organomegaly and no edema. A 1-cm diameter, reddish nodular lesion was seen on the palate. A white blood cell count reveals marked lymphopenia, but normal neutrophil, red cell, and platelet numbers. What is the most likely virus that could be identified within the lesions?

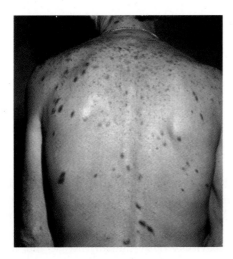

(A) Epstein–Barr virus
(B) Hepatitis C virus
(C) Human herpes virus type 8
(D) Molluscum contagiosum virus
(E) Papillomavirus

76 Which antiviral therapy is most frequently recommended as a first step in treating these lesions?

(A) Acyclovir
(B) Antiretroviral therapy
(C) Imiquimode
(D) Lamivudine
(E) Ribavirin

77 A 32-year-old woman is worked up for an abnormal Papanicolaou test result. Colposcopy reveals aceto-white lesions in the cervix. A sample was taken to test for the DNA of specific viruses belonging to which group?

(A) Enterovirus
(B) Herpes virus
(C) Papillomavirus
(D) Polyomavirus
(E) Retrovirus

78 A 36-year-old woman is preparing for an adventure trip down the Amazon River in Brazil by receiving recommended vaccinations. Against which arbovirus should she be vaccinated?

(A) Arenavirus
(B) Dengue virus
(C) Venezuelan equine encephalitis virus
(D) West Nile virus
(E) Yellow fever virus

79 A 22-year-old woman is diagnosed with condyloma acuminatum and treated with imiquimode. What is the mechanism of action of this drug?

(A) Activates macrophages
(B) Acts as nucleoside analog to block DNA synthesis
(C) Induces secretion of interferon-α
(D) Inhibits cyclooxygenases
(E) Inhibits neovascularization

80 Which vaccine is made from reassorted bovine and human viruses?

(A) Hepatitis A vaccine
(B) Influenza vaccine
(C) Mad cow disease vaccine
(D) Poliovirus vaccine
(E) Rotavirus vaccine

81 A 30-year-old elementary school teacher presents with low-grade fever and symmetrical polyarthritis of the metacarpophalangeal and interphalangeal joints of 3 days duration. The joints are mildly inflamed and tender. She has no family history of rheumatic disease and no risk factors for hepatitis B virus. The cause is suspected to be viral. Which virus is most likely?

(A) Echovirus
(B) Measles
(C) Papillomavirus
(D) Parvovirus B-19
(E) Polyomavirus

82 A 37-year-old AIDS patient develops an insidious onset of cognitive, motor, and visual problems and is diagnosed with progressive multifocal leukoencephalopathy. What is the viral etiology of this condition?
(A) Cytomegalovirus
(B) Endogenous retrovirus
(C) Human herpes virus type 6
(D) Human immunodeficiency virus
(E) JC virus

83 Prior to deployment to Iraq in 2003, a 22-year-old marine was vaccinated against smallpox. What kind of vaccine is given to protect against this agent?
(A) Heat inactivated smallpox virus
(B) Killed vaccinia virus
(C) Live, attenuated variola virus
(D) Live vaccinia virus
(E) Smallpox immune globulin

84 A 34-year-old man, an avid hiker from New Jersey, presents with a fever, fatigue, headache, malaise, myalgia, and arthralgia. The patient reported that the fever had first occurred 1 week ago and lasted for 3 days, then resolved for 3 days, and returned, at which time he sought medical attention. His history is significant for a recent hiking trip in Utah during which he experienced a tick bite. Which tick-borne viral disease might this man have contracted in his hiking trip?
(A) Colorado tick fever
(B) Lyme disease
(C) Relapsing fever
(D) Rocky Mountain spotted fever
(E) Tick-borne encephalitis

85 A 12-year-old girl is brought to her family physician to receive the vaccine that helps prevent cervical cancer and genital warts. Protection against infection with which specific viruses is afforded by this vaccine?
(A) Adenovirus serotypes 7, 10, 22, and 43
(B) Herpes simplex viruses types 1 and 2
(C) Human immunodeficiency viruses types 1 and 2
(D) Human papillomaviruses (HPV) types 6, 11, 16, and 18
(E) Parainfluenza viruses 1, 2, 3a, and 3b

86 An outbreak of a hemorrhagic virus occurs in a village in Uganda, Africa. Clinical manifestations included hemoptysis, bleeding from the eyes, skin, and gastrointestinal tract. The mortality rate exceeded 70%. The virus appeared to be transmitted in the village by contact with the blood and bodily secretions of affected individuals; thus, infection rates were highest among those caring for the sick. Which viral disease was involved in this outbreak?
(A) Dengue hemorrhagic fever
(B) Ebola
(C) Hantavirus pulmonary syndrome
(D) West Nile fever
(E) Yellow fever

87 A 67-year-old male in Minnesota is hospitalized in August with fever, lethargy, and disorientation. Cerebral spinal fluid analysis reveals a WBC count of 100 with 65% mononuclear cells, elevated protein, and normal glucose. IgM antibodies to the most common arbovirus in the United States are found in his serum. With which virus is he infected?
(A) Eastern equine encephalitis virus
(B) LaCrosse virus
(C) St Louis encephalitis virus
(D) Western equine encephalitis virus
(E) West Nile virus

88 Protease inhibitors are useful drugs against HIV by preventing maturation of the budding virion. This maturation process involves proteolytic cleavage of which HIV protein?
(A) Env
(B) Pol
(C) Gag
(D) Matrix
(E) Nef

89 In 2003, a previously unknown viral disease arose in China and spread to five countries around the world, causing thousands of cases with about a 10% overall mortality rate. The disease was attributed to a novel Coronavirus. What human disease did this newly described Coronavirus cause?
(A) Aseptic meningitis
(B) Bird flu
(C) Hantavirus pulmonary syndrome
(D) Meningoencephalitis
(E) Severe acute respiratory syndrome

90 Four days after returning to the United States from a trip to the Caribbean, a 34-year-old man presents with fever that had been as high as 39°C two days previously but had returned to normal, severe headache, and severe pain behind the eyes, in the joints, and in the muscles. Physical exam reveals a macular rash seen on the trunk and extremities, hepatomegaly, petechiae on mucous membranes of the mouth and induced on the arm following a tourniquet test. Laboratory tests reveal a white blood cell count of 6,720 with 30% neutrophils, 50% lymphocytes, 16% monocytes, and 4% atypical lymphocytes and 65,000 platelets. IgM to which virus was found in his serum?
(A) Dengue virus
(B) Ebola virus
(C) Epstein–Barr virus
(D) Hepatitis A virus
(E) Parvovirus B-19

91 Which method is best for prevention of this infection?
(A) Avoiding places with poor public hygiene when visiting endemic areas
(B) Drinking only bottled water
(C) Taking prophylactic ribavirin
(D) Use of insect repellent
(E) Vaccination

92 The 6-week-old infant shown in the photograph is brought to the emergency department with poor feeding, irritability, and rapid breathing. Studies reveal hepatosplenomegaly, bilateral deafness, and patent ductus arteriosus. The infant's mother, an undocumented immigrant, reported experiencing fever and joint pain that lasted a few days during her second month of pregnancy. The maternal illness is determined to be related to the infant's condition. What is the most likely diagnosis for the infant?

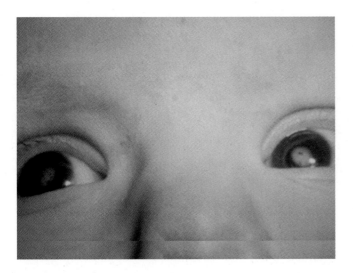

(A) Congenital cytomegalovirus
(B) Congenital rubella syndrome
(C) Congenital varicella
(D) Neonatal enterovirus infection
(E) Neonatal herpes

93 A 65-year-old woman refuses to be vaccinated against influenza virus because she was vaccinated the previous year. What changes in the virus necessitate annual vaccination?
(A) Acquisition of new genes through coinfection of cells with parainfluenza viruses
(B) Antigenic changes in the viral matrix protein
(C) Changes in the level of expression of the envelope fusion proteins
(D) Mutations in the genes for the envelope glycoproteins
(E) Reassortment of RNA strands between animal and human strains

The next two questions are linked.

94 One month after receiving a heart transplant, a 43-year-old man develops fever, malaise, abdominal pain, weight loss, and bloody diarrhea. Endoscopy reveals an erythematous, hemorrhagic colonic mucosa with multiple erosions and ulcerations. Histopathology of biopsied colonic mucosa reveals several large cells with prominent intranuclear inclusion bodies typical of the viral etiologic agent. With which antiviral should this man be treated?
(A) Acyclovir
(B) Azidothymidine
(C) Ganciclovir
(D) Ribavirin
(E) Voriconazole

95 In making a definitive diagnosis in cases such as the one above, which one of the following techniques is appropriate for detection of the viral DNA in the blood?
(A) Direct fluorescent antibody assay
(B) Enzyme-linked immunoassay
(C) Northern blot
(D) Polymerase chain reaction (PCR)
(E) Western blot

96 Why do polio eradication programs in developing countries utilize the oral polio vaccine (OPV) rather than the inactivated polio vaccine (IPV)?

(A) Persons immunized with IPV can still become infected with and shed wild-type virus.

(B) The vaccine strain of IPV can be shed from the feces and cause disease in susceptible individuals.

(C) The IPV cannot be used in immune deficient patients.

(D) The IPV does not contain all strains of poliovirus.

(E) Vaccine-induced cases of paralytic polio have occurred with IPV.

97 A 14-month-old girl presents with a low-grade fever and rash on her hands and feet as seen in the accompanying photographs. Vesicular lesions were also present on the tongue, palate, and buccal mucosa. The lesions resolved spontaneously within 1 week. What is the most likely etiology of this infection?

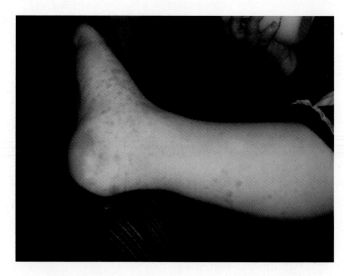

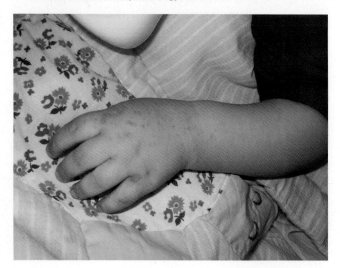

(A) Adenovirus

(B) Coxsackievirus

(C) Cytomegalovirus

(D) Papillomavirus

(E) Rotavirus

ANSWERS

1 **The answer is B: Low infectious dose required for infection.** The human Calicivirus, better known as Norwalk virus, is an important cause of viral gastroenteritis, tends to occur in outbreak fashion, and can cause infection with as few as 10 virus particles. Caliciviruses are nonenveloped viruses and are thus more resistant to environmental conditions than are viruses surrounded by a lipid envelope. Caliciviruses are resistant to desiccation and to levels of chlorine as high as 10 ppm. Immunity is short-lived and there is no vaccine. Outbreaks of Norwalk virus are associated most commonly with ingestion of contaminated food. Person-to-person transmission through a fecal–oral route or infection via contaminated fomites also leads to outbreaks. The virus can become aerosolized from fecal material or vomitus, and infection can occur following such exposure, but this route of transmission is not common.

2 **The answer is C: Attachment, Penetration, Uncoating, Replication, Assembly, Release.** Viruses must attach to host cells via the viral attachment protein and then penetrate the cell either by endocytosis or, in the case of enveloped viruses, fusion of the envelope with the host cell membranes. Following penetration, the genetic material must be released from the capsid in a process called uncoating. The viral genome can then be replicated and its proteins transcribed and translated by the host cell. Once viral structural proteins are produced and the genome replicated, assembly of new virions can occur and the virus is released from the cell by budding or cell lysis.

3 **The answer is A: Activation of natural killer cells.** As part of the innate immune response, natural killer (NK) cells are one of the earliest defenses mounted by the body against viral infections. Following infection of a cell, viruses typically down-regulate the cellular expression of MHC class I molecules. MHC-deficient virally infected cells are recognized and killed by NK cells. The remaining choices listed are part of the adaptive immune response, which require a number of days for activation before they can participate in host defense. Adaptive immune defenses are mediated by T and B cells, and their activation begins with the interaction of dendritic cells and T cells in lymph nodes draining sites of infection. Tissue dendritic cells pick up virus and/or viral antigens and transport them to local lymph nodes, maturing as they travel in the lymph. Mature dendritic cells present antigen to T cells. Activated T helper cells can assist in the activation of B cells. Cytotoxic T cells kill virally infected cells and secrete certain cytokines following activation.

4 **The answer is C: Northern blot.** This technique is used for the identification of RNA sequences separated by gel electrophoresis, transferred (blotted) to a nitrocellulose or similar substrate, and then hybridized with known radiolabeled probes. The southern blot is similar, except that it identifies DNA sequences. The western blot identifies proteins separated by gel electrophoresis, blotted, and probed with specific antibodies. Similarly, the dot blot technique is used to detect and identify proteins applied directly to a membrane. The FISH is a technique used to detect DNA from tissue samples, not from fluid samples.

5 **The answer is B: Hydrops fetalis.** Erythema infectiosum is caused by human parvovirus B-19. This virus is also known as erythrovirus B-19. Erythema infectiosum is a mild rash illness commonly occurring in school-aged children. When a seronegative pregnant woman becomes infected, her fetus has a 10% chance of developing hydrops fetalis, a condition with a high intrauterine mortality rate. This is particularly true if she is less than 20 weeks gestation. Intrauterine parvovirus B-19 is not associated with the other manifestations of congenital infection listed.

6 **The answer is E: Pre-erythrocytes.** Parvovirus B-19 replicates in mitotically active cells of the erythroid linage. This cellular tropism is true regardless of the age of the patient. The result of viral infection in the fetus is death of infected erythrocyte progenitor cells, leading to profound anemia and subsequent congestive heart failure. The virus does not replicate in the other cells listed.

7 **The answer is C: Flow cytometry.** In this method, mononuclear cells are separated from the blood and incubated with fluorescence-conjugated anti-CD4 antibodies. CD4+ cells are stained and the number of fluorescing cells is determined as the cells are passed singly in a fluid stream by a series of detectors in the flow cytometer. The direct fluorescent antibody test utilizes fluorescent-tagged monoclonal antibodies to detect specific pathogen antigens in patient tissues. Enzyme immunoassay is a technique whereby antibodies are utilized to detect antibodies or antigens from patient samples—detection made possible by coupling an enzymatic reaction to a detection antibody. Immunoprecipitation is a procedure using antibodies to bind antigens for extraction from tissue samples. Quantitative polymerase chain reaction is a method used to measure the amount of pathogen DNA in patient samples. It is used to determine viral load in HIV-infected individuals, and is part of an initial evaluation to determine if a patient should be placed on antiretroviral drugs.

8 **The answer is E: Uncoating.** Influenza virus A attaches to the host respiratory epithelium cell and is subsequently endocytosed into the cell. In order for viral replication to occur, the viral genome must be released from the surrounding protein coat or capsid. The viral envelope protein M_2 serves to translocate hydrogen ions from the endosome into the internal compartment of the virus. This maneuver facilitates the fusion of the viral envelope with the endosomal membrane, thereby releasing the viral RNA from the capsid in a process called uncoating. Amantadine and a related compound, rimantadine, block the activity of the M_2 protein. Resistant strains of influenza A have been found to have single amino acid substitutions at four sites in the M_2 protein.

9 **The answer is C: Rabies immune globulin plus rabies vaccine.** See next answer for explanation.

10 **The answer is D: The immune globulin provides immediate but short-lived protection and the vaccine generates long-lasting neutralizing antibodies.** Because the incubation period of rabies is usually long (more than 2 weeks—unless bitten on the face) and the disease is completely preventable with neutralizing antibodies, vaccination is used to generate those antibodies. The first dose of rabies prophylaxis consists of both the immune globulin for immediate protection and active rabies vaccine to promote the generation of neutralizing antibodies. Four additional doses of the active vaccine are given at least 1 week apart. Rabies prophylaxis is given to prevent disease in the exposed individual; it is not given to prevent spread of the virus from the exposed individual. The vaccine is not administered along with interferon. There is no antiviral therapy for rabies.

11 **The answer is D: Activated cells express transcription factors and polymerases required for transcription of HIV genes.** While reduction of cell surface viral receptors might reduce virus retention from infected host cell surface (choice A), activated CD4 T cells increase in surface expression of CD4, CCR5, and CXCR4. Activated cells are not likely to be impaired in the potential to induce the antiviral state (choice B). While TLR can bind viral RNA (including HIV), this binding does not induce the antiviral degradation of integrated DNA (choice C). HIV is not limited to infection of activated cells due to a lack of coreceptors on resting cells (choice E). HIV requires host factors, in particular, transcription factors in order to optimize gene expression for viral replication to occur. In fact, HIV produces a protein, negative factor, which promotes the activation of macrophages (M-tropic disease).

12 **The answer is D: Penciclovir.** The photograph shows a cold sore, a vesicular lesion that recurs on the face around the lips and nose. It is due to latent infection with herpes simplex type 1. Penciclovir is available as a topical crème and inhibits viral replication. Topical acyclovir can also be used to reduce symptoms and duration of cold sores. Azidothymidine is an antiretroviral drug. Foscarnet is used for treatment of cytomegalovirus infections. It also has activity against herpes simplex viruses, and can be used to treat serious, acyclovir-resistant infections. It is not used to treat cold sores. Ganciclovir is used to treat cytomegalovirus infections. Ribavirin is used to treat hepatitis C virus infections.

13 **The answer is C: Macrophages.** An M-tropic HIV isolate binds to CD4 and the coreceptor CCR5 which are both expressed on macrophages, monocytes, and dendritic cells. These cells carry the virus to draining lymph nodes, where the virus infects other cells. Activated T cells express CCR5 as well as CD4 and are infected as they pass through the lymph nodes. As the disease progresses, the virus mutates to a T-trophic strain, infecting T cells expressing CD4 and a different coreceptor, CXCR4. HIV has been shown to infect mucosal epithelial cells and mast cells; however, these cells are not the primary cellular targets for virus replication and systemic spread.

14 **The answer is D: HIV peptides have alterations which do not permit efficient CTL TCR interactions.** The CTL response to HIV is quite robust; however, HIV employs a number of evasion maneuvers to avoid clearance, including downregulation of class I MHC molecules and upregulation of FasL on target infected cells. Also, infection of dendritic cells results in inhibited maturation and limited professional Ag presentation. These infected dendritic cells can also serve as taxis for the virus to invade monocytes and T cells. HIV cannot infect CTL (choices A and B) due to a lack of the appropriate viral receptors (CD4 and chemokine receptor). Since CTLs recognize antigens presented only by class I MHC molecules, any impact on class II MHC is irrelevant (choice C). One of the reasons HIV is so elusive is that the high error rate of the reverse transcriptase produces differences in the virus during the course of infection within the same patient (choice E). In many cases, these mutations alter HIV proteins to the point that either they do not bind to the class I MHC properly or cannot be recognized by the responding CTL.

15 **The answer is B: Influenza virus.**

16 **The answer is B: Prevents the release of mature virions from the infected host cell.** Oseltamivir (Tamiflu) is a neuraminidase inhibitor. Neuraminidase is an enzyme which functions to cleave sialic acid, a monosaccharide derivative common on host cells and serving as a component of many surface receptors. In the case of influenza virus, sialic acid serves as the viral receptor. In order for a successful viral replication cycle to occur, the new virion must bud from the surface of the infected cell. If the new virions encounter sialic acid in abundance, they will bind and not be released to infect naïve cells. In order to facilitate the release of new virions, neuraminidase on the surface of influenza virus cleaves the sialic acid. As for naïve cell infections, neuraminidase action allows for the bound virus to penetrate the cell and proceed with infection. Thus, oseltamivir operates to prevent the action of neuraminidase, thereby trapping the virus on the surface of the naïve or infected host cells. Therefore, oseltamivir does not directly prevent viral replication (choice A), uncoating (choice C), nuclear translocation (choice D), or bind to the viral polymerase (choice E).

17 **The answer is B: Increases degradation of mRNA of infected host cells.** Type I interferons (IFN-α and INF-β) are secreted in response to viral challenges and induce the antiviral state in neighboring uninfected cells. Two events result as a consequence of antiviral state: (1) inhibition of protein synthesis and (2) degradation of mRNA of both host and viral products. While viral presence tends to reduce class I MHC expression (choice A), type I IFNs act to upregulate its expression. Type I IFNs also do not decrease viral receptors (choice C), directly lyse free virion (choice D), nor do they promote opsonization (choice E).

18 **The answer is E: Varicella-zoster virus.** The photograph shows a rash with papules, vesicles, and crusting scabs with a dermatomal distribution consistent with zoster, otherwise known as shingles. This infection is due to reactivation of varicella-zoster virus. Most latently infected people acquire the virus in childhood when it manifested as chickenpox. The virus remains latent in ganglion cells for several decades and may recur as zoster. Recurrence is associated with a decrease in T-cell immunity specific for the virus. Zoster tends to occur in people over 60 year of age, or individuals who are immune suppressed. The other viruses listed are causes of viral exanthems. Herpes simplex is the only one listed that causes vesicular lesions. Herpes simplex virus causes clusters of lesions in the genital area (HSV-2 or HSV-1), or gingivostomatitis and cold sores (HSV-1).

19 **The answer is A: Acyclovir/postherpetic neuralgia.** Postherpetic neuralgia (PNH) is the most troublesome aspect of shingles. It is a persistent, often severe and incapacitating pain that can last for months to years. The risk of PNH, as well as the duration of PNH, increases with age. Treatment of shingles with

acyclovir or the related compounds, valacyclovir and famciclovir, has been shown to reduce the duration and severity of PNH should it occur in a patient with shingles. Antivirals are not used to prevent cutaneous spread of the infection as this is not a problem. CNS involvement can occur in patients with shingles, particularly those who are immune suppressed; however, varicella-zoster immune globulin (VZIG) is not used to prevent this. Rather VZIG can be used to prevent primary VZV infection in the immune suppressed following exposure. Corticosteroids have been used along with antivirals to prevent PNH; however, this is not commonly accepted practice. Ganciclovir has no effect on varicella-zoster virus and is not used to treat shingles.

20 **The answer is E: HIV Vpr stops cell cycling in G2.** Based upon the HIV replication cycle, the virus buds from the infected cell and does not lyse it for release (choice A). Rev or regulator of viral gene expression (choice B) is a protein which serves to enhance translation by facilitating transfer of viral mRNA across the nuclear pore complex into the cytoplasm (or ER). Thus, Rev does not impact host cell mitosis. Nef can promote apoptosis of cells but generally it accomplishes this task by upregulating FasL on infected cell surface providing a type of immune privilege. Nef has many other functions but does not upregulate Bax expression (proapoptotic molecule) (choice C). HIV promotes activation of host cells to utilize host transcription factors for viral gene expression, and employs Vpr to arrest the infected cells in the G2 stage. The infected host cell does not detect the integrated HIV DNA at least according to our current understanding (choice D).

21 **The answer is C: Substitute for nucleosides resulting in replication termination (chain termination).** Nucleoside analogs are structures that mimic natural nucleosides used in the elongation of DNA during replication. These analogs have altered structures at points where phosphodiester bonds are to form between nucleosides in the growing DNA chain. Without the proper structure, chain elongation is terminated. Nucleoside analogs do not insert into the DNA helix; these agents are called intercalating agents (choice A). Some antimicrobial agents, such as tetracycline, bind to components of ribosomes and prevent protein synthesis (choice B). There is no binding of analogs to DNA or RNA polymerase recognition sites in the viral genome (choices D and E).

22 **The answer is E: Perinatally.** In general, developing countries are places where HBV is endemic. This is particularly true for Africa, Southeast Asia, and the Indian subcontinent. In endemic countries, HBV is most commonly transmitted from a chronically infected mother to her newborn during birth. The infant is exposed to virus present in vaginal secretions and blood. HBV does not cross the placenta. Infection of newborns most commonly leads to chronic infection; whereas infection of adults (as typically occurs in nonendemic countries) most commonly leads to acute infection. Prevention of infection in infants born to infected women includes administration of hepatitis B immune globulin as well as the active, recombinant vaccine. Infants begin the vaccination series against HBV in the United States at the time of birth. The other mechanisms of transmission listed occur more commonly in developed countries in which HBV is not endemic and infection occurs in adults.

23 The answer is B: Increased expression of MHC-I on infected cells. Interferon-α (or type 1 interferon) has multiple and poorly understood mechanisms by which it acts to treat certain chronic viral infections. In addition to upregulation of genes that interfere with viral replication, interferon-α also upregulates MHC class I gene expression, thereby enhancing antigen presentation by infected cells. Cytotoxic T cells are better able to recognize and thus destroy infected cells. Therapy with α-interferon often leads to an initial increase in liver cell damage as seen by elevated serum liver enzymes. This is due to the increased clearance of infected hepatocytes by cytotoxic T cells. None of the other activities listed are mechanisms of action of type 1 interferon.

24 The answer is E: Lamivudine. The replication cycle of HBV includes the viral enzyme reverse transcriptase; thus, inhibitors of this enzyme are being investigated as potential therapeutic agents. The currently approved drugs that inhibit HBV reverse transcriptase are: lamivudine, adefovir, entecavir, and telbivudine. None of the other antiviral drugs listed are used for HBV. Acyclovir is used to treat infections with herpes simplex virus or varicella-zoster virus; fomivirsen and ganciclovir are used to treat cytomegalovirus infections; and amprenavir is a protease inhibitor used to treat HIV.

25 The answer is B: Human herpes virus type 6. The case describes the typical presentation of the childhood disease roseola. The other viruses listed cause rash illnesses, but are not the cause of roseola.

26 The answer is A: Acute infection with HBV. The finding of surface antigen and IgM to the core antigen of hepatitis B virus is consistent with acute infection. Antibodies to the surface antigen are not found in the presence of detectable surface antigen. The "e" antigen of HBV may or may not be detected in acute

infections. The IgG to HAV indicates either a past infection or vaccination.

27 The answer is E: Unprotected sex with multiple partners. Sexual activity is the most common mode of transmission of HBV in the United States. Intravenous drug abuse, while another important mode of transmission of HBV, is less common than sexual activity. Donated blood is screened for the presence of HBV and HCV as well as other bloodborne pathogens; thus, transfusion-associated infections are rare in the United States. While alcoholism and cocaine addiction can lead to unprotected sex, they are not independent risk factors for transmission.

28 The answer is B: Chronic infection with HBV. The finding of surface antigen in the serum for over 6 months is indicative of a chronic infection with HBV. By this time, IgM to the core antigen would be replaced with IgG antibodies (referred to as total anti-HBcAg). The presence of the "e" antigen is indicative of a greater degree of virus replication and higher transmissibility. However, it may or may not be present in chronic infections. The presence of IgG to HAV indicates a past infection or vaccination.

29 The answer is E: Zanamivir. This case involves infection with either influenza A or influenza B virus, since both are circulating in the area. Of the drugs listed, only oseltamivir can be used for either influenza A or B. Zanamivir along with oseltamivir are neuraminidase inhibitors which block the release of the virus from infected cells. Amantadine and rimantadine block the release of the influenza A nucleic acid from the nucleocapsid, thereby preventing viral replication. These two drugs have no effect on the replication of influenza B viruses. Foscarnet is used for cytomegalovirus infections; ribavirin is used in combination therapy for hepatitis C virus; and ritonavir is a protease inhibitor used against HIV.

30 The answer is E: Western blot for HIV. Several rapid screening tests for antibodies to HIV have been approved by the FDA with the intent of offering HIV testing in more medical sites as well as community sites where persons who do not regularly seek medical care may be tested. The CDC estimates that as many as 25% of persons infected with HIV are unaware of their infection status. Thus, offering testing in more sites is an essential part of an overall prevention strategy by making people aware of their infection and offering counseling on medical care and ways to prevent transmission to others. These rapid screening tests can use saliva, blood, or plasma and can give results in 20 min. The results of all positive HIV screening tests must be confirmed with western blot, regardless of whether the test was done by conventional laboratory based methods or by point-of-care rapid tests.

31 **The answer is C: 50%.** Sensitivity of a test is defined as the probability that the test result will be positive if the patient truly is positive. Specificity of a test is defined as the probability that the test result will be negative if the patient truly is negative. The positive predictive value is the ratio of true positives over the number of total positives. Thus, if 1,000 people in this area with a prevalence of 0.5% were screened with this test, five would be true positives because the sensitivity of the test is 100%. However, five additional people would be false positives because the specificity of the test is 99.5%. The positive predictive value is thus five true positives/ten total positives, or 50%.

32 **The answer is C: Croup.** The case described is typical for this disease. Croup occurs most commonly in children less than 3 years of age. The symptoms, particularly the barklike cough and the steeple sign, are indicative of croup. Several respiratory viruses can cause croup; however, the most common cause is a parainfluenza virus (PIV 1, 2, or 3). Bronchiolitis and pneumonia can be ruled out due to the lack of infiltrates on chest radiographs. Epiglottitis is an inflammation of the epiglottis, most commonly bacterial in origin. It is included in the differential diagnosis of croup; however, it is a medical emergency with a distinct clinical presentation. Bronchitis is a cause of cough in young children; however, radiological findings are usually negative.

33 **The answer is E: Some individuals who receive a single dose of mumps vaccine do not respond adequately.** Mumps vaccine, combined with measles and rubella has been in use in the United States since 1967 when it was approved by the FDA. A single dose of the live, attenuated trivalent vaccine was recommended at about 15 months of age. Children 15 months of age and even younger respond well to protein antigens. The efficacy of a single dose of MMR is 90%; thus, on a college campus of 10,000 students who received a single dose of MMR, 1,000 would still be susceptible to all three viruses. There is only a single strain of mumps virus, and the virus does not undergo rapid antigen variation. In 1989, following outbreaks of measles virus in vaccinated populations, a second dose of the vaccine was recommended for children 4 to 6 years of age.

34 **The answer is D: Epstein–Barr virus.** All the choices listed can cause pharyngitis; however, only Epstein–Barr virus (EBV) fits the entire picture presented in the case. HIV can cause a similar clinical presentation as well as atypical lymphocytes. Only EBV induces heterophil antibodies. Heterophil antibodies are usually

of the IgM class and bind to red blood cells of other mammals. They are detectable during the acute phase of infectious mononucleosis caused by EBV. Following the acute illness, heterophil antibodies rapidly decline in titer. Not all patients with EBV-associated mononucleosis develop heterophil antibodies, and for those cases, definitive diagnosis is made by demonstrating IgM to viral capsid antigen.

35 **The answer is D: Nasopharyngeal epithelial cells and B cells, respectively.** EBV infects cells expressing CD21, also known as complement receptor 2. B cells and epithelial cells of the upper respiratory tract and parotid gland epithelial cells express CD21. The virus produces a lytic infection with virus production in epithelial cells, but is only semipermissive in B cells. Semipermissive means that the virus can replicate in only a small percentage of infected B cells. B cells in which viral proteins are produced but replication is not complete may be stimulated to proliferate, and viral proteins may upregulate expression of cellular genes involved in cytokine secretion and prevention of apoptosis. These B cells may become transformed. EBV is associated with B cell lymphomas including those occurring in the central nervous system of immune suppressed individuals, as well as Burkitt lymphoma and at least some Hodgkin lymphomas.

36 **The answer is A: Adenovirus.** This DNA virus family is associated with a variety of respiratory illnesses including pharyngitis, conjunctivitis, colds and flu-like illness, and pneumonia in persons with underlying lung disease or immune suppression. The other viruses listed also cause pneumonia; however, they are RNA viruses.

37 **The answer is A: Anti-HCV antibodies would not be demonstrable.** The window period is defined as the period of time during which HCV is present in the blood but antiviral antibodies are not detectable. Thus, a person in the window period could conceivably donate contaminated blood. A window period also occurs with hepatitis B virus infection. The window period explains why there remains a small but measurable risk of transfusion-associated infection.

38 **The answer is B: Measles.** The symptoms, including the prodromal signs, fever, and rash are typical of measles virus infection. In addition, the lack of vaccination supports this suggestion. The signs and symptoms described are not consistent with any of the other choices. Mumps typically presents as parotitis. Echoviruses can cause a mild summer rash illness. Rubella, also rare in the United States due to vaccination, is generally a mild illness with low-grade fever. The rash in varicella is itchy and consists of maculopapular eruptions, vesicles, and scabs, accompanied by a low-grade fever.

39 **The answer is D: Neutralizing IgG antibodies specific for the agent.** Although all the immune mechanisms listed can play a role in defense against viruses, viral neutralizing antibodies are the most important defense mechanism against reinfection. Natural killer cells and interferon-α are important innate defenses which come into play following viral infections. Naïve, viral-specific cytotoxic T cells must be activated, but play an essential role in recovery from viral infections. Activated macrophages can phagocytize viral particles, secrete proinflammatory cytokines, and kill viral-infected cells, but do not play a role in prevention of infection.

40 **The answer is D: Respiratory syncytial virus.** All the viruses listed can cause pneumonia; however, by far, the most common cause of pneumonia in children less than 1 year of age is respiratory syncytial virus.

41 **The answer is C: Demonstration of IgM antibodies against the agent.** The case describes an outbreak of an infectious cause of acute hepatitis. The most common infectious cause of acute hepatitis in the United States is hepatitis A virus. This agent is diagnosed by the demonstration of IgM antiviral antibodies in the patient's serum. Although virus is shed in the stool, most viral shedding occurs prior to the onset of symptoms. Thus, demonstration of virus in stool is not a method of diagnosis. Hepatitis A virus is also not isolated from the blood. Bacteria and parasites are not commonly associated with acute hepatitis outbreaks in the United States.

42 **The answer is C: His CD4 cells cannot activate CD8 cells.** The pictures show herpes zoster or shingles due to a recurrence of varicella-zoster virus (VZV). This virus is latent in ganglia, and prevented from recurring by a strong antiviral T-cell immune response. As CD4 cells decline in number, the ratio of CD4:CD8 cells decreases. In addition, the functional capacity of noninfected CD4 cells also declines in HIV-infected patients; thus, immune responses dependent on these cells decline. Latent herpes viruses tend to recur because cytotoxic T cells cannot be adequately activated by CD4-positive cells. B cells play no role in the control of viral latency. The patient's ability to make antibodies to HIV or to VZV, or the ability to activate complement are not affected in HIV nor do they have a role in the occurrence of shingles. Shingles can occur in immune compromised patients regardless of their levels of antibody or complement.

43 **The answer is B: Enfuvirtide.** This drug represents a novel treatment modality that blocks the ability of HIV to enter cells following binding of the viral gp120 with host cell CD4 molecules. Normally, a conformational change in the viral gp41 allows the viral envelope to fuse with the host cell plasma membrane. Enfuvirtide (Fuzeon) blocks the conformational change in gp41, thereby inhibiting the virus from entering the cell. Enfuvirtide was approved in 2003 for use in adults and children with advanced HIV disease resistant to several reverse transcriptase inhibitors and protease inhibitors, and for whom there are limited treatment options. It is still used in combination with other classes of antiretroviral drugs. No HIV medication is used as monotherapy due to the rapid appearance of resistant mutants.

44 **The answer is C: Reverse transcriptase polymerase chain reaction.** Although the finding of elevated serum liver enzymes in a patient with antibodies to hepatitis C virus (HCV) is sufficient to make a diagnosis of ongoing infection, demonstration of the virus by reverse transcriptase polymerase chain reaction (RT-PCR) does confirm active viral replication. In addition, a quantitative RT-PCR should be done prior to treatment to assess viral load. Culture of HCV is not possible at this time due to a lack of susceptible cell lines. ELISA and western blot were most likely used to determine her positive serology. Indirect fluorescent antibody tests are not used in the diagnosis of HCV infection.

45 **The answer is A: Predicts response to therapy.** According to the World Health Organization, there are 11 genotypes of HCV around the world. Many of these genotypes also have subtypes. Genotypes 1 to 3 are most common globally including the United States, where genotype 1 is far more common than 2 and 3 combined. Unfortunately, genotype 1 responds poorly to standard antiviral therapy. In fact, a genotype other than 1 is a better predictor of response to therapy than is viral load, histopathological staging, age, or race. Some studies have found variations in virulence with different genotypes; however, this is still controversial.

46 **The answer is D: Pegylated interferon and ribavirin.** This combination of drugs is currently the standard therapy for HCV-infected patients regardless of genotype. In general, those patients with genotypes 2 or 3 are treated for 24 weeks whereas those patients with genotype 1 are treated for 48 weeks.

47 **The answer is B: Fusion protein.** Respiratory syncytial virus (RSV) is a paramyxovirus. The envelope proteins of this virus involved in attachment and entry into the cell are the G protein and the fusion protein, respectively. The G protein attaches to the receptor on the host cell membrane and the fusion protein mediates the fusion of the viral envelope with the cell's plasma membrane, delivering the nucleocapsid directly into the cytoplasm. Palivizumab is a humanized monoclonal antibody directed against the fusion protein. It is used as prophylaxis in infants born during the RSV season (winter to spring), who are at high risk of lower respiratory tract disease due to RSV. Infants at highest risk include premature infants and infants born with cardiopulmonary disease. RSV does have capsid and matrix proteins; however, unlike the closely related parainfluenza viruses, it lacks hemagglutinin–neuraminidase protein.

48 **The answer is E: Vaccinated against HBV and HAV.** Vaccines are available for both hepatitis A virus (HAV) and hepatitis B virus (HBV). Vaccination of healthcare workers against HBV is highly recommended if not required. The presence of antibodies to HAV indicates either vaccination or previous infection and is not related to the needlestick injury. Vaccination against HBV results in antibodies to the surface antigen, but not to the core antigen of the virus. Conversely, acute infection with HBV would be supported by the finding of IgM antibodies to the core antigen. These antibodies would not be demonstrable for weeks after exposure. Chronic infection with HBV would be supported by the finding of surface antigen as well as antibodies (IgG or total) to the core antigen. Past infection with HBV would be supported by the finding of antibodies (IgG) to both the surface and the core antigens. The student is not at risk for infection from HAV or HBV due to the fact that he has IgG antibodies to both viruses. In addition, it is highly unlikely that HAV would be in the blood of the patient from whom the needlestick occurred. HAV is generally not transmitted though blood, but rather through fecal contamination of food or water. Another possible infectious risk for the student is HCV, since the reason for the patient's jaundice has not been determined.

49 **The answer is E: Latency with periodic recurrences.** The case describes gingivostomatitis due to herpes simplex virus type 1. The most common age for acquisition of HSV-1 is during early childhood, and the most common clinical manifestation of primary infection in young children is gingivostomatitis. The virus is most commonly transmitted to young children from caregivers with apparent or inapparent shedding of recurrent virus. Thus, the mother transmitted HSV-1 to the child when she had the cold sore. Following recovery from gingivostomatitis, the child remains infected with HSV-1. The virus remains latent in ganglia through out life and can periodically reactivate to cause cold sores or be shed asymptomatically. HSV-1 can also cause encephalitis and keratitis in immune competent individuals, although these outcomes

are fortunately rare. Esophagitis may occur in T-cell immune suppressed individuals. Acute infection with complete recovery (i.e., ridding the body of the virus) does not occur in herpes virus infections.

50 **The answer is A: Adenovirus.** Outbreaks of viral conjunctivitis are common, particularly in crowded situations like camps, families, and schools. The most common viral cause is adenoviruses. This virus is able to remain viable in swimming pools particularly if they lack adequate chlorination and have noticeable organic matter that creates turbidity in the water. The other viruses listed are not common causes of conjunctivitis.

51 **The answer is A: Acyclovir.** The case describes a patient with genital herpes, most likely a primary episode, as suggested by the extragenital symptoms of meningitis. Genital herpes can be treated with acyclovir or famciclovir or valacyclovir. The latter two drugs have better oral bioavailability than acyclovir. Imiquimod is used topically for the treatment of genital and anal warts. Ketoconazole is an antifungal drug. Lamivudine is a nucleoside reverse transcriptase inhibitor used for HIV and chronic hepatitis B virus infections and zanamivir is a neuraminidase inhibitor used to treat influenza virus infections.

52 **The answer is B: Resting cells have unphosphorylated nucleosides which are phosphorylated by the viral kinases in order to be usable for viral replication by viral DNA polymerase.** Resting cell nucleosides, used during DNA replication, are unphosphorylated. Upon activation, these nucleosides are phosphorylated and can be used in DNA elongation. Since the virus infects a resting cell and does not induce activation, in order to replicate the viral genome, the virus must have the capacity to phosphorylate the nucleosides. That is, the virus does not encode a polymerase of its own for viral genome replication and requires the host polymerase activity. Thus, the viral kinase acts much like host kinases when the host cell is active and dividing.

Levels of viral receptors on host cell surfaces are usually increased upon activation (choice A). Viral kinases have no function associated with viral transmigration into the nucleus (choice C). Viral kinases do not influence the binding of small and large ribosomal subunits for protein expression (choice D). Cell permeability has no impact upon already infected cells or cells in which viruses will bud or lyse (choice E).

53 **The answer is B: A strong antiviral cell mediated immune response.** Much evidence suggests that antiviral T cell immunity is essential for the maintenance of latency. The mechanism by which T cells prevent viral recurrence may involve γ-interferon-induced suppression of viral replication. In addition, T-cell immune suppression such as in HIV infection is associated with an increased frequency and severity of recurrence. Studies also suggest that significant stress may decrease T-cell immune function and allow virus to become reactivated. Antiviral medication can reduce, but does not prevent viral recurrence. It is important for physicians and patients to have a clear understanding of the limitations of antiviral medications. High levels of interferon-α, natural killer cells, and antiviral antibody are involved in the body's response to herpes simplex virus infection; however, they play little or no role in maintenance of herpes latency.

54 **The answer is A: Birds; mosquitoes.** Equine encephalitis virus is transmitted among the bird reservoir by mosquitoes. Transmission of the virus to humans typically occurs in the late summer or early fall after a large number of birds and mosquitoes have become infected. Although horses can be sickened by this virus, they do not develop a sufficient level of viremia necessary to infect another mosquito. The same is true for humans; thus, horses and humans are considered "dead-end hosts" for the virus. Of the mammals listed, only rodents such as the rat serve as reservoirs for arboviral encephalitides (i.e., the California group viruses such as LaCrosse virus) Fleas serve as vectors for *Yersinia pestis*, the causative agent of the plague. In the United States, ticks serve as vectors for the bacteria causing Lyme disease, Rocky Mountain spotted fever, and ehrlichiosis, and the virus causing Colorado tick fever. Ticks transmit encephalitic viruses in Europe, Russia, and other areas of the world.

55 **The answer is D: CXCR4 or CCR5.** These molecules are chemokine receptors. Attachment and entry of HIV into infected cells involves the initial binding of viral gp120 to CD4 and then to one of the chemokine receptors. This binding induces a conformational change in the viral gp120/gp41 complex which brings gp41 (also called the fusion protein) in contact with the host cell plasma membrane, and allows the viral envelope to fuse with the cell membrane. CCR5 is the coreceptor for strains of HIV which infect macrophages; whereas CXCR-4 is the coreceptor for strains of the virus which infect T cells. HIV also binds to the dendritic cell membrane molecule DC-SIGN, which may enable dendritic cells to carry the virus into secondary lymphoid tissues to infect T cells. Binding of HIV to DC-SIGN does not appear to facilitate infection of dendritic cells. The other molecules listed are not involved in the attachment or entry of HIV into target cells. Both CD3 and CD25 are found on T cells, whereas CD80/86 is an essential costimulatory molecule on antigen presenting cells.

56 **The answer is A: Intravenous drug abuse.** Epidemiological surveys of acute hepatitis indicate that intravenous drug abuse is the most common mode of transmission of hepatitis C virus (HCV) in the United States. Of newly diagnosed cases in 2006, 54% were attributed to intravenous drug use. Sexual transmission of the virus is possible, particularly among persons engaging in unprotected sex with multiple partners. Persons involved in monogamous sexual relationships do not appear to be at increased risk of infection when one partner is infected. Transmission by needlestick injury is uncommon. Transfusion associated infections are rare since the development of sensitive tests to screen donated blood.

57 **The answer is D: Inhibits synthesis of guanosine triphosphate (GTP).** Ribavirin is an analog of guanosine. It has several possible mechanisms of action including the inhibition of inosine monophosphate dehydrogenase, the enzyme involved in the synthesis of guanine nucleotides. Ribavirin also inhibits the capping of viral transcripts and may be incorporated by viral RNA-dependent RNA polymerase, leading to lethal mutations of the viral genome. It does not enhance immunity, and may in fact cause immune suppression. None of the other options describe the mechanisms of action of ribavirin.

58 **The answer is D: 1/100 live births.** It is important for physicians to recognize the high incidence of congenital cytomegalovirus (CMV) infections in the United States. About 1% of infants born each year in the United States are infected with CMV. Of these, only a minority (5% to 10%) will show symptoms at birth.

59 **The answer is C: Mental retardation and deafness.** While only 5% to 10% of infants congenitally infected with cytomegalovirus are symptomatic at birth, the symptoms and permanent sequelae can be devastating. Reversible manifestations at birth include low birth weight, microcephaly, petechial rash, hepatosplenomegaly, jaundice, and retinitis. The majority of symptomatic infants later develop permanent neurological complications. The most notable of these nervous system complications are sensorineural deafness and mental retardation. Congenital CMV is reported to be the most common cause of nonhereditary sensorineural deafness, and second to Down syndrome as a cause of mental retardation. The other neurologic conditions listed are not typical for congenital CMV infection.

60 **The answer is E: 2.5 million.** The World Health Organization estimates that 2.5 million people became infected with HIV in 2007. It is important for physicians to recognize the global impact of this virus.

61 **The answer is C: 40,000.** It is important for physicians to recognize the impact of this virus in the United States. The CDC estimates that the number of new infections with HIV in the United States has remained stable at 40,000 for a number of years. In 2006, 35,180 newly diagnosed cases were reported from 33 states with long-term, confidential name-based HIV reporting.

62 **The answer is D: Sub-Saharan Africa.** According to the World Health Organization, almost 70% of people currently living with HIV/AIDS reside in Sub-Saharan Africa. In this area, about 5% of adults are infected. By comparison, the estimated prevalence of infection in 2007 in the other regions included in the question is as follows:
South and Southeast Asia—0.3%
Eastern Europe and Central Asia—0.9%
North America—0.6%

63 **The answer is A: Heterosexual sex.** The majority of HIV infections globally result from heterosexual sex. In contrast, only 33% of newly diagnosed cases of HIV/AIDS in the United States in 2006 were attributed to heterosexual sex; whereas 50% were attributed to men having sex with men.

64 **The answer is D: Male-to-male sexual contact.** Of the new infections among adults and adolescents diagnosed in 2006, 50% occurred in male homosexuals; 33% occurred in people who engage in high-risk heterosexual sex; and 13% occurred in intravenous drug users. Less than 1% of infections diagnosed in 2006 occurred in persons less than 13 years of age.

65 **The answer is C: Increase in CD4 cells, decrease in viral load.** Acute retroviral syndrome refers to the clinical manifestations that may develop within weeks of infection with HIV. The virus during this time is replicating rapidly in T cells and a decreased number of T cells is seen along with a peak in plasma viral load. Following recovery from acute retroviral syndrome, virus is sequestered in lymph nodes; thus the viral load typically declines. In addition, T-cell proliferation is thought to raise T-cell numbers in order to maintain homeostasis.

66 **The answer is B: Invasive cervical cancer.** Of the options listed, only invasive cervical cancer is considered an AIDS-defining illness. Zoster; pelvic inflammatory disease; recurrent fever, night sweats, and generalized lymphadenopathy; and recurrent, severe vaginal yeast infections are conditions that indicate diminished T-cell immunity and/or are complicated by the presence of HIV; however, they do not fit the case definition of AIDS as defined by the CDC.

67 **The answer is D: Replication of viral DNA.** The replication of herpes viruses following entry of the DNA into the host cell nucleus involves the production of three sets of proteins: immediate early, early, and late. Immediate early proteins, transcribed and translated by host enzymes, regulate transcription of the remaining viral genes. Early proteins include the viral DNA polymerase which replicates the viral DNA. Late proteins are the structural proteins of the viral capsid and envelope.

68 **The answer is B: Chronic.** Persistent viral infections are distinguished from acute infections in that virus is not cleared from the body in persistent infections. There are several types of persistent infections, including latent, chronic, and "slow." Latent infections are those in which there is intermittent viral replication. In contrast, in chronic infections, the virus is constantly replicating. Thus, the person in this case has a chronic infection. A slow viral infection is one in which the manifestations of infection are not apparent for years to decades following initial infection. Prion diseases are sometimes described as slow viral infections; however, this is not accurate as prions are not viruses. A localized infection is one in which the virus does not spread from the initial site of infection.

69 **The answer is B: Coxsackievirus B.** This case is descriptive of myocarditis. This inflammatory condition can result from infectious or noninfectious causes. Viruses are the most common cause of myocarditis when a cause can be identified. The fact that the virus was identified using reverse transcriptase PCR indicates that the viral genome is RNA. Of the viruses, coxsackie B viruses are most frequently involved. These RNA viruses are members of the enterovirus group of the family Picornaviridae. Influenza virus and measles virus are also RNA viruses; however, they are rarely involved in viral myocarditis. Adenovirus, particularly serotypes 2 and 5 are important causes of myocarditis; however, they are DNA viruses. Cases of parvovirus B19 associated myocarditis have been reported; however, it too is a DNA virus and thus not the etiologic agent of this case.

70 **The answer is A: Adsorption.** The first step in virus replication is adsorption, in which a specific viral protein binds to a specific protein on the membrane of the host cell. In the case of HIV, the viral protein is gp120. Neutralizing antibodies are defined as those which bind to the specific viral protein involved in adsorption, thereby directly preventing the virus from entering the cell. The other options are steps in the replication cycle of viruses, and certainly would not occur if the virus does not enter the cell.

71 **The answer is B: Cytomegalovirus.** This virus causes retinitis in AIDS patients with CD4 cell counts below 100/cmm. Of the other viruses listed, only adenoviruses cause eye infections; however, these viruses are associated with conjunctivitis. Human herpes virus type 8 is associated with Kaposi sarcoma. Lymphocytic choriomeningitis virus causes a febrile meningitis. Metapneumovirus causes respiratory illness ranging from pneumonia and bronchiolitis to colds and croup.

72 **The answer is C: Ganciclovir.** Of the drugs listed, only ganciclovir is approved for use in cytomegalovirus infections. Acyclovir, famciclovir, and valacyclovir are used for herpes simplex and varicella-zoster virus infections. Zanamivir is used to treat influenza virus infections.

73 **The answer is E: Poxvirus.** Molluscum contagiosum is caused by a poxvirus.

74 **The answer is C: _pol._** The _pol_ gene codes for reverse transcriptase. This enzyme has a high error rate, and rapidly generates mutant viruses which can be selected for resistance to antiviral medications. The _env_ gene codes for the envelope glycoproteins gp120/gp41. Nef, tat, and vpu are viral regulatory proteins.

75 **The answer is C: Human herpes virus type 8.** The lesions in the case fit the description of Kaposi sarcoma, a vascular tumor caused by human herpes virus type 8 (HHV-8). This virus was first described in 1994. It affects about 5% of the general population but 30% to 60% of male homosexuals. It has been shown to be transmitted by sexual contact, shared needles, and transfusion. Kaposi sarcoma in the United States is most frequently associated with AIDS. The man in the case is at high risk for HIV infection due to his homosexuality and IV drug use and his lymphopenia is suggestive of AIDS. More rarely, KS can occur in patients with immune suppression due to other causes, such as transplantation. Although associated with lymphoproliferative diseases which may manifest in the skin, Epstein–Barr virus does not typically cause skin lesions. Chronic hepatitis C virus is associated with numerous skin lesions, many of which are due to immune complex-mediated vasculitis. The skin lesions of molluscum contagiosum are flesh-colored, umbilicated papules. Papillomaviruses cause warts.

76 **The answer is B: Antiretroviral therapy.** The form of Kaposi sarcoma seen in the United States occurs primarily in AIDS patients not receiving or not responding adequately to antiretroviral therapy. Kaposi sarcoma in AIDS patients may respond to antiretroviral therapy (ART) alone. Other treatment modalities depend on the extent of disease and include surgery, chemotherapy, and radiation therapy. The other antiviral therapies listed are not effective against the tumor or its viral cause. Acyclovir is used for diseases caused by herpes simplex viruses and varicella-zoster virus. Imiquimode is used to treat genital warts. Lamivudine is an inhibitor of reverse transcriptase used in some ART regimens and used for chronic hepatitis B virus infections. Ribavirin is used most frequently in combination with α-interferon to treat chronic hepatitis C virus infections.

77 **The answer is E: Papillomavirus.** Human papillomavirus (HPV) are highly associated with invasive cervical carcinoma. The initial signs of this neoplasia are abnormal cells seen in the Papanicolaou test or Pap smear. Colposcopy can be used as a follow-up to detect the presence of cervical intraepithelial neoplasia (CIN), a precursor to invasive cervical carcinoma. Cervical infection with HPV-16 or HPV-18 is more likely to progress to cervical carcinoma than is infection with HPV-6 or HPV-11. Thus, typing of HPV in women with abnormal Pap smears yields important prognostic information. Enteroviruses are RNA viruses and are not associated with genital infection, cervical carcinoma, or any other cancer. Both herpes simplex virus types 1 and 2 can cause genital lesions but they are not causally linked with cervical carcinoma. Infection with the retrovirus, human immunodeficiency virus, another RNA virus, can increase the severity of cervical carcinoma due to its suppression of immunity, but does not cause the disease. Polyomaviruses are in the same taxonomic family as papillomaviruses, but are not associated with genital lesions.

78 **The answer is E: Yellow fever virus.** The term arbovirus is used for those viruses transmitted by arthropods, such as mosquitoes or ticks. Yellow fever virus, a mosquito-borne virus, is endemic in South America and Africa. This is the only arbovirus for which a human vaccine is available. Vaccination against Yellow fever is recommended for travelers to endemic areas. Arenaviruses are not transmitted by arthropods, therefore are not arboviruses. Although this woman will be at risk for dengue virus, Venezuelan equine encephalitis virus, and possibly West Nile virus, there are no human vaccines routinely available for these agents.

79 **The answer is C: Induces secretion of interferon-α.** Imiquimode is an immunomodulator that acts via stimulation of toll-like receptor 7 to induce the secretion of interferon-α. It is used topically to treat condyloma acuminatum caused by papillomaviruses, especially types 6 and 11.

80 **The answer is E: Rotavirus vaccine.** The RotaTeq vaccine was licensed in 2006 and is recommended for use in children, beginning at 2 months of age. It consists of the five most common strains of rotavirus recombined with a bovine strain of rotavirus. Vaccines are available for all other diseases listed, except mad cow disease. No other available vaccines are made by recombining human and animal strains of viruses.

81 **The answer is D: Parvovirus B-19.** Viral causes of arthritis include hepatitis B virus, HIV, rubella virus, and most commonly, human parvovirus B-19 (HPV-B19). This virus causes a mild rash illness in school-aged children. Many people are infected with HPV-B19 in childhood; however, approximately 65% of adults are seronegative. Susceptible adults in close contact with school-aged children can acquire the infection. Adults who become infected may or may not develop the characteristic rash seen in children. An acute onset of transient, symmetrical polyarthritis occurs in up to 60% of infected adults. The arthritis, which resembles early rheumatoid arthritis, typically affects the joints of the wrists, hands, knees, and ankles, and can last for weeks to months. Echovirus can cause a rash in children and adults but is not associated with arthritis. Similarly, measles causes a rash illness, but is not considered a mild disease, nor is it associated with arthritis. Papillomaviruses cause warts. Polyomaviruses are not associated with rash illness.

82 **The answer is E: JC virus.** Progressive multifocal leukoencephalopathy (PML) is caused by JC virus, a ubiquitous human polyomavirus. Most people carry this virus latently in the kidney, from which it is periodically reactivated. Seroprevalence of this viral infection is about 90% among adults. Initial infection is not linked to any particular disease. In severely T cell-immune compromised individuals, the virus is reactivated and enters the brain where it replicates and damages glial cells. Damage to oligodendrocytes leads to areas of demyelination within the brain and subsequent clinical manifestations of neurologic disease. No specific treatments exist for PML. The disease is addressed by attempting to improve the immune status of the patient. In AIDS patients, suppression of virus replication with antiretroviral therapy has reduced mortality from PML from about 90% to about 50% by improving the patient's T-cell immunity. Cytomegalovirus and human herpes virus type 6 can cause encephalitis in AIDS patients. Human immunodeficiency virus also causes neurologic disease in AIDS. Endogenous retroviruses are found in the DNA of all cells in the body, but have not to date been linked with any disease.

83 **The answer is D: Live vaccinia virus.** Vaccinia virus is antigenically similar to smallpox virus and was used in the global smallpox eradication effort. The virus replicates locally at the site of inoculation and induces protective immunity in 95% of vaccinees. The origin of vaccinia virus is unclear; however, vaccination against smallpox has been ongoing since Edward Jenner's first studies with cowpox virus in 1796.

84 **The answer is A: Colorado tick fever.** Although all the diseases listed are tickborne, Colorado tick fever (CTF) and tick-borne encephalitis are the only ones caused by a virus. Tickborne encephalitis occurs in Europe and Russia. Lyme disease, caused by the bacterium *Borrelia burgdorferi*, typically occurs in the northeast and northern Midwest and presents with a rash and arthritis. Tickborne relapsing fever, caused by *Borrelia hermsii*, is found in coniferous forests of the western United States and Canada. It can present as recurring episodes of fever along with a variety of nonspecific symptoms including headache, myalgia, and arthralgia. Rocky Mountain spotted fever is caused by *Rickettsia rickettsii*. This disease was first described in the Rocky Mountain area; however, the majority of cases occur in North and South Carolina, Missouri, Arkansas, and Oklahoma.

85 **The answer is D: Human papillomaviruses (HPV) types 6, 11, 16, and 18.** Genital warts, a benign condition, are most commonly caused by HPV-6 and HPV-11, and invasive cervical carcinoma is most commonly caused by HPV-16 and HPV-18. All four types are associated with cervical intraepithelial neoplasia (CIN). Several other HPV types can cause genital warts, CIN, and cervical cancer, thus the vaccine does not provide complete protection from these diseases. Adenoviruses are associated with respiratory or gastrointestinal diseases, not genital diseases. Herpes simplex viruses cause vesicular lesions in the orofacial region (HSV-1) or genital region (HSV-2 >>> HSV-1). Neither is causally associated with cervical cancer or CIN. Human immunodeficiency virus causes profound immune suppression, which can allow cervical cancer to become more highly aggressive; however, HIV itself does not induce genital growths. Parainfluenza viruses are associated with respiratory disease.

86 **The answer is B: Ebola.** Ebola virus has one of the highest mortality rates of any viral disease affecting humans. The clinical manifestations described are typical for Ebola virus. Outbreaks of this viral infection occur periodically in sub-Saharan Africa, and typically spread from the index patient to the care givers through contact with blood and body fluids. Dengue virus, Yellow fever virus, and West Nile virus are transmitted by mosquitoes, and, although they cause serious morbidity, their mortality rate is much lower than that of Ebola virus. Hantavirus pulmonary syndrome occurs in the Americas, is transmitted by inhalation of virus in rodent urine and feces, and is not transmitted person-to-person.

87 **The answer is E: West Nile virus.**   Prior to the introduction of West Nile virus (WNV) into the United States in 1999, St Louis encephalitis virus was the most common arbovirus in the United States. WNV entered the United States in New York City, causing 66 cases in 1999. It spread rapidly across the United States, causing an average of 3,000 cases every year since its introduction (range of 21 cases in 2000 to 9,862 cases in 2003). Very few cases of arbovirus encephalitis other than that attributable to WNV occur annually in the United States.

88 **The answer is C: Gag.**   HIV protease serves to make cuts in the polyprotein, group-specific antigen or Gag, in three areas releasing the matrix, capsid, and nucleocapsid proteins. This release allows proper formation of the virion for infection (maturation). Without these splices, the virion would have limited ability to infect new cells. Env or envelope proteins (choice A), pol or polymerase (choice B), and Nef or negative factor (choice E) are spliced by other enzymes. Matrix (choice D) is spliced by protease but is only one of the proteins released during maturation as discussed above.

89 **The answer is E: Severe acute respiratory syndrome.** The severe acute respiratory syndrome (SARS) outbreak began in the Guangdong region of southern China where it killed over 300 people before it came to the attention of the World Health Organization. It was spread to other countries by infected persons traveling by air during the incubation period. The virus generally caused a high fever with chills, headache, malaise followed by severe respiratory signs including unproductive cough, hypoxia, and dyspnea. Neurologic disease was not typically associated with this disease. Bird flu, another viral disease originating in China in the late 1990s, is caused by a novel influenza A virus termed A/H5N1. This virus has caused a few hundred human cases so far with about a 60% mortality rate. Hantavirus pulmonary syndrome was first described in the 1993 in the Four Corners area of the western United States. It is a zoonotic infection caused by several strains of rodent Hantaviruses.

90 **The answer is A: Dengue virus.**   This case is descriptive of dengue hemorrhagic fever. The high fever, severe body aches and petechiae are typical for this viral disease. Hemorrhagic manifestations usually appear after the fever has spiked and returned to normal.

A positive tourniquet test demonstrates the formation of at least 20 petechiae per square inch on the skin of the arm elicited by inflating a blood pressure cuff on the upper arm for 5 min. This test is one of the criteria for clinical diagnosis of dengue hemorrhagic fever. Dengue virus is endemic in most tropical and subtropical areas around the world and a few cases of dengue are reported almost every year among travelers returning to the United States from those areas. The outcome of infection with this virus ranges from asymptomatic infection to fever and severe body aches to hemorrhagic disease with or without shock. There are four strains of the virus, and infection with one strain does not protect against infection with the others. Indeed, reinfection with a second strain is associated with more severe disease including hemorrhage and shock, particularly in children. Ebola virus causes a highly fatal hemorrhagic fever and has only been found in sub-Saharan Africa. Epstein–Barr virus (EBV) typically causes low grade fever, pharyngitis, cervical lymphadenopathy, and profound fatigue. The white blood cell count in EBV-associated mononucleosis does show lymphocytosis as in the present case; however, atypical lymphocytes are usually more than 10%. Hepatitis A virus presents as an acute onset of abdominal pain with nausea and vomiting. Parvovirus B-19 is a mild rash illness most commonly seen in school-aged children.

91 **The answer is D: Use of insect repellent.**   Dengue virus is transmitted by mosquitoes of the genus *Aedes*. Two species of *Aedes* mosquitoes capable of serving as a vector for dengue virus are found in the southern United States, and have on occasion transmitted the virus from a returned traveler to people in the community. The virus is not transmitted in fecal contaminated water, thus avoiding places with poor public hygiene and drinking only bottled water when visiting endemic areas will not prevent infection with dengue virus. There is no prophylactic medication to prevent dengue, as there is to prevent malaria. No vaccine is available to prevent dengue.

92 **The answer is B: Congenital rubella syndrome.**   This disease has been virtually eliminated from the United States by vaccination. Cases occasionally occur among unvaccinated immigrants. The photograph shows an infant with cataracts. While many signs and symptoms reflecting involvement of multiple organs are seen in this disease, the classic triad of congenital rubella syndrome (CRS) is cataracts, deafness, and patent ductus arteriosus. Postnatal rubella is a mild febrile rash illness that may present without a rash, and with arthralgia, particularly in adult women. Classic signs and symptoms of congenital cytomegalovirus infection include petechial rash, microcephaly, chorioretinitis, and sensorineural hearing loss. Symptomatic infection of the mother during pregnancy would most likely have been manifested as a mononucleosislike syndrome. Congenital varicella usually manifests as limb deformities, and infection of the mother during pregnancy would have caused severe chickenpox with a heightened risk of varicella pneumonia. Neonatal enterovirus infection could present as poor feeding, irritability, and rapid breathing, consistent with cardiac problems; however, cataracts are not seen in this disease. Neonatal herpes most commonly manifests as vesicular lesions on the skin and mucous membranes and keratoconjunctivitis. Disseminated disease could present as irritability, poor feeding, and rapid breathing in addition to other manifestations. Symptomatic infection of the mother during pregnancy would have manifested as vesicular genital lesions.

93 **The answer is D: Mutations in the genes for the envelope glycoproteins.** Influenza viruses are noted for their high degree of antigenic variation, arising from point mutations in the genes for the envelope glycoproteins hemagglutinin (HA) and neuraminidase (NA). This type of antigenic variation in influenza viruses is called antigenic drift, and occurs in both group A and group B viruses. As the viruses circulate around the world each year, isolates are antigenically typed and the predicted predominant serotypes of H1N1, H3N2, and B virus are propagated and incorporated into vaccines. New vaccines are made each year due to differences in predominant serotypes from one year to the next. Reassortment of RNA strands between animal and human strains is an example of another, fortunately rare type of antigenic change that occurs in influenza A viruses. Influenza A viruses can infect several different species of animals, whereas influenza B viruses are species specific. If an animal gets infected with two different influenza A viruses, the eight separate strands of RNA that make up the genome of each virus can be combined such that virions emerge from the infected cell containing RNA strands from both viruses and representing a new influenza A subtype. This process is called antigenic shift. Subtypes of influenza A, including those currently in circulation (A/H1N1 and A/H3N2) have emerged by antigenic shift and have caused pandemics leading to the death of hundreds of millions of people. Because antigenic shift is an infrequent event, it does not contribute to the need for annual vaccination. Worldwide surveillance to detect the emergence of new influenza A viruses by antigenic shift or other mechanisms is an important function of the World Health Organization, the Centers for Disease Control and Prevention, and similar organizations around the world. Influenza viruses do not acquire genes from parainfluenza viruses, nor does antigenic variation occur in the matrix protein. The HA protein contains a segment called a fusion peptide, but its level of expression does not change.

94 **The answer is C: Ganciclovir.** This case is descriptive of cytomegalovirus colitis. This disease occurs in immune suppressed individuals such as solid organ transplant patients and individuals with AIDS. The use of highly active antiretroviral medications has reduced the incidence of this disease in AIDS patients. Ganciclovir is the recommended drug for treatment of this condition. Cytomegalovirus does not respond to the other antiviral medications listed: acyclovir (used for genital herpes) and ribavirin (used for hepatitis C infections) or azidothymidine (an antiretroviral drug). Voriconazole is an antifungal drug.

95 **The answer is D: Polymerase chain reaction (PCR).** This technique amplifies pathogen DNA in samples with the use of cDNA probes specific for the pathogen in question. It is useful in the diagnosis of many viral pathogens. Direct fluorescent antibody assays are used to detect viral proteins in tissue samples. Enzyme-linked immunoassays are also serologic tests that can be used to detect viral proteins in patient samples, or to detect antibodies to specific pathogens in patient serum. Northern blot is a technique that can be used to detect viral RNA sequences in patient samples. The western blot is used to detect antibodies in patient serum to specific viral proteins separated by gel electrophoresis and blotted onto nitrocellulose paper.

96 **The answer is A: Persons immunized with IPV can still become infected with and shed wild-type virus.** Polio virus is spread by a fecal–oral route. In the vast majority of infected individuals, the virus replicates asymptomatically in the intestinal tract and is shed in the feces. Paralytic polio occurs in less than 1% of infected individuals and results from a viremia that allows the virus access to the central nervous system (CNS). Vaccination with both the OPV and IPV results in the production of neutralizing IgG antibody that blocks viral entrance into the CNS, thereby protecting against paralytic disease. The IPV, given by injection, only stimulates systemic immunity. Thus, a vaccinated individual can still develop an asymptomatic intestinal infection with the wild-type virus and shed the virus in the feces to other susceptible individuals in the community. In contrast, the OPV is a live, attenuated vaccine which replicates in the intestine and stimulates both systemic and intestinal immunity. The advantage of the OPV in areas where poliovirus is endemic is that, by stimulating intestinal immunity, a vaccinated individual is not only protected from paralytic disease, but also from asymptomatic intestinal infection. The use of the OPV stops asymptomatic transmission of the virus in the community.

The disadvantages of the OPV are that it can be shed in the feces and cause disease in susceptible immune compromised family members. More importantly, there is a small risk of vaccine-induced paralytic polio. Reduction of wild-type poliovirus transmission in the United States has been so dramatic since the development of OPV that the occurrence of poliomyelitis in recent years has been due to imported cases or OPV-associated cases. The use of IPV has replaced the use of OPV in countries free from wild-type poliovirus transmission such as the United States.

97   **The answer is B: Coxsackievirus.** The case is descriptive of hand-foot-and-mouth disease caused by coxsackieviruses. Coxsackieviruses belong to the Enterovirus group and are transmitted by a fecal–oral route. They are common childhood infections. None of the other viruses listed cause this constellation of symptoms. Adenoviruses are associated with respiratory and diarrheal illnesses. Cytomegalovirus is associated with various diseases in the immune compromised. Papillomaviruses cause warts. Rotavirus is a cause of diarrhea.

Chapter 3

Mycology

QUESTIONS

Select the single best answer.

1 A severely immunosuppressed man in hospice is transported to the local ER because of episodes of unusual behavior. On physical examination, cutaneous lesions on his arms, torso, and legs are noted. In addition, he is febrile, seems to be suffering from a severe headache and is clearly unresponsive when asked simple questions about his condition. A spinal tap is ordered. India ink wet mount of the CSF reveals the microbial cells shown in the photograph. With which organism is he infected?

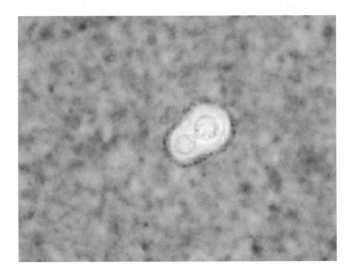

(A) *Acanthamoeba* spp.
(B) *Balamuthia mandrillaris*
(C) *Cryptococcus neoformans*
(D) *Naegleria fowleri*
(E) *Toxoplasma gondii*

2 A patient who has been diagnosed with sarcoidosis experiences severe hemoptysis. Imaging studies are strongly suggestive of bronchiectasis and cavitation. In addition, several movable masses are detected within the cavitation. Surgical resection of the affected area is preformed and the contents of these cavitary masses are cultured. Microscopic view of the 3-day culture is shown in the image. Which of the following microbes was isolated?

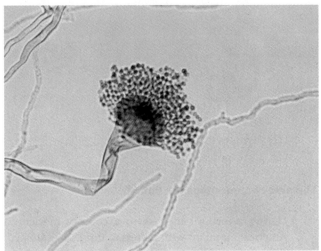

(A) *Aspergillus*
(B) *Candida*
(C) *Cryptococcus*
(D) *Pneumocystis*
(E) *Rhizopus*

3 A 56-year-old woman is brought to the emergency department with a 5-day history of fever, facial pain, and headache and a 1-day history of epistaxis, visual disturbances, and increasing lethargy. Physical examination reveals a toxic appearing woman with proptosis (forward bulging) of the left eye. Erosive lesions of the sinus and orbit are seen on CT of the head. Culture of material from a sinus aspirate grew the organism seen in the photo. What underlying condition most likely predisposed the woman to this infection?

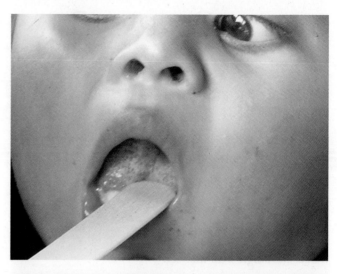

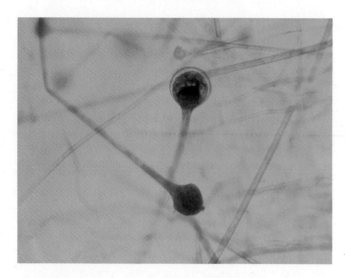

(A) Diabetes
(B) Graves disease
(C) HIV infection
(D) Hypothyroidism
(E) Osteoporosis

The next two questions are linked.

4 During a medical mission to a country in Central America, an infant with failure to thrive is evaluated. The mother indicates that the child has a poor appetite and is resistant to breast feeding. A white pseudomembranous coating seen in the child's mouth is shown in the photograph. A scraping of the material, observed under the microscope, is also shown. Which antimicrobial is the most appropriate treatment for this condition?

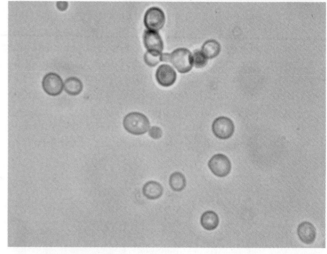

(A) Albendazole
(B) Metronidazole
(C) Nalidixic acid
(D) Nystatin
(E) Tetracycline

5 A teenager in the same community suffers from the same general condition but, despite treatment, the infection returns every month. This patient should be evaluated for which of the following conditions?
(A) Acute glomerulonephritis
(B) Chronic giardiasis
(C) Chronic hepatitis B
(D) HIV infection
(E) Rheumatic fever

6 A kitten is taken to the veterinarian because of crusty lesions on its head and ear. The vet, recognizing the infectious nature of the lesion, suggests culture of the lesion and treatment of the kitten to prevent possible transmission of the organism to family members. A 3-week culture of the organism is shown in the photograph. What is the etiologic agent?

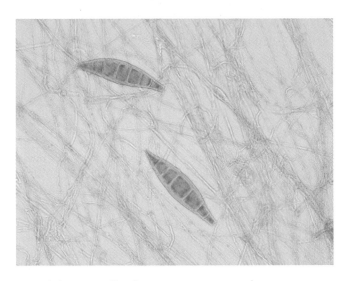

(A) *Aspergillus fumigatus*
(B) *Blastomyces dermatidis*
(C) *Cryptococcus neoformans*
(D) *Microsporum canis*
(E) *Sporothrix schenckii*

The next two questions are linked.

7 A high school wrestler develops a superficial lesion as shown in the photograph. Which description or term is frequently used to describe the fungal group responsible for this infection?

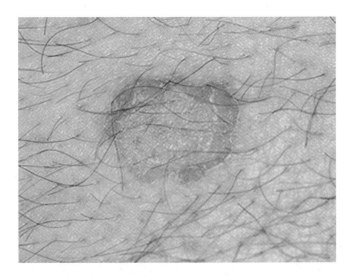

(A) Diatomaceous fungi
(B) Dermatophyte
(C) Endemic dimorphic fungi
(D) Opportunistic fungi
(E) Thermally dimorphic fungi

8 Two of the patient's teammates also have similar lesions. If cultures are taken to identify the causative agent, which laboratory media would be most useful for this purpose?

(A) Chocolate agar
(B) Lowenstein–Jensen medium
(C) MacConkey agar
(D) Sabouraud dextrose agar
(E) Sheep blood agar

The next two questions are linked.

9 A patient presents with a nail problem as shown in the photograph. Extended treatment with an antifungal agent is recommended for the patient. Which of the following drugs is most commonly prescribed to treat this condition?

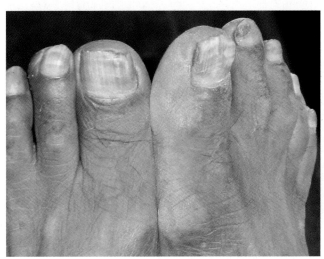

(A) Amphotericin B
(B) Caspofungin
(C) Flucytosine
(D) Terbinafine
(E) Voriconazole

10 What is the mechanism of action of the antimicrobial used to treat the patient in the above case?
(A) Inhibits ergosterol synthesis
(B) Inhibits glucan synthesis
(C) Inhibits mitosis through microtubule disruption
(D) Inhibits nucleic acid synthesis
(E) Inhibits protein synthesis

11 A patient, who is being treated for a squamous cell carcinoma of the lungs, develops pneumonia. A sputum sample cultured on routine laboratory media at 37 °C grows cream-colored colonies within 24 hours. Characteristic cellular growth in rabbit plasma is shown in the photograph and confirms the identification of the organism. With which of the following fungal species is the patient infected?

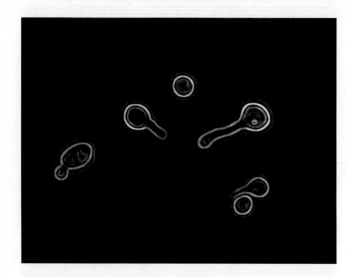

(A) *Aspergillus flavis*
(B) *Candida albicans*
(C) *Coccidioides immitis*
(D) *Cryptococcus neoformans*
(E) *Pneumocystis jiroveci*

12 A neutropenic patient is hospitalized because of high fever and periods of delirium. Unfortunately, the patient dies later that day. Two-week blood culture yields the fungus shown in the photograph. Which fungal structure is plainly visible in the photograph and aids in the identification of the organism?

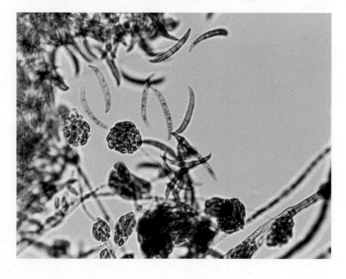

(A) Arthrospores
(B) Basidiospores
(C) Macroconidia
(D) Microconidia
(E) Sporangia

The next two questions are linked.

13 A 32-year-old female greenhouse worker seeks medical care for an ulcerative nodule on her right distal forearm that has persisted for over a month. The lesion began as a reddish bump above the right hand where the patient had received multiple scratches from moving thorn-covered bayberry plants. It had been subsequently diagnosed empirically as a staph infection and treated with antibiotics without improvement. At this visit, the patient is afebrile and in no significant pain. Cultures of the lesion yield a thermally dimorphic fungus. A photograph of the fungus grown at ambient temperature is shown. With which organism is the patient infected?

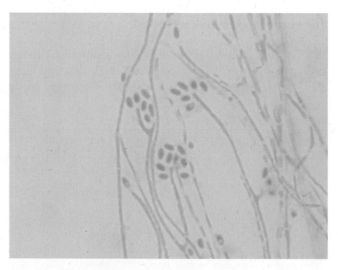

(A) *Acremonium* spp.
(B) *Blastomyces dermatitidis*
(C) *Candida tropicalis*
(D) *Cladosporium carrionii*
(E) *Sporothrix schenckii*

14 With which antimicrobial should the woman in the above case be treated?
(A) Amphotericin B
(B) Caspofungin
(C) Itraconazole
(D) Nystatin
(E) Topical bacitracin

15 Dimorphic fungi are most likely to be in which of the following fungal forms when observed in a sample from a patient?

(A) Pseudohyphae
(B) Mycelium
(C) Hyphae
(D) Endospores
(E) Yeasts

16 Many antifungal agents target the fungal cell membrane. Which of the following is found in fungal cell membranes and not in mammalian cell membranes?

(A) Chitin
(B) Cholesterol
(C) Ergosterol
(D) Peptidoglycan
(E) Teichoic acid

17 A 12-year-old female who recently emigrated from Central America with her parents presents with a rather large black macular lesion on the palm of her hand. The parents were not initially concerned until the lesion increased in size to cover about half of the palm. Fearing skin cancer, they decided to have the lesion examined. Skin scrapings treated with 10% KOH revealed the presence of numerous hyphal fragments that were branched and dark in color with elongated budding cells along their length. Which of the following organisms is most likely the cause of the child's skin lesion?

(A) *Hortaea wernickii*
(B) *Malassezia furfur*
(C) *Piedraia hortae*
(D) *Sporothrix schenckii*
(E) *Trichophyton* spp.

18 A 31-year-old female cancer patient presents with fever and difficult and painful swallowing. Endoscopy reveals multiple raised white plaques on the esophagus. Brushings of the plaques viewed under the microscope reveal pseudohyphae and budding yeasts as shown in the accompanying photograph. With which of the following organisms is this patient infected?

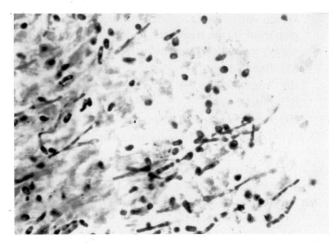

(A) *Actinomyces israelii*
(B) *Aspergillus flavus*
(C) *Candida albicans*
(D) *Cryptococcus neoformans*
(E) *Blastomyces dermatidis*

19 A 24-year-old male presents with fever, headache, chills, cough, and chest pain a few weeks after visiting caves in the Ozark Mountains of northern Arkansas. A chest radiograph reveals patchy lung infiltrates and hilar lymphadenopathy. An immunodiffusion test detects antibodies in the patient's serum to the H antigen of the causative fungal agent. Which organism caused the patient's clinical manifestations?

(A) *Candida albicans*
(B) *Histoplasma capsulatum*
(C) *Blastomyces dermatitidis*
(D) *Coccidioides immitis*
(E) *Cryptococcus neoformans*

20 Which one of the following represents the general transmission route of endemic dimorphic fungi to humans?

(A) Ingestion of fungal hyphae
(B) Inhalation of fungal hyphae
(C) Ingestion of fungal yeast cells
(D) Inhalation of fungal spores
(E) Ingestion of fungal spores

21 Which one of the following represents the mechanism of action of caspofungin?

(A) Inhibits translocation of t-RNA and ribosomes along the mRNA during translation
(B) Inhibits of the activity of the enzyme, chitin synthase
(C) Interaction with fungal ergosterol to form pores in the fungal cell
(D) Inhibits the activity of the enzyme, β-glucan synthase
(E) Inhibits mRNA synthesis by deamination of 5-flourouracil

22 Which one of the following antifungals is specifically employed in the treatment of cryptococcosis and is always used in combination with other antifungals?
(A) Itraconazole
(B) Amphotericin B
(C) Flucytosine
(D) Ketoconazole
(E) Trimethoprim–sulfamethoxazole

23 Which one of the following represents the mechanism of action of the antifungal azoles?
(A) Inhibition of GTP hydrolysis carried out by elongation factor-2 (EF-2).
(B) Inhibition of the activity of the enzyme, chitin synthase.
(C) Interaction with fungal ergosterol to form pores in the fungal cell.
(D) Inhibition of the activity of the enzyme, β-glucan synthase.
(E) Inhibition of the activity of the enzyme, 14-α-demethylase.

24 While on a medical mission trip to Africa, you encounter a 35-year-old male who presents with a series of pruritic, warty papules ("cauliflowerlike" lesions) which extend from the foot to the knee. You learn that this patient has had these lesions for some time and that he is employed by the region's forest agency. Microscopy of the biopsied lesions reveals the presence of characteristic "muriform bodies" that are pigmented yeastlike cells. Which one of the following clinical syndromes most likely accounts for this clinical presentation?
(A) Zygomycosis
(B) Sporotrichosis
(C) Dermatophytosis
(D) White Piedra
(E) Chromoblastomycosis

25 A 67-year-old male from Michigan presents with fever, cough, night sweats, dyspnea, and weight loss. His history indicates a recent vacation which included travel through the desert southwest. Shortly thereafter he experiences a illness and worsening influenza has difficulty in breathing. Microscopic examination of the patient's sputum reveals the presence of endosporulating spherules. In addition, chest radiograph reveals the presence of multiple, small, thin-walled apical cavities. Which of the following is most likely the fungus responsible for this clinical syndrome?
(A) *Candida albicans*
(B) *Coccidioides immitis*
(C) *Blastomyces dermatitidis*
(D) *Histoplasma capsulatum*
(E) *Cryptococcus neoformans*

26 Which one of the following represents the mechanism of action of amphotericin B?
(A) Inhibition of GTP hydrolysis carried out by elongation factor-2 (EF-2).
(B) Inhibition of the activity of the enzyme, chitin synthase
(C) Interaction with fungal ergosterol to form pores in the fungal cell
(D) Inhibition of the activity of the enzyme, β-glucan synthase
(E) Inhibition of the activity of the enzyme, 14-α-demethylase

27 A little girl presents with a bald spot on the scalp as shown in the photograph. The mother indicates that despite her objections, her daughter sleeps with a newly acquired puppy. Which of the following procedures would be most appropriate in aiding the physician to make a immediate diagnosis in the office?

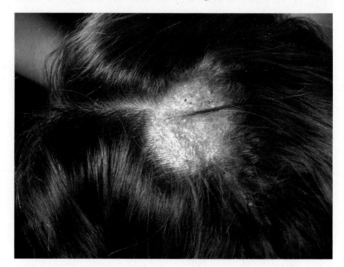

(A) Culture of a skin scraping on Sabouraud dextrose agar
(B) Detection of antibodies to dermatophytes by latex agglutination
(C) Gram stain of a skin scraping
(D) Polymerase chain reaction
(E) Wood lamp to detect fluoresence

28 A 45-year-old migrant agricultural worker in the sugar cane fields of southern Florida seeks treatment for an elephantoid condition of the foot and ankle as shown in the photograph. He has been a resident of the United States for the past 10 years. Grossly, the affected tissue is firm and noticeably swollen. The patient believes that the lesions are "getting bigger" each year. Furthermore, he complains of bone pain, mostly during the night. On close inspection, granulomatous lesions are diffusely distributed over the surface. A micrograph of a lesion is also shown. From which of the following infectious conditions is this man suffering?

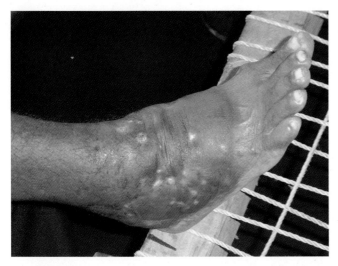

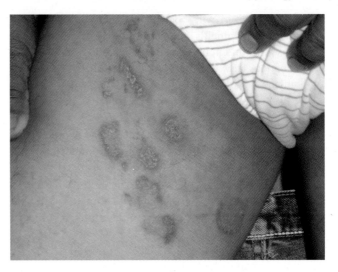

(A) Arthroconidia
(B) Ascospores
(C) Sporangiospores
(D) Yeast cells with germ tubes
(E) Zygospores

30 A 23-year-old female, who just finished a 2-week course of a fluoroquinolone, now complains of vulvar pruritis and a white cottage cheese-like vaginal discharge. The Gram stain result of the exudate is shown in the image. What is the probable agent responsible for her symptoms?

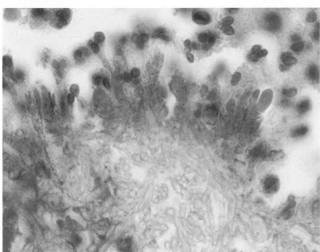

(A) Aspergillosis
(B) Dermatophytosis
(C) Eumycotic mycetoma
(D) Paracoccidioidomycosis
(E) Zygomycosis

29 A 20-year-old male presents with a pruritic rash on the thigh and groin as shown in the photograph. Microscopic examination of a skin scraping from the lesions are cleared in 10% KOH and reveal fungal structures. Of the following, which fungal structure would likely to be seen microscopically?

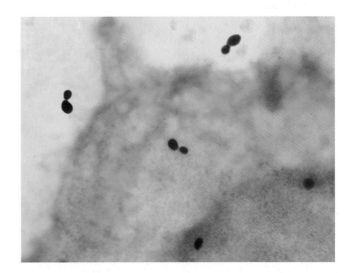

(A) *Candida albicans*
(B) *Gardnerella vaginalis*
(C) *Klebsiella granulomatis*
(D) *Mycoplasma hominis*
(E) *Trichomonas vaginalis*

31 A 56-year-old AIDS patient presents with fever and signs of meningitis. Antigens of *Cryptococcus neoformans* are found in his cerebral spinal fluid by latex agglutination. How did this patient most likely acquire this infection?

(A) Consumption of spores in contaminated food or water

(B) Immune suppression-induced reactivation of previously acquired organisms contained within lung granulomas

(C) Inhalation of infectious particles in respiratory secretions from a person with similar symptoms

(D) Inhalation of oocysts from the cat feces while cleaning a litter box

(E) Inhalation of yeast-like cells from soil contaminated with pigeon droppings

The next two questions are linked.

32 A Mexican patient who works as a landscaper in Phoenix presents with a buccal abscess at the extraction site of a molar. The molar was removed 30 days earlier and now an adjacent molar has started to loosen. Microscopic views of the infected tissue, one stained with Periodic Acid Schiff (PAS), are shown in the images. What is the most likely fungal agent causing this patient's condition?

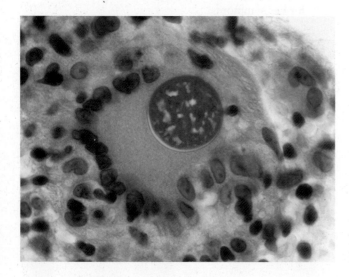

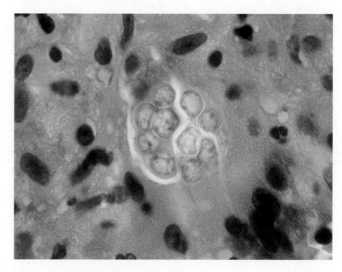

(A) *Aspergillus flavis*
(B) *Blastomyces dermatitidis*
(C) *Coccidioides immitis*
(D) *Cryptococcus neoformans*
(E) *Histoplasma capsulatum*

33 The patient in the above case is managed with long-term antifungal therapy. Which of the following antifungal agents is most appropriate for this condition?

(A) Amphotericin B
(B) Flucytosine
(C) Griseofulvin
(D) Ketoconazole
(E) Metronidazole

34 A competitive swimmer at a university, who has the habit of cleaning his ears with cotton-tipped swabs, develops an otitis externa. Inspection of the canal reveals a fuzzy growth in the canal and a slight discharge. Stained microbial elements taken directly from the auditory canal are shown in the image. Which microbe is responsible for otitis externa in this patient?

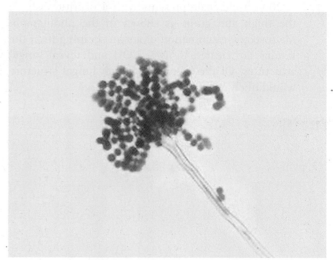

(A) *Aspergillus fumigatus*
(B) *Candida albicans*
(C) *Nocardia asteroides*
(D) *Pseudomonas aeruginosa*
(E) *Staphylococcus aureus*

35 A 5-year-old, hospitalized neutropenic cancer patient develops fever, respiratory distress, and hemoptosis. Imaging studies reveal cavitary lung lesions and are strongly suggestive of angioinvasive disease. Septate hyphae are visualized in the histopathology studies and microbiologic culture as shown in the photograph. How did the child acquire this nosocomial infection?

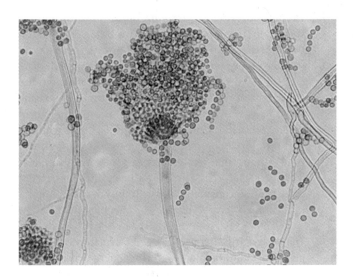

(A) Fungal spore contamination of the tips of catheters used to deliver anticancer drugs
(B) From normal intestinal flora
(C) From normal oropharyngeal flora
(D) From the hands of health care workers
(E) Inhalation of ubiquitous conidia in the air

36 Which of the following antimicrobial agents is most appropriate for the treatment of the patient in the above case?
(A) Amphotericin B
(B) Isoniazid
(C) Penicillin G
(D) Pentamidine
(E) Voriconazole

37 An elderly patient with a history of uncontrolled hyperglycemia is hospitalized because of fever, purulent nasal discharge, and recurrent epistaxis. Sinus culture produces the microbe shown in the photograph. Nonseptate hyphae in the histological sections confirm the physician's fear of tissue invasion. From which of the following infectious diseases is this patient suffering?

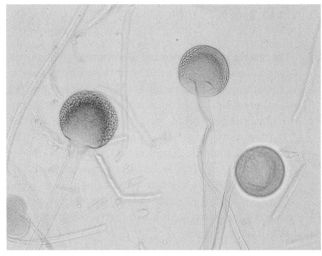

(A) Disseminated coccidioidomycosis
(B) Invasive aspergillosis
(C) Pneumocystis pneumonia
(D) Rhinocerebral mucormycosis
(E) Sporothrichosis

38 A 49-year-old patient with advanced HIV disease presents with fever, dyspnea, nonproductive cough, and moderate chest pain. His history includes noncompliance with medication. His CD4 count is 120/cmm. Chest radiographs reveal diffuse bilateral infiltrates. Lactate dehydrogenase levels are elevated. Cystlike structures are recovered in the bronchoalveolar lavage fluid (shown in the image). Which of the following antimicrobial agents represents the best treatment option for this patient?

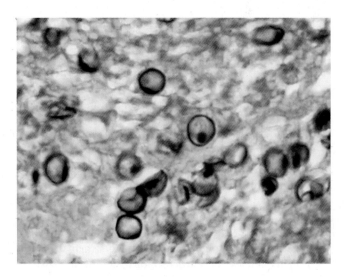

(A) Amphotericin B
(B) Diethylcarbamazine
(C) Itraconazole
(D) Ketoconazole
(E) Trimethoprim–sulfamethoxazole (TMP/SMZ)

ANSWERS

1 **The answer is C: *Cryptococcus neoformans.*** The photograph shows budding yeast surrounded by a polysaccharide capsule that excludes the India ink stain. The other organisms listed are parasites. *Acanthamoeba* spp., *B. mandrillaris,* and *N. fowleri* are free-living amebae. The former two can cause a granulomatous encephalitis in the immune compromised, whereas *N. fowleri* causes an acute, highly fatal meningoencephalitis in persons regardless of their immune status. *T. gondii* is a sporozoite organism that causes encephalitis in severely immune compromised individuals or congenitally infected infants.

2 **The answer is A: *Aspergillus.*** Movable cavitary mass and hemoptysis in a patient with a history of sarcoidosis is strongly suggestive of aspergillomas. Pre-existing conditions, such as tuberculosis, emphysema, or sarcoidosis, which promote pulmonary cavitation, are linked to the condition. Usually, the infection is noninvasive and may spontaneously resolve when the underlying condition is corrected. Itraconazole may be indicated, however, if the patient does not prove to be a viable candidate for surgery. The microscopic structure in the image is a conidiophore characteristic of *Aspergillus.* By contrast, *Rhizopus* features a sporangium; *Candida* and *Cryptococcus* produce budding yeast cells; and a diagnosis of *Pneumocystis* would be supported only if cysts and trophozoites were observed in stained sections of lung tissue.

3 **The answer is A: Diabetes.** The case describes an individual with rhinocerebral zygomycosis, a fungal infection involving the nasal cavity, sinuses, eye, and even the brain and meninges. The fungi involved belong to the group Zygomycetes, which includes *Rhizopus* spp. and *Mucor* spp. among others. These organisms produce the characteristic sporangium seen in the photograph. These opportunistic fungi readily invade blood vessels, entering tissues and producing necrotic lesions. Infection with these organisms is rapidly progressive, with a high mortality rate despite appropriate treatment. The most common predisposing factor for this infection is diabetic ketoacidosis. Other predisposing conditions include persons with acidosis due to other causes such as renal failure or diarrhea. Patients with solid organ transplants, hematological malignancies, or corticosteroid therapy are also at risk. This infection has been reported in HIV-infected patients. Poorly controlled diabetes is, however, the most important risk factor for this infection.

4 **The answer is D: Nystatin.** The child in this case has oral thrush due to an overgrowth of *Candida.* The lack of appetite is more than likely associated with dysphagia in this case. Thrush is common in children who are poorly nourished. Most commonly, the condition is self-limiting. Nystatin, the best first choice, will speed the healing process and allow the child to comfortably feed. None of the other choices listed in this question have antifungal activity.

5 **The answer is D: HIV infection.** Recurrent candidiasis is an early marker of HIV disease. Acute glomerulonephritis and rheumatic fever are complications of streptococcal disease; giardiasis is childhood intestinal parasitic disease; and chronic hepatitis B is not linked to candidiasis.

6 **The answer is D: *Microsporum canis.*** The structures shown in the image are macroconidia, characteristic of *Microsporium canis,* a common dermatophytic fungus of puppies and kittens. Pets, when discovered infected, should be treated to avoid a zoonotic transmission to children. None of the other organisms listed cause crusty lesions on pets, nor do they form macroconidia. In culture, *Aspergillus* forms conidia that **sit** atop a conidiophore. *Blastomyces* is a dimorphic fungus that grows as yeast when cultured at 37°C. *Cryptococcus* also grows in culture and in tissues as an encapsulated yeast. In culture, the conidia of *Sporothrix* have a "daisy-petal" arrangement.

7 **The answer is B: Dermatophyte.** Dermatophytes are a group of fungi belonging to the genera *Trichophyton,* *Microsporum,* and *Epidermophyton.* They cause an infection of the outer, keratinized layers of the skin as well as hair and nails. The skin infections are commonly known as ringworm, or tinea corporis. This question involves a simple case of ringworm, probably *Trichophyton rubrum,* as this species commonly occurs in body-to-body contact sports like wrestling. The skin lesions characteristically appear as oval-shaped, scaly plaques with erythematosus, raised borders, as seen in the photograph. Diatomaceous fungi are pigmented fungi associated with subcutaneous mycoses, chromoblastomycosis, and phaeophomycosis. Endemic dimorphic fungi include *Histoplasma,* *Blastomyces,* and *Coccidioides.* They typically cause pulmonary or systemic infections in a person's living or visiting endemic areas. The opportunistic fungi include *Candida, Aspergillus, Cryptococcus, Rhizopus, Mucor,* and *Pneumocystis* and cause severe, systemic infections in the immune-suppressed.

8 **The answer is D: Sabouraud dextrose agar.** The three high school students in this case have a fungal infection called tinea corporis, also known as ringworm. Although the fungi will grow on many of the media used for the isolation of bacteria, it is preferable to use media specifically enriched for fungal growth. Sabouraud dextrose agar is a medium that is routinely employed for the isolation of fungi. The low pH inhibits the growth of most clinically significant bacterial species. The addition of chloramphenicol will enhance the antibacterial activity of the medium. The other agars listed are used to isolate bacteria and are ones with which students should be familiar. Sheep blood agar is very commonly used for the isolation of a wide variety of bacteria. It is especially useful for distinguishing various groups of hemolytic bacteria, such as streptococci. Chocolate agar is sheep blood agar that has been heated to lyse the red blood cells, releasing nutrients from the cells. This agar is used for more fastidious organisms such as *Haemophilus*. Lowenstein–Jensen medium is used to isolate *Mycobacterium* spp. MacConkey agar is used to isolate Gram-negative enteric bacteria.

9 **The answer is D: Terbinafine.** This drug, along with itraconazole, has been shown to have higher rates of cure compared to the previous oral antifungal agents used for this condition. Terbinafine is available in oral and topical formulations and is useful for many types of dermatophyte infections. The other drugs listed are generally used for serious, invasive fungal infections.

10 **The answer is A: Inhibits ergosterol synthesis.** Terbinafine works by inhibiting the enzyme squalene epoxidase involved in ergosterol synthesis. Ergosterol is a unique and essential component of the cell membrane of fungi. Echinocandins such as caspofungin inhibit glucan synthesis and are used for invasive candidiasis or aspergillosis. Griseofulvin inhibits mitosis through microtubule disruption. Its use in dermatophytic skin infections has been largely replaced by the topical azoles. Flucytosine inhibits nucleic acid synthesis. It is often used in combination with amphotericin B to treat serious respiratory or systemic fungal infections with *Cryptococcus* or *Candida*. The sordarins are promising investigational drugs which inhibit fungal protein synthesis.

11 **The answer is B: *Candida albicans*.** The fungal structure seen in the image is a germ tube characteristic of *C. albicans*. This fungal structure is a virulence factor and has a role in adherence and invasion. None of the other fungi listed form germ tubes.

12 **The answer is C: Macroconidia.** The fungus in question is *Fusarium*, an opportunistic, environmental species that afflicts immunodeficient patients. The banana-shaped macroconidia are characteristic to this genus. The point of this question is not so much the identification of *Fusarium* as being familiar with fungal structures and stages.

13 **The answer is E: *Sporothrix schenckii*.** Infection with this organism causes a disease known as cutaneous or lymphocutaneous sporotrichosis. It occurs in farm or nursery workers or others handling thorny plants, baled hay, or sphagnum moss. The progression of the lesion occurs slowly with the initial lesion resembling an insect bite and progression to nodules and open ulcers. Diagnosis can be made by finding characteristic fungal forms in cultures from the lesions. The distinctive arrangement of the conidia on the conidiophore and the characteristic thermal dimorphism (i.e., mold at 25 °C and yeast at 37 °C) are consistent with *S. schenckii*. The fungus is described as a geophilic species, and traumatic inoculation into the subcutaneous layer is the means by which a person becomes infected. None of the other fungal diseases listed manifest similar symptoms, nor do their fungal etiologies show fungal structures as described in this case. *Acremonium* spp. are causes of eumycotic mycetoma, a fungal disease found in the tropics. Similarly, *C. carrionii* is found in the tropics and causes a subcutaneous fungal infection called chromoblastomycosis. *B. dermatitidis* is an endemic, dimorphic fungus found in the Ohio and Mississippi river valleys and causes a pulmonary disease that can be accompanied by skin lesions. *C. tropicalis* is an opportunistic fungus that causes a variety of diseases.

14 **The answer is C: Itraconazole.** The CDC recommends this antifungal as the drug of choice for cutaneous or lymphocutaneous sporotrichosis. Amphotericin B is reserved for serious systemic fungal infections; caspofungin is used for invasive candidal infections, while nystatin is a topical agent used for treatment of cutaneous or mucocutaneous candidal infections. Bacitracin has no activity against fungal disease.

15 **The answer is E: Yeasts.** Dimorphic fungi are organisms that can exist in two different morphologies based upon the environment in which they are thriving. Generally, this morphology is dictated by temperature. That is, when a dimorphic fungus is growing at room temperature (25 °C), the morphology is usually hyphal or mycelium in nature. However, when the dimorphic fungus is growing at 37 °C, as would be the case in patient tissues, the morphology is yeast. Pseudohyphae is a characteristic morphological finding for *Candida albicans* infections. Mycelium is a collection of hyphae and as indicated above, would not be the finding in a typical patient. Endospores are a dormant stage of bacteria resistant to environmental insults.

16 **The answer is C: Ergosterol.** Although fungi are eukaryotic, fungal cells are unique in several ways. Their cell membranes contain ergosterol, rather than cholesterol found in mammalian cell membranes. The antifungal azoles inhibit ergosterol synthesis and amphotericin B binds to ergosterol, leading to membrane damage. Fungi cell walls contain chitin, the synthesis of which can be inhibited by the investigational drug nikkomycin. Peptidoglycan and teichoic acid are components of bacterial cell walls.

17 **The answer is A: _Hortaea wernickii_.** The case is descriptive of tinea nigra, a fungal disease caused by _H. wernickii_ and found most commonly in tropical areas of Central and South America and Africa. Detection of dark colored hyphal fragments and arthroconidia in skin scrapings aids in the diagnosis. _M. furfur_ causes pityriasis versicolor, a superficial fungal infection that leads to hypopigmented macular lesions on the skin of the arms, trunk, shoulders, face, and/or neck. _P. hortae_ causes black piedra, a fungal infection of hair shafts. _S. schenckii_ causes a lymphocutaneous mycosis following traumatic inoculation of the skin with fungi present on plant thorns. _Trichophyton_ spp. belong to a group of fungi collectively called the dermatophytes that are responsible for the development of various cutaneous fungal infections including athlete's foot and jock itch.

18 **The answer is C: _Candida_ spp.** This case is descriptive of esophagitis. This disease is most commonly secondary to gastroesophageal reflux disease; however, in immune compromised patients, it can have a microbial cause. Infectious causes of esophagitis are numerous; however, _Candida_ spp. are most common. The finding of pseudohyphae and budding yeasts is typical for _Candida_. Although cases of esophagitis due to _Aspergillus_, _Cryptococcus_, and _Mycobacterium avium-intracellulare_ have been reported, none of these organisms have the morphological features shown in the photograph. The filamentous bacteria _Actinomyces_ are not associated with esophagitis.

19 **The answer is B: _Histoplasma capsulatum_.** The case is descriptive of acute pulmonary histoplasmosis. This condition occurs following inhalation of large numbers of fungal spores of _H. capsulatum_. This endemic, dimorphic fungus is found in much of the eastern United States associated with soils enriched with bird or bat droppings. Caves inhabited by bats are examples of places in which exposure to _H. capsulatum_ is a risk. Diagnosis of acute pulmonary histoplasmosis can best be accomplished by serology, using either immunodiffusion or complement fixation tests. Both tests can be used to detect antibodies in the patient's serum to either or both the M antigen and the H antigen of this organism. _B. dermatitidis_ and _Coccidioides immitis_ are also endemic dimorphic fungi that cause pulmonary symptoms. The geographic location of _B. dermatitidis_

and _H. capsulatum_ overlap; however, _B. dermatitidis_ is found in soil and leaf litter. _Coccidioides immitis_ is found in the southwestern United States. _Candida albicans_ causes serious respiratory disease in the immune compromised, thus would not be included in the differential for this patient. _Cryptococcus neoformans_ typically causes neurological disease in the immune compromised.

20 **The answer is D: Inhalation of fungal spores.** Based upon the dimorphic behavior of these fungi, hyphal forms at temperatures around 25 °C and yeast forms at temperatures around 37 °C; humans have a greater chance of obtaining disease upon contact with environmental (hyphal) forms. Hyphal growths in the soil generate spore-containing structures as part of their life cycle (asexual reproduction). Spores released by the mycelium can be inhaled and gain access to the respiratory system. Ingestion of fungal forms does not result in disease due to the action of gastric acids. While inhalation of hyphae may cause disease, these structures are often secured in the soil or the structure on which the fungus is growing. Thus, inhalation of fungal spores represents the most likely method of inoculation of dimorphic fungi in humans for disease development.

21 **The answer is D: Inhibits the activity of the enzyme, β-glucan synthase.** Echinocandins such as caspofungin directly inactivate the activity of β-glucan synthase preventing the construction of the fungal cell wall. Sordarin and derivatives prevent fungal growth by inhibiting t-RNA and ribosome translocation along the mRNA through direct binding to elongation factor-2 (EF-2). Nikkomycin Z acts to inhibit the function of chitin synthase, which synthesizes chitin in the fungal cell wall. Polyenes such as amphotericin B directly bind to ergosterol in the fungal membrane destroying osmotic integrity. Flucytosine deaminates 5-fluorouracil, which then competes with uracil during RNA synthesis.

22 **The answer is C: Flucytosine.** Cryptococcosis is caused by _Cryptococcus neoformans_, an opportunistic pathogen. It is the most common cause of fungal meningitis and AIDS patients are at high risk of developing this disease. In addition, cryptococcosis can present initially as pneumonia that may quickly disseminate depending upon the immune status of the patient. Neurological infection is 100% fatal if left untreated. In this setting, amphotericin B is the most appropriate treatment. Flucytosine appears to be highly effective against this fungus, however, resistance can develop when this drug is used alone for therapy. Therefore, treatment of cryptococcal meningitis initially involves 2 weeks of amphotericin B in combination with flucytosine. Following this, an 8-week treatment with an azole is recommended. Amphotericin B can also be administered for other fungal infections without the aid of another antifungal. Itraconazole, TMP–SMZ, and ketoconazole can be used alone against susceptible fungi.

23 **The answer is E: Inhibition of the activity of the enzyme, 14-α-demethylase.** 14-α-methylase synthesizes ergosterol from the intermediate lanosterol. The lack of ergosterol production disrupts cell membrane integrity. Azoles such as fluconazole, itraconazole, or miconazole function to inhibit this enzyme. Sordarin and its derivatives inhibit GTP hydrolysis important for ribosome function in protein synthesis. Nikkomycin Z inhibits the function of chitin synthase. The polyenes directly bind ergosterol and promote formation of pores in the fungal cell membrane. Echinocandins inhibit the activity of β-glucan synthase thereby weakening fungal cell walls.

24 **The answer is E: Chromoblastomycosis.** There are several clues to answer this question—cauliflowerlike lesions, patient employment with forest agency, muriform bodies in the biopsy, etc. Chromoblastomycosis is a disfiguring disease occurring in rural areas of the tropics and is common among men—seen on the arms and legs—especially those working in the forest. It is transmitted by contact with woody plants and soil. The disease is caused by numerous fungal species, however, all of these form muriform bodies in the tissue lesions. These muriform bodies tend to be brown in coloration due to the presence of melanin in the cell walls. White piedra is a soft mold growth on hairs in the groin area. Zygomycosis is similar to this disease in terms of gross disfiguring lesions, however, there is no cauliflowerlike appearance. Sporotrichosis is characterized by the development of skin ulcerations along a lymphatic pathway. Dermatophytosis represents the different tineas or ringworm infections characterized as erythematosus, annular, scaling patches.

25 **The answer is B: *Coccidioides immitis*.** This case is descriptive of coccidioidomycosis. This organism is an endemic dimorphic fungus found in the desert southwest. Its arthroconidia are spread in blowing dust and transmission occurs by inhalation. Those at risk of serious infection include the elderly and immune compromised individuals. In these persons, a progressive pulmonary infection with cavitary lesions can result. Diagnosis can be accomplished by the finding of characteristic spherules containing endospores in the sputum. None of the other fungi listed form these characteristic spherules, although all of them can cause pulmonary infections.

26 **The answer is C: Interaction with fungal ergosterol to form pores in the fungal cell.** Amphotericin B operates by binding directly with ergosterol. This interaction results in the formation of pores within the fungi which alters the osmotic integrity between the inner and outer membrane areas. In addition, oxidative damage can occur to the cell as a by-product of drug oxidation. This drug is most useful in systemic, life-threatening fungal infections and nephrotoxicity is a potential side effect. Sordarin and its derivatives inhibit protein synthesis by action on EF-2. Nikkomycin Z inhibits the function of chitin synthase. Echinocandins inhibit the activity of β-glucan synthase to weaken fungal cell walls. Azoles inhibit the action of 14-α-methylase which synthesizes ergosterol from the intermediate, lanosterol.

27 **The answer is E: Wood lamp to detect fluoresence.** In children, tinea capitis or ringworm of the scalp is a pediatric condition that is regularly diagnosed in a primary care practice using a Wood lamp. This lamp shines UV light on the lesion and many dermatophyte fungi causing this condition will fluoresce under UV light. Fungal elements can be detected in hair follicles cleared with potassium hydroxide (KOH). Gram stain is used for bacterial infections. The fungi can also be cultured on Sabouraud dextrose agar; however, this is time consuming. Dermatophyte infections are not diagnosed serologically, or by PCR.

28 **The answer is C: Eumycotic mycetoma.** The case is descriptive of eumycotic mycetoma, a type of subcutaneous fungal infection found in tropical areas and caused by a number of fungal genera. Fungi that produce subcutaneous mycosis like the one this patient is suffering from are residences of the environment. Many are associated with plants or are saprobes in natural environments. Infections most commonly involve the extremities and follow traumatic inoculation of soil fungi. A puncture wound from a thorn or an abrasion may not be that innocuous, especially if the wound is allowed to become dirty and contaminated. Eumycotic mycetoma is a chronic infection in which granulomatous lesions grow slowly and abscess over time leading to lymphedema and possible secondary bacterial infection. As the fungus spreads subcutaneously, involvement of bone in the area of the lesion is also possible. The micrograph shows a mycelial aggregate mass. The exact species has little relevance with regards to therapeutic management. Actinomycete bacteria can also produce a mycetoma, but there is no evidence of bacterial cells in the biopsy. Therapy is more successful with bacterial than fungal causes of mycetoma, hence identification of the microbial group is paramount when considering management of this disease. Early diagnosis and treatment of eumycotic mycetomas have the greatest chance for success. The infection, which takes years to develop, is most common among the poor who can afford neither shoes nor medical care. None of the other fungal infections listed are associated with this type of lesion.

29 **The answer is A: Arthroconidia.** The lesions shown in the photograph are consistent with tenia cruis or "jock itch." This condition is usually diagnosed clinically; however, hyphal elements, especially chains of arthroconidia, are easily visualized with a KOH wet mount. Yeast cells are characteristic of *Candida*, and the germ tube outgrowths of the cell are usually viewed in enriched culture media. Zygospores, ascospores, and sporangiospores are also fungal structures viewed in specimens cultured in the laboratory.

30 **The answer is A: *Candida albicans.*** This case is descriptive of a vaginal yeast infection. Predisposing factors for vaginal thrush, an overgrowth of *Candida* are plentiful, including hormonal issues, diabetes, and broad-spectrum antibiotic use. In this case, it is likely that the fluoroquinolone was the precipitating factor. The budding cells seen in the photograph are yeast, and *C. albicans* is the most likely species. The other organisms listed also cause vaginal discharge; however, the discharge associated with yeast infections is thick and described as cottage cheese-like. Bacterial vaginitis is associated with a thin milky-white discharge, and that of *T. vaginalis* is also thin and often frothy. Neither motile flagellated protozoa nor the distinctive clue cell (epithelial cell covered with bacterial cells) that is a microscopic marker for Gardnerella vaginosis is present in this case.

31 **The answer is E: Inhalation of yeast-like cells from soil contaminated with pigeon droppings.** *C. neoformans* is an opportunistic fungus that is found worldwide as a saprophyte in soil enriched with bird droppings. Although immune competent persons can be infected, the result is often a flulike illness with complete recovery. The organism is not walled off in the lung as is the case with *Histoplasma capsulatum* or *Mycobacterium tuberculosis*. Infection of persons with T cell immune suppression, such as AIDS patients or patients with hematological malignancies, most commonly leads to meningoencephalitis.

32 **The answer is C: *Coccidioides immitis.*** This case is descriptive of osteomyelitis due to disseminated *C. immitis*. Valley fever or coccidioidomycosis is a disease endemic to the desert landscape of the southwestern United States. The disease is extremely common in the Phoenix, Arizona area and is transmitted by inhalation of the soilborne mold stage (i.e.,

arthroconidium). The above case is a classic example of disseminated *C. immitis*, a relatively rare condition that is influenced by race, gender, age, and immune status. Hispanics, Asians, American Indians, African-Americans, pregnant women, middle-aged and older men, and immunocompromised persons are most likely to have serious complications with the fungus. This is an osteomyelitis related to a *C. immitis* systemic infection. The images show spherules, endospores, and a chronic inflammatory response with giant cells. These histological findings are consistent with infection with *C. immitis*.

33 **The answer is A: Amphotericin B.** Disseminated infections with *Coccidioides immitis,* such as described in the present case, are best treated with amphotericin B. Azoles are useful for mild-to-moderate disease; itraconazole may be better absorbed into skeletal lesions than fluconazole. Ketoconazole is not routinely used for this infection. Flucytosine is used in combination with amphotericin B or fluconazole for cryptococcal meningitis or serious candidal infections. Griseofulvin is used for the treatment of dermatophytes. Metronidazole is used to treat anaerobic bacterial infections and *Trichomonas vaginalis*.

34 **The answer is A: *Aspergillus fumigatus.*** There are numerous reasons not to clean the ears with cotton-tipped swabs, aspergillosis being one of them. Undoubtedly, a swimmer would be more predisposed to this infection. Otic acidifying agents in the form of eardrops are useful to control this type of fungal infection. Of the choices, only *Aspergillus* produces conidiophores as illustrated.

35 **The answer is E: Inhalation of ubiquitous conidia in the air.** The case is descriptive of invasive aspergillosis. The photograph shows a conidial head typical of *Aspergillus*. Neutropenic patients are particularly susceptible to infection with *Aspergillus* as well as *Candida* and various extracellular bacteria. *Aspergillus* is common in hospital environments, with conidia found in the air, water sources (sinks, showers), and in the soil of potted plants. The organism is not part of the normal flora as is the case for *Candida* and several important extracellular bacterial infections that can cause serious disease in neutropenic patients. Thus, infection would not result from normal flora or on contaminated hands or medical implements such as catheters.

36 **The answer is E: Voriconazole.** Voriconazole, a newer azole, is the preferred drug, especially when compared to the renal toxicity issues associated with amphotericin B. Pentamidine has activity against *Pneumocystis*, and penicillin and isoniazid are antibacterial agents.

37 **The answer is D: Rhinocerebral mucormycosis.** The micrograph plainly shows sporangial structures, which would point in the direction of *Rhizopus* or a closely related species. Histological identification of nonseptate hyphae would also lead to the same identification. *Rhizopus* and *Mucor* account for many of the cases of rhinocerebral mucormycosis. The other species listed are not characterized with sporangia. Diabetic patients, especially those with acidosis, are more at risk because of impaired neutrophil chemotaxis and a generalized decrease in phagocytosis. Mortalities have been reported. The hyperglycemia must be brought under control. Therapy consists of amphotericin B and possibly extensive surgical debridement.

38 **The answer is E: Trimethroprim–sulfamethoxazole (TMP/SMZ).** This case is descriptive of pneumocystis pneumonia. *Pneumocystis jiroveci* (formally *carinii*) is the causative agent of this condition. The micrograph depicts the cystic stage of the organism. It is found in the respiratory tracts of healthy individuals where its growth is controlled by macrophages. Without sufficient CD4$^+$ cells that secrete γ-interferon to activate macrophages, these phagocytic cells will have difficulty in killing the microbe. *Pneumocystis* infection can be prevented by TMP/SMZ given prophylactically to HIV-infected individuals with CD4 counts of less than 200/cmm. The patient in this case was noncompliant with medication, thereby increasing his risk for this and other opportunistic infections. *P. jiroveci* was once thought to be a protozoan; however, genetic evidence supports its categorization as a fungus. Nevertheless, antifungal drugs are not effective either as chemoprophylactic agents or in treating a full-blown infection. TMP/SMZ is the preferred choice, assuming of course that the AIDS patient can tolerate the drug. Pentamidine, clindamycin plus primaquine, atovaquone, and dapsone have also been shown to have activity against this organism.

Chapter 4
Parasitology

QUESTIONS

Select the single best answer.
The next two questions are linked.

1 Within 2 weeks of eating jerky that is made from a mountain lion, a Montana man develops intense vomiting and diarrhea, followed shortly by a fever of 103°F, throbbing headache, and achy muscles. After a few more days of these unrelenting symptoms, he seeks medical attention. His white blood cell count at presentation is 16,100/mm³, with 22% eosinophils. Which of the following laboratory tests would be most helpful to make the correct diagnosis?
(A) Creatine kinase serum level
(B) Creatinine clearance level
(C) Examination of a wet mount of fresh stool
(D) Enzyme-linked immunosorbent assay (ELISA)
(E) Inspection of a Giemsa-stained blood smear

2 What is the best therapeutic option available for the patient?
(A) Mebendazole
(B) Albendazole plus a corticosteroid
(C) Corticosteroid alone
(D) Metronidazole
(E) Praziquantel plus a hydrochlorothiazide

3 Public health officials investigate an onset of febrile gastrointestinal illness in a member of a family who recently emigrated from a Southeast Asian country. A raw pork dish is implicated, and the meat was purchased from an owner of a small farm. A micrograph of stained tissue from the meat is shown in the image. What is the correct term that properly describes the encysted larval stage?

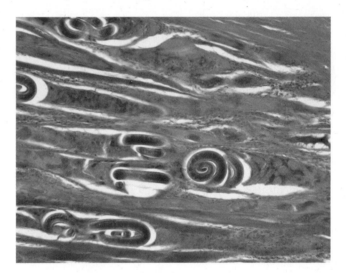

(A) Encapsulated cysticercus
(B) Metacercaria
(C) Nurse cell
(D) Onchocercoma
(E) Pseudocyst

4 A 55-year-old man undergoes a colonoscopy. A biopsy and a mucosal scraping of a suspicious area are positive for a parasite. The wet mount specimen is particularly impressive (shown in the image). The patient works in a slaughterhouse. He has no clinical manifestations associated with the parasite. What is the identification of this parasite?

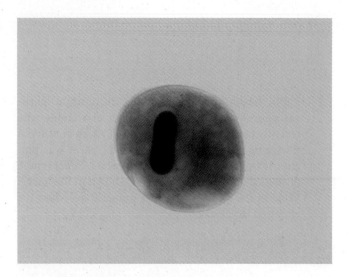

(A) *Balantidium coli*
(B) *Cryptosporidium parvum*
(C) *Entamoeba coli*
(D) *Entamoeba dispar*
(E) *Entamoeba histolytica*

5 A child undergoes an appendectomy, and the pathologist identifies a parasite in the surgical biopsy (shown in the image). What is the most likely parasitic diagnosis?

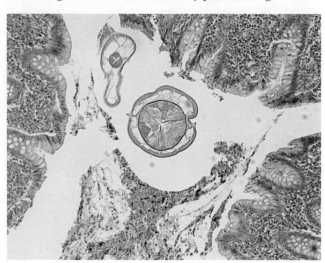

(A) Amebiasis
(B) Ascariasis
(C) Enterobiasis
(D) Giardiasis
(E) Hookworm disease

6 A medical student, who is completing a pathology rotation, is given an assignment to review the collection of parasite specimens taken from patients with gastrointestinal disease. On one of the slides, the label is faded and unreadable. Even so, the specimen (shown in the image) is well preserved and, according to the attending pathologist, easy to identify. What is the identification of this parasite?

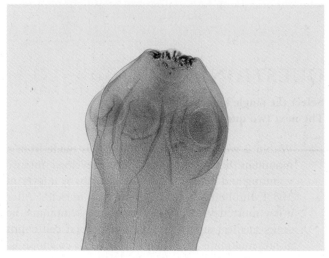

(A) *Ascaris lumbricoides*
(B) *Echinococcus granulosum*
(C) *Fasciola hepatica*
(D) *Taenia solium*
(E) *Toxocara canis*

The next three questions are linked.

7 The nurse of an emergency shelter for young children reports that several are suffering from a gastrointestinal illness, presumably a viral illness characterized with colicky intestinal pain and loose stools. To be safe, fecal specimens from each of the children are analyzed for pathogenic bacteria and parasites. A sample from one of the symptomatic children tests positive for ova (shown in the image) and for worm fragments. The fragments measure approximately a centimeter long and are similar to the stained specimen shown. Additional stool samples from several children who are not experiencing colitis also prove positive for the same parasite. What is the correct identification?

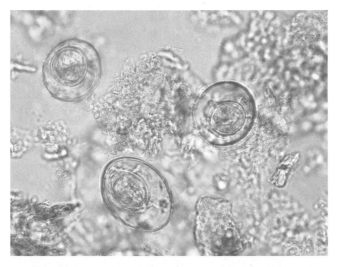

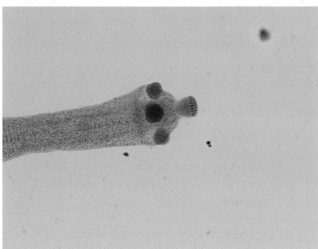

10 A 70-year-old man who has roots in a farming community in Canada undergoes a cholecystectomy, and during the procedure a liver cyst is discovered (shown in the image). The decision is made to remove it, but unfortunately during the procedure, an error allows for a significant amount of cyst fluid (contents shown) to spill out into the abdominal cavity. Epinephrine averts an anaphylactic attack, and his immediate recovery proves uneventful. But, what is his long-term prognosis as a result of the surgical mishap?

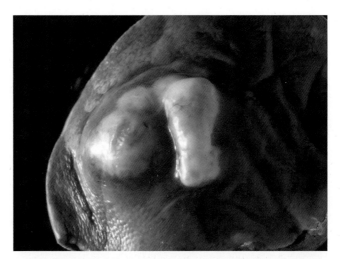

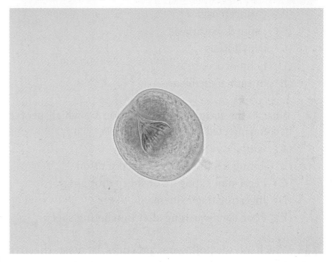

(A) *Ancylostoma duodenale*
(B) *Enterobius vermicularis*
(C) *Hymenolepis nana*
(D) *Strongyloides stercoralis*
(E) *Taenia saginata*

8 The attending physician decides to treat in an effort to control the infections in the facility. Which of the following antiparasitics would be most effective?
(A) Chloroquine
(B) Mebendazole
(C) Metronidazole
(D) Praziquantel
(E) Tetracycline

9 Which of the following practices would be most relevant and crucial in an effort to reduce the risk of a future outbreak at the shelter?
(A) Drink only filtered or purified water
(B) Exterminate cockroaches and other insect pests
(C) Thoroughly cook all pork and beef products
(D) Uphold good hygiene practices
(E) Wash all vegetable and salad greens

(A) Excellent but only if he undergoes additional abdominal surgeries for anisakiasis
(B) Good but only if he undergoes long-term therapy for visceral larva migrans
(C) Guarded because of the development of secondary echinococcosis
(D) He will die in less than a month as a result of spread of cryptosporidiosis
(E) Poor because of likelihood of disseminated amebiasis

The next three questions are linked.

11 Several dogs that work Native American sheep ranches in a community of New Mexico undergo their yearly purges for intestinal worms. Examination reveals that all the stools are positive for tapeworms, including a tiny tapeworm species that measures <10 mm (shown in the image). Which medically important disease is linked to this worm?

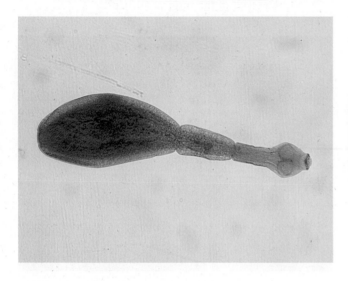

- (A) Cysticercosis
- (B) Diphyllobothriasis
- (C) Dipylidiasis
- (D) Echinococcosis
- (E) Intestinal taeniasis

12 What is the means of transmission by which people become infected with this parasite?
- (A) Eating raw sheep liver
- (B) Eating insufficiently cooked mutton
- (C) Fecal-oral exposure of sheep droppings
- (D) Ingesting dog excrement
- (E) Poor hand washing after butchering sheep

13 Which of the following practices is most effective in order to prevent these sheepdogs from becoming infected with the same tapeworm species next year?
- (A) Periodically worm the sheep
- (B) Stop feeding raw sheep livers to dogs
- (C) Vaccinate dogs against round worms
- (D) Vaccinate dogs against tapeworms
- (E) Vaccinate sheep against intestinal worms

The next two questions are linked.

14 A woman who emigrated from Asia undergoes a spontaneous abortion, and in the recovery room she passes numerous proglottids. The medical technologist injects one of the proglottids with India ink to delineate the uterus (shown in the image). How did she become infected with this tapeworm?

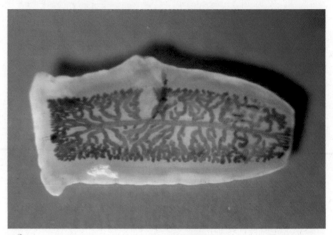

- (A) Person-to-person or direct fecal-oral exposure
- (B) Consumption of insufficiently cooked sirloin
- (C) Consumption of insufficiently cooked pork sausage
- (D) Consumption of sushi
- (E) Fecal contamination of food or drink

15 What is an appropriate therapy for the woman in the above case?
- (A) Chloroquine
- (B) Ivermectin
- (C) Metronidazole
- (D) Praziquantel
- (E) Piperazine

16 A 65-year-old woman in Finland suffers from a macrocytic anemia. Her history is significant for frequent consumption of pickled fish. A stool sample reveals parasite ova like the one shown in the first image. Upon treatment, she expels a tapeworm similar to the stained specimen shown in the second image. With which tapeworm was she most likely infected?

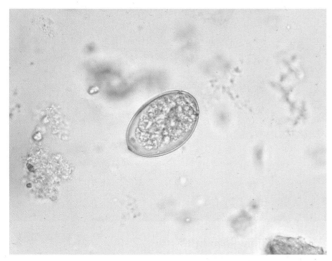

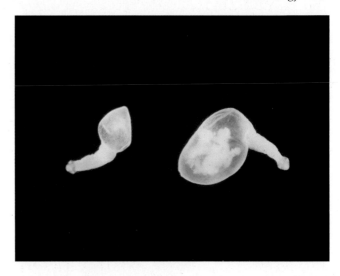

(A) *Echinococcus granulosus*
(B) *Onchocerca volvulus*
(C) *Taenia saginata*
(D) *Taenia solium*
(E) *Toxocara canis*

18 What was the probable source or vehicle of infection for the child in the above case?
(A) Autoinfection from her own feces
(B) Consuming rare hamburgers
(C) Consuming undercooked pork
(D) Drinking fecal contaminated water at the farm labor camp
(E) Ingestion of fecal-contaminated salad vegetables

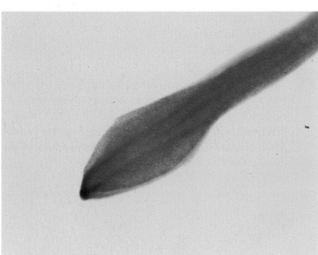

(A) *Diphyllobothrium latum*
(B) *Echinococcus granulosus*
(C) *Hymenolepis nana*
(D) *Taenia saginata*
(E) *Taenia solium*

The next two questions are linked.

17 A 9-year-old patient—a daughter of a migrant farm laborer—experiences onset of epileptic seizures. The family has recently arrived in the United States from Mexico. A few pea-sized lipomalike lesions are undeniably palpable in her subcutaneous tissue of her torso and limbs. Excision of two of these lesions reveals parasites (shown in the image). These parasites are active when placed in warm saline. MRI demonstrates similar lesions in the CNS, and an immunoblot assay is positive for the suspected parasitic disease. Of interest is the discovery of taeniid ova in the stool of her father. Which parasite is most likely the cause of the child's illness?

19 A mother becomes alarmed when she discovers a serpiginous reddish rash on the foot of her child who just returned from a 2-week summer camp on a beach in South Florida. The child reports that the lesion "itches a lot." Their family physician prescribes a topical preparation of thiabendazole and, within 2 weeks, the condition resolved. What is the most likely diagnosis?

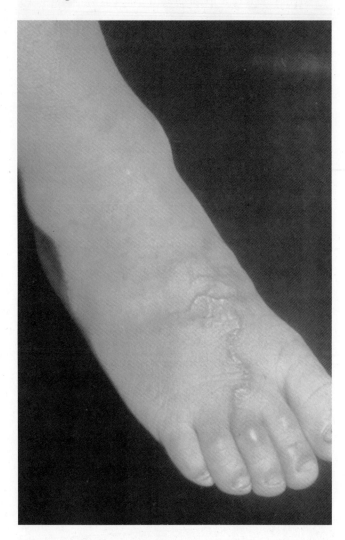

(A) Cercarial dermatitis
(B) Chigger dermatitis
(C) Cutaneous larva migrans
(D) *Demodex follicularis* infesation
(E) *Dracunculus medinensis* infection

20 A filet of sea bass, a marine fish, is heavy infected with worms (shown in the image). If eaten raw, which of the following diseases is the person most at risk of acquiring?

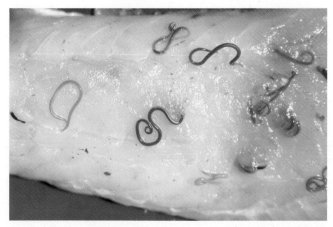

(A) Diphyllobothriasis
(B) Clonorchiasis
(C) Paragonimiasis
(D) Schistosomiasis
(E) Anisakiasis

21 A nurse, who appears somewhat anxious, acknowledges an infestation of bugs on her pubic area. As evidence, she produces a bug (shown in the image). What relevant advice should be offered to this patient when considered the overarching ramifications of the case?

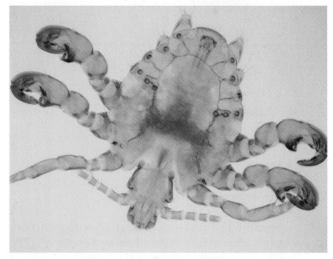

(A) Avoid hot tub use, especially facilities with inadequate chlorination
(B) Submit to a thorough screening for common sexually transmitted infections
(C) Treat pet dog or cat with shampoo containing insecticide
(D) Wash all clothing that has been stored for more than 2 months
(E) Wear insect repellent when in wooded areas or when gardening

22 During an international outreach operation, a medical student examines a young teenager who complains of a scaly and itchy rash on the postauricular area. The student quickly notes that the hairs on the occipital region are heavily contaminated with casts or minute granular objects (shown in the photograph). Of the following, which is the most logical presumptive diagnosis that should be presented to the attending physician?

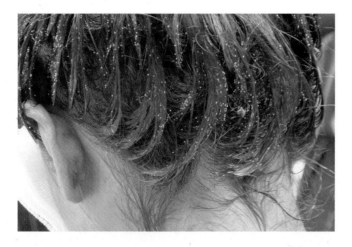

(A) Demodicidosis
(B) Dermatobiasis
(C) Flea-bite hypersensitivity
(D) Pediatric scabies
(E) Pediculosis capitis

23 A 6-year-old boy, who has a history of eating dirt while playing in a New York City park, develops a vision problem in one eye. An opaqueness of pupil or leukokoria is readily discernable by the parents, and this prompts a visit to the ophthalmologist. Funduscopic examination reveals a single granulomatous lesion of the retina. Assuming that his ocular condition is caused by a parasitic worm, what is most likely the etiologic agent?
(A) *Ancylostoma caninum*
(B) *Loa loa*
(C) *Onchocerca volvulus*
(D) *Toxocara canis*
(E) *Trichuris trichiura*

24 A college exchange student from Korea is hospitalized because of chest pain and night sweats. He has had a productive cough since arriving in the United States. The sputum sample is speckled with brown granules, which upon microscopic examination are identified as parasite ova. These same ova are present in the stool (shown in the image). What is the diagnosis?

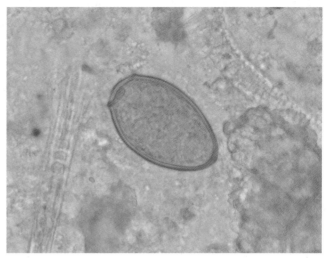

(A) Ascariasis
(B) Clonorchiasis
(C) Paragonimiasis
(D) Taeniasis
(E) Visceral larva migrans

25 A Taiwanese patient dies from complications of cholangiocarcinoma. Postmortem examination determines parasite bile duct involvement. Which of the following is the most likely species?

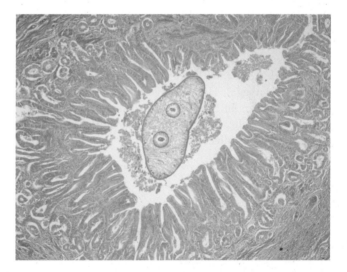

(A) *Ascaris lumbricoides*
(B) *Clonorchis sinensis*
(C) *Entamoeba histolytica*
(D) *Fasciola hepatica*
(E) *Taenia solium*

26 The photograph depicts a group of intestinal worms that is endemic to the Far East. How do humans acquire the parasites within this group?

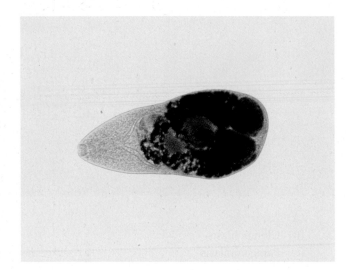

(A) Consuming water contaminated with miracidia
(B) Eating cysticerci in insufficiently cooked beef
(C) Eating metacercariae in raw or partially cooked fish
(D) Finger-to-mouth or direct fecal-oral exposure to ova
(E) Wading in water polluted with cercariae

27 A man in his twenties experiences a burning sensation upon urination. Microscopic examination of centrifuged, clean-catch urine reveals parasite eggs (shown in the image). He has traveled and lived abroad for many years in countries in the Americas, Caribbean, South Pacific, and Africa. Where did he most likely acquire this infection?

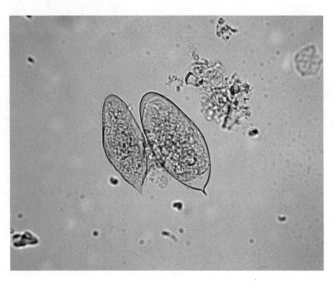

(A) Africa
(B) Caribbean Islands
(C) Central America
(D) South America
(E) South Pacific Islands

28 A resident expatriate who is now employed as a river guide for a safari and adventure enterprise in a central African nation returns to the United States for treatment of hepatic disease and dysentery. Surgical biopsy reveals granulomas (shown in the first image). Parasite ova are also noted in the stool examination (shown in the second image). What is the most likely parasite agent responsible for this patient's clinical presentation?

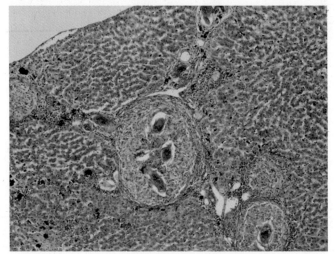

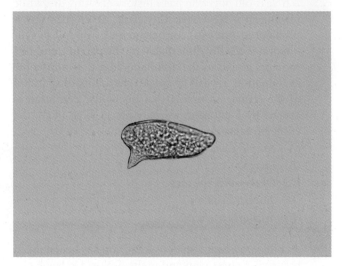

(A) *Schistosoma hematobium*
(B) *Schistosoma intercalatum*
(C) *Schistosoma japonicum*
(D) *Schistosoma mekongi*
(E) *Schistosoma mansoni*

29 Ova, similar to the one shown, are discovered in a microscopic examination of a stool specimen. The patient is a missionary who has resided in remote villages of Brazil for approximately 2 years. His only symptom is an occasional bout of mild diarrhea. A positive ELISA, performed by the CDC, confirms the diagnosis. What course of action should be taken by the physician at this point?

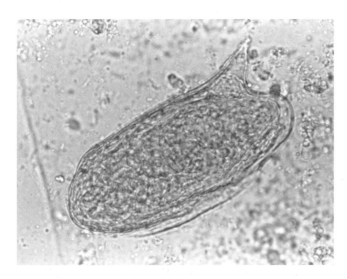

(A) Bismuth subsalicylate only
(B) Metronidazole
(C) Praziquantel
(D) Supportive therapy to prevent dehydration
(E) No therapy required as the diarrhea will spontaneously resolve

30 Tourist backpackers, visiting a primitive tropical island, are assured that the untreated water supply is safe for bathing because it originates from a pristine river. However, water analysis reveals infestation with the organism shown in the image. Based on the photo, what are tourists who bathe in unheated water from this river at risk for?

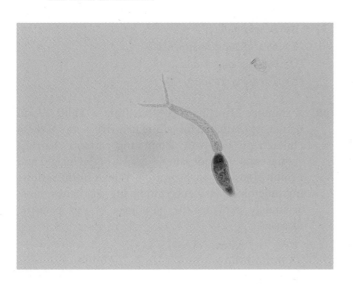

(A) Amebiasis
(B) Ascariasis
(C) Fasciolopsiasis
(D) Giardiasis
(E) Schistosomiasis

31 A Brazilian man presents with an enlarged scrotum (shown in the first photograph). The man reports that his scrotum is gradually "getting bigger." During the medical history, he also expresses alarm that his urine appears milky—giving the physician the impression that he is also suffering from chylous urine. A thick blood film stained with Giemsa is shown in the second image. With which organism is he most likely infected?

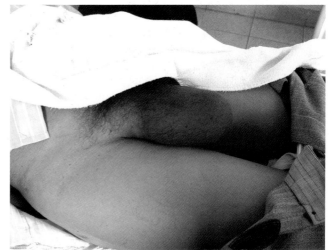

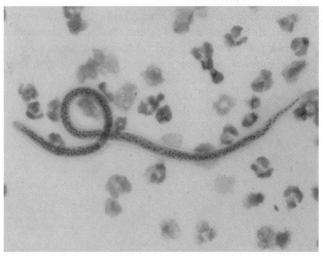

(A) *Ancylostoma brasiliense*
(B) *Loa loa*
(C) *Onchocerca volvulus*
(D) *Trichinella spiralis*
(E) *Wuchereria bancrofti*

32 An ophthalmologist makes the diagnosis of sclerosing keratitis in a patient who immigrated to the United States from a Pacific coastal community of Ecuador. Of note are many filariform juveniles (similar to the one shown in the image) in the chambers of the eye. Which of the following parasites is the causative agent?

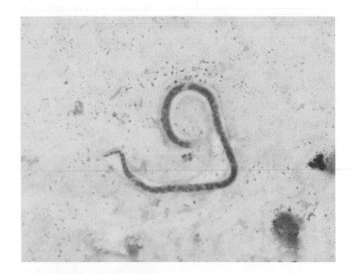

(A) *Dracunculus medinensis*
(B) *Loa loa*
(C) *Onchocerca volvulus*
(D) *Toxocara canis*
(E) *Wuchereria bancrofti*

33 Over a 1-week period, several elementary age children, who are involved in a summer camp in the Pocono Mountains of Pennsylvania, contract a gastrointestinal illness (i.e., they all exhibit similar manifestations like painful bloating and the passage of loose stools). A common microbe is present in fresh stool smears (example shown under oil immersion). Of the following means of transmission, which one is the most likely way each of these children became infected?

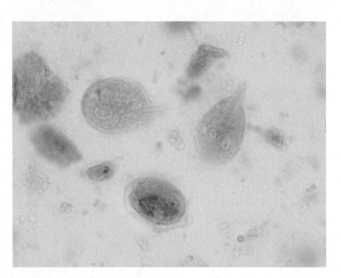

(A) Breathing (and swallowing) dust laden with bird droppings
(B) Drinking contaminated lake or stream water
(C) Eating rare or insufficiently cooked hamburger
(D) Eating salad that contains dandelion flowers grown in nature
(E) Poor hygiene practice of urinating while wading in streams

34 A 30-year-old male, who recently emigrated from Asia, presents at the emergency room with severe intestinal spasms and cramps. The abdominal pain has persisted for almost 2 days. Physical examination reveals bowel sounds and localized tenderness of the right lower quadrant with rebound tenderness. An appendectomy is performed. The pathology report does not describe associated inflammation but does mention that the anterior or head end of a parasitic worm is embedded in the mucosa. The cross section of the parasite at the level of its esophagus is shown in the image. Which of the following is the probable offending agent in this case?

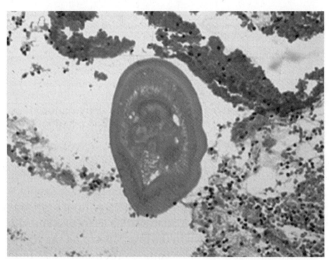

(A) *Ancylostoma duodenale*
(B) *Brugia malayi*
(C) *Dracunculus medinensis*
(D) *Necator americanus*
(E) *Trichuris trichiura*

35 A number of orphan children from a Third World nation are evaluated for failure to thrive. Some of these children present with debilitating parasitic diarrhea (representative stool sample shown in the image) and exhibit signs of malabsorption. Which of the following microbial virulence-producing attributes most accurately explains the pathology of this parasitic disease?

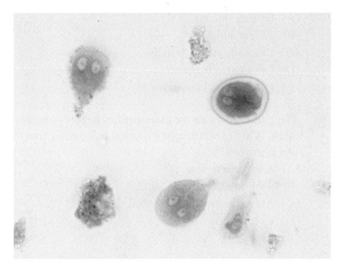

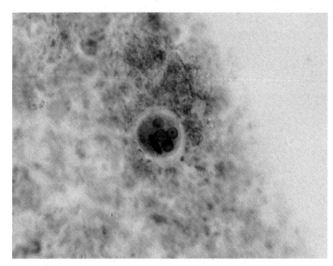

(A) Development of macrocytic iron-deficiency anemia

(B) Heavy parasite burden covering the epithelial surface of the duodenum

(C) Lysis of the epithelial lining in the colon, resulting in blood in the stools

(D) Massive infections, resulting in intestinal blockage and peritonitis

(E) Perforation of the small intestine and hepatic abscess formation

36 A missionary returns home from South America because of health problems. Principally, the patient is suffering from weeks of acute colitis. The diarrheic stool sample submitted for analysis is positive for occult blood, trophozoites with ingested erythrocytes (shown in the first image), and quadrinucleate cysts (shown in the second image). Based on these clinical findings, what is the most likely diagnosis?

(A) Amebiasis

(B) Balantidiasis

(C) Cryptosporidiosis

(D) Cyclosporiasis

(E) Giardiasis

37 A young child from Louisiana is seen because of lower abdominal pain and blood-streaked diarrhea. The stool sample shows an abundance of eggs, like the one in the micrograph, suggesting a heavy worm burden. Considering these findings, what is the correct course of action that should be taken by the physician?

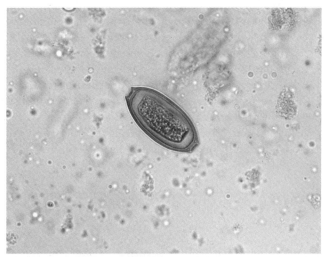

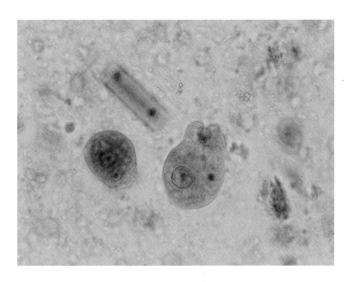

(A) Order a fresh sample to test for amebic dysentery

(B) No treatment necessary since the infection will spontaneously resolve

(C) Prescribe albendazole for trichuriasis

(D) Prescribe metronidazole for hookworm disease

(E) Treat for pernicious anemia but not intestinal parasites

38 A 9-year-old child is observed repeatedly scratching herself around the anal canal. Distinctive microscopic eggs (shown in the image) are detected via the cellophane tape technique. What is the correct diagnosis?

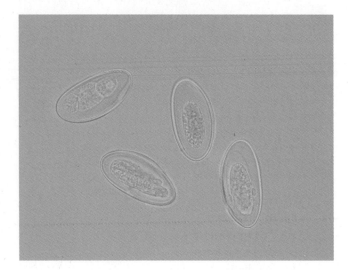

(A) Ascariasis
(B) Enterobiasis
(C) Strongyloidiasis
(D) Trichinosis
(E) Trichuriasis

The next three questions are linked.

39 A 5-year-old child, who lives with his missionary parents in a rural locality in Sierra Leone, Africa, contracts an illness that is initially characterized by vomiting and periods of moderate fever. Over the next few days, his condition dramatically worsens, he becomes markedly lethargic, and his fever intensifies to the point of delirium and convulsions. At the aid station, a blood smear reveals the infective agent (shown in the image). What is the cause of this child's illness?

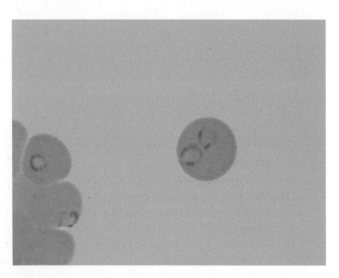

(A) *Babesia microti*
(B) *Brugia malayi*
(C) *Cryptosporidium parvum*
(D) *Leishmania tropica*
(E) *Plasmodium falciparum*

40 The child in the above case requires aggressive treatment. Which antimicrobial is suitable for treatment of this organism?
(A) A carbapenem
(B) Amphotericin B
(C) Atovaquone plus proguanil (Malarone)
(D) Chloroquine
(E) Foscarnet

41 The child in the above case makes a full recovery following treatment. But, when the family is transferred to another region of Africa a year later, the child is again diagnosed with the same infection. What is the most likely explanation for the second infection?
(A) The child was infected with a different strain of the same organism.
(B) The child is deficient in complement components C5–C9 and could not clear the organism despite appropriate treatment.
(C) The child was inadequately treated a year ago, and was not completely cleared of the organism.
(D) The infection is chronic for up to 20 years, and an annual recrudescence is to be expected.
(E) This is a relapse and is attributed to the activation of the dormant liver stage or hypnozoite.

42 With the exception of one, all peace corps volunteers assigned to a remote village in African contract vivax malaria. Which of the following volunteers is the person who did not become infected with *Plasmodium vivax*?
(A) West African man
(B) Italian-American woman
(C) Mexican-American man from Texas
(D) Asian-American woman
(E) Central American man

The next three questions are linked.

43 A 40-year man, who recently returned from a vacation in Brazil, seeks medical care at an urgent care clinic because of an incapacitating febrile illness of 4 days duration. On examination, the patient has a temperature of 104°F and complains of generalized body aches and pains. Laboratory blood work reveals pancytopenia and decreased hemoglobin. A blood smear is shown in the image. Chloroquine was prescribed and, within days, the patient made a dramatic recovery. What is the diagnosis?

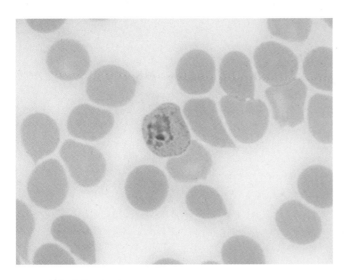

(A) Babesiosis
(B) Chagas' disease
(C) Ovale malaria
(D) Visceral leishmaniasis
(E) Vivax malaria

44 How was the infection in the above case acquired?
(A) Bite of an infected mosquito
(B) Drinking contaminated water
(C) Inhalation of agent shed in rodent urine
(D) Person-to-person via respiratory droplets
(E) Swimming in contaminated streams or lakes

45 Why would the infectious disease resident caring for the patient in the above case recommend a combination therapy that included primaquine?
(A) To treat the exoerythrocytic stages and reduce the chance of relapse
(B) To prevent the emergence of resistant strains of this organism
(C) To treat coinfection with a related organism
(D) To prevent central nervous system manifestations
(E) To prevent development of renal disease

46 An undocumented 18-year-old Guatemalan male, who currently lives in South Florida, is evaluated for a febrile illness. Specimens are taken for laboratory analysis; he is treated symptomatically and sent home for recuperation. Later that day, the physician is notified that the CBC blood smear reveals an irregularity (shown in the image). The patient is, therefore, advised to return promptly to the medical center for treatment. However, presumably for fear of deportation, he does not return and instead departs from the area. What is the most likely outcome of his illness in view of the fact that he did not receive treatment?

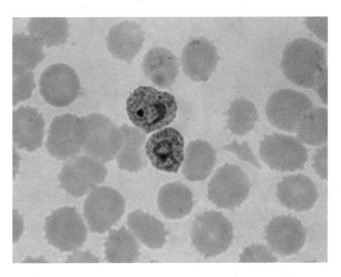

(A) Cerebral involvement with psychotic behavior and convulsions
(B) Death secondary to kidney failure
(C) Multiple organ dysfunction secondary to generalized capillary obstruction resulting in poor tissue perfusion
(D) Spontaneous resolution within several months to a few years
(E) Unremitting pernicious anemia

47 During the winter, an immigrant farm laborer in Missouri seeks medical care from a family practice clinic for a pruritic, vesicular rash on his abdomen (shown in the first image). The physician places a few drops of mineral oil on the skin and gently scraps the lesions with a scalpel blade. Microscopy reveals numerous objects (shown in the second image). What is the most likely diagnosis?

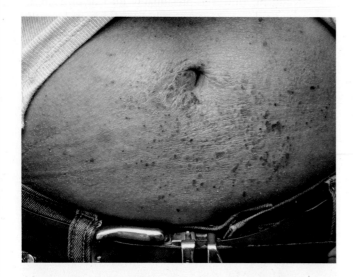

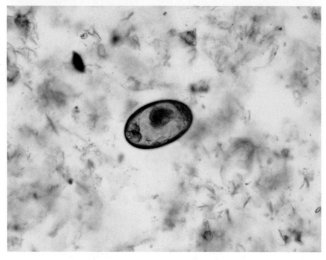

(A) Chigger dermatitis
(B) Demodicidosis
(C) Pediculosis corporis
(D) Pediculosis pubis
(E) Scabies

48 A young Haitian boy is brought to an aide station by his mother. She is seeking vitamins for her son. She indicates that her son "does not eat" and sometimes complains of nausea. He apparently has no diarrhea and no significant gastrointestinal pain. A fecal concentration is positive for parasite ova (shown in the image). How did this child become infected?

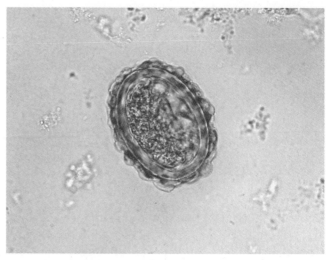

(A) Drinking water polluted with the cystic forms
(B) Eating insufficiently cooked meat infected with cysticerci
(C) Ingesting soil contaminated with embryonated eggs
(D) Wading in streams that harbor snails and cercariae
(E) Walking barefoot, thus allowing larvae to penetrate the skin

49 An immigrant from eastern Asia develops a cholangiocarcinoma. A fecal sample shows evidence of a parasitic infection which the physician believes to be linked to malignancy. What did the specimen reveal that led to this conclusion?
(A) Ameba cyst
(B) *Cryptosporidium* oocysts
(C) Flagellated protozoan trophs
(D) Fluke eggs
(E) Nematode larvae

50 Which of the following modes of transmission accounts for the development of neurocysticercosis in humans?
(A) Ascarid eggs from soil
(B) Bladderworms in raw beef
(C) Cyclosporan oocysts in water
(D) Fecal-oral taeniid eggs
(E) *Toxoplasma* zoitocysts in raw pork

51 Surgical removal of a liver cyst about the size of a tennis ball from a 45-year-old man reveals the presence of protoscolices, allowing for a definitive diagnosis. The patient likely acquired this infection by ingesting what?
(A) Cyst-contaminated raspberries grown in Guatemala
(B) Food or water contaminated with tapeworm eggs
(C) Undercooked calf liver containing hydatid sand
(D) Undercooked fish or shellfish containing larvae
(E) Viable cysticerci in pork or pork products

52 A child is taken to the doctor because of a 2-week bout of abdominal discomfort and diarrheic stools. A fecal concentration reveals scores of bipolar eggs like the one shown, indicating a heavy parasite burden. Which of the following complications might occur if the child is not treated for this parasite?

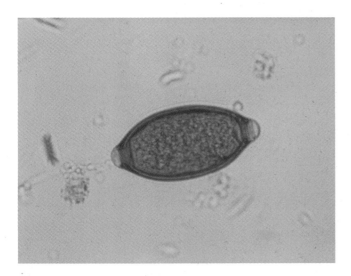

(A) Asthmalike manifestations
(B) Blockage of the duodenum
(C) Extraintestinal infection
(D) Prolapse of the rectum
(E) Severe pernicious anemia

The next two questions are linked.

53 A businessman who recently returned from a trip to Scandinavia goes to the clinic because of intestinal distress. Based on positive stools, a diagnosis of diphyllobothriasis is made. Which of the following diagnostic stages would support this conclusion?
(A) Armed scolex and segments
(B) Elongated eggs with a thin shell
(C) Operculated eggs with an anopercular knob
(D) Rhabditiform juveniles
(E) Thick, corrugated oval eggs

54 What is the most likely vehicle for infection in the above case?
(A) Drinking water
(B) Raw fish
(C) Raw hamburger
(D) Salad greens
(E) Soil or sewage

55 Several individuals present with explosive watery diarrhea, mild fever, and profound fatigue. Epidemiologically, the common link is the eating of imported salad greens. Acid-fast preparations of fresh stools reveal large oocysts. Furthermore, the illness responds to TMP–SMZ treatment. What is the most likely pathogen?
(A) *Blastocystis*
(B) *Cryptosporidium*
(C) *Cyclospora*
(D) *Entamoeba*
(E) *Giardia*

56 A child with a helminth parasite is found to be anemic. Which parasitic worm is linked to microcytic anemia in children?
(A) Broad fish tapeworm
(B) Hookworm
(C) Pinworm
(D) Pork tapeworm
(E) Schistosome blood fluke

57 Which of the following microbiologic properties distinguishes *Entamoeba. histolytica* from nonpathogenic ameba like *E. dispar*?
(A) Ability to produce cytotoxins
(B) Characteristic shape of the cyst
(C) Colonization of the colon
(D) Fecal-oral route of transmission
(E) Number of nuclei in the troph

58 A young child, who was adopted from an orphanage in Asia, routinely experiences loose stools. An abundance of microscopic worms (shown in the image) are noted in a fecal preparation smear. What is the correct diagnosis?

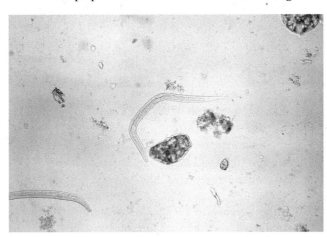

(A) Ascariasis
(B) Enterobiasis
(C) Hookworm disease
(D) Strongyloidiasis
(E) Trichuriasis

59 A resident performs a skin scraping on a child suspected of being infested with *Sarcoptes scabiei*. Which of the following microscopic findings would be most supportive of a scabies diagnosis?

(A) Mesocercariae

(B) Mite ova and scybala

(C) Nematode microfilariae

(D) Nits and louse fragments

(E) Nurse cells and larvae

The next two questions are linked.

60 An 8-year-old child, who recently emigrated with the family from Central America, is taken to the emergency department because of a stomach ache that has persisted for about 24 hours. In fact, the mother indicates that the pain did not lessen even after the child vomited up two worms (shown in the image) the night before. The mother further indicates that for the past several weeks the child has had little desire to eat and often complains of diarrhea. Physical examination reveals that the pain is more pronounced in the right upper quadrant region and directly radiates to the scapular area of the back. Based on these findings, what is the most likely diagnosis?

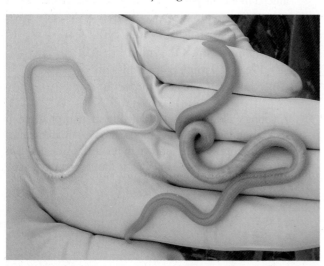

(A) Ascariasis with biliary involvement

(B) Disseminated strongyloidiasis

(C) Hemolytic uremic syndrome

(D) Intestinal and hepatic amebiasis

(E) Salmonella enterocolitis

61 With reference to the above question, how did the child most likely become infected?

(A) Direct fecal contamination from a sibling

(B) Eating raw or insufficiently cooked hamburger

(C) Ingestion of contaminated soil or water

(D) Swimming in cercariae-infested lake water

(E) Walking barefoot on moist soil or grass

62 A patient, who lives on Long Island, presents with fever and hemoglobinuria. The lab reports that the CBC is remarkable for a parasite (shown in the image). Of note, the patient has not traveled abroad for at least 10 years, except for an occasional trip to Canada. What is the most likely diagnosis?

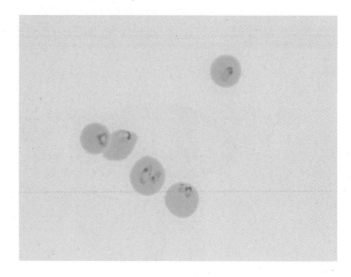

(A) Babesiosis

(B) Benign tertian malaria

(C) Falciparum malaria

(D) Ovale malaria

(E) Quartan malaria

63 While completing a public health rotation in an urban clinic in Peru, a US medical student is given an academic assignment to study a cluster of acute febrile cases in young children. Incident to each case is an acute regional lymphadenitis, myalgia, and a characteristic bloodborne parasite (shown in the image). Which of the following diseases is the most reasonable diagnosis?

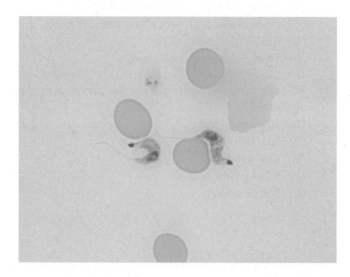

(A) Acute Chagas' disease
(B) Benign tertian malaria
(C) Blackwater fever
(D) Chronic sleeping sickness
(E) Disseminated leishmaniasis

64 A middle-aged man who emigrated from South America unexpectedly dies of cardiac failure. A histological section of myocardial tissue reveals numerous bodies as shown in the image. How did the man most likely become infected with this disease?

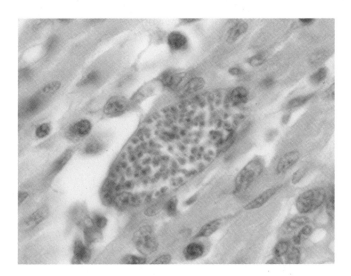

(A) A sand fly injected the parasite into the blood stream while feeding
(B) An infected anopheline mosquito introduced the parasite during a blood meal
(C) He inoculated himself by rubbing infected reduviid feces into the bite site
(D) The man inadvertently ingested infected feces from a house cat
(E) The parasite was transmitted to the man during a tick bite

65 A flight attendant, who works trips to Latin America, presents with fever, right upper abdominal pain, fever, and blood-streaked diarrhea. A stained sample under oil immersion reveals the diagnostic stage (shown in the image). If treatment were to be withheld, what would the flight attendant be in danger of developing?

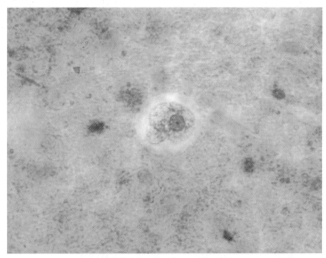

(A) A liver abscess
(B) Aplastic anemia
(C) Bladder cancer
(D) Malignancy of the bile duct
(E) Pancreatitis

66 A patient presents with a malodorous vaginal discharge, which according to the patient is significantly worse during menstruation. A motile microbe that is considerably smaller than an epithelial cell is detected in the saline wet microscopic preparation and also a stained preparation (shown in the image). What is the diagnosis?

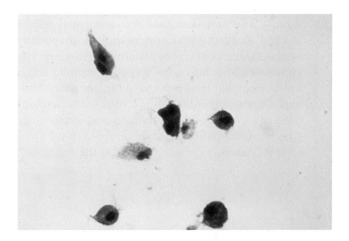

(A) Bacterial vaginosis
(B) Candidiasis
(C) Chlamydia
(D) Gonorrhea
(E) Trichomoniasis

67 The Red Cross sends a relief team to visit a refugee camp in central Africa. It is noted that most of the people have not been able to bathe for weeks, generally appear unkempt, and many complain of dermatitis and bug bites. In fact, the clothing seems to be infested or "crawling" with bugs (shown in the image). With respect to the conditions described above, which of the following diseases is of paramount concern for the inspecting physicians?

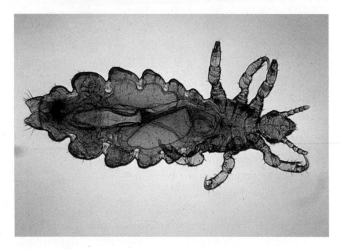

(A) Cholera
(B) Ebola
(C) Epidemic typhus
(D) Q fever
(E) Typhoid fever

68 A nurse who works part time in an elementary school in rural southern Mississippi notes loss of appetite, weakness, and poor school performance in a boy. The child's weight is below the second percentile, and a low hemoglobin level is noted in the laboratory find ings. Of note, the child lives in a rural setting without adequate toilet or latrine facilities and customarily goes barefoot. Parasite eggs are observed in the stool sample (shown in the image). What is the diagnosis?

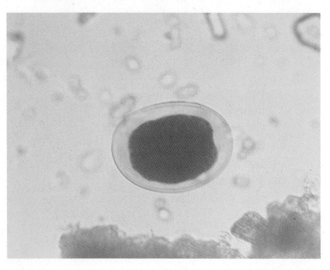

(A) Ascariasis
(B) Hookworm disease
(C) Intestinal amebiasis
(D) Strongyloidiasis
(E) Taeniasis

69 A wildlife photographer travels to a big game park in East Africa and returns home with intermittent fever and a painless chancrelike sore on his neck. A Giemsa-stained blood smear is positive for a flagellated microbe (shown in the image). Which of the following mechanisms gives the microbe the ability to evade humoral defense responses?

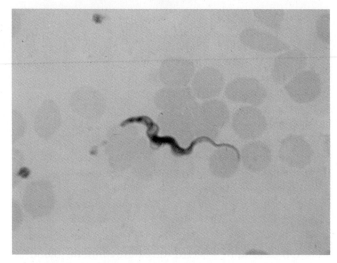

(A) Cysteine proteinase production
(B) Host antigenic mimicry
(C) Glycoprotein switching
(D) Lectin adhesion
(E) Phospholipase activity

70 A US Army Special Forces unit is considering establishing a training center in a tropical forested region of Central America. A reconnoiter team of army physicians and public health officers note that a substantial number of children and young adults are afflicted with chronic sores like the ones shown in the photographs. Which of the following measures is most relevant in preventing this disease from becoming a problem in the US soldiers?

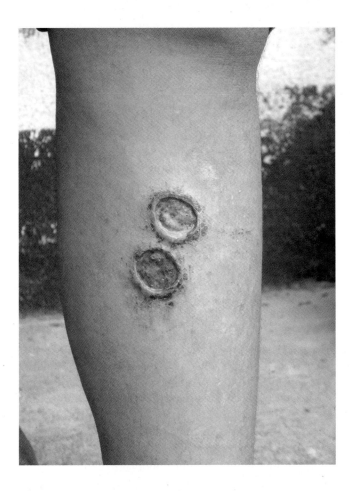

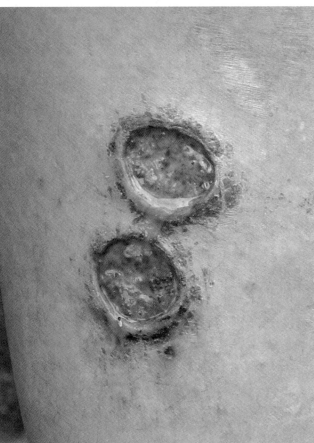

(A) Avoid swimming or wading in waters that contain snails

(B) Control the anopheline mosquito larval population with insecticides

(C) Frequent inspection of the body and prompt removal of tick

(D) Soldiers protecting themselves from the bites of sand flies

(E) Washing clothing in hot water to kill attached nits

71 A 24-year-old emigrant from Belize presents with an insidious but nontender skin condition that on casual inspection appears to be lepromatous leprosy (shown in the photographs); however, scraping from the skin lesions do not produce acid-fast bacilli when stained. Consequently, the attending physician believes that his patient is infected with a parasite common to tropical areas of Central America. Of the following diseases, which is the most reasonable diagnosis?

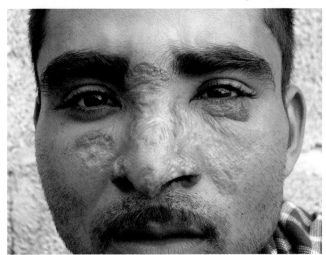

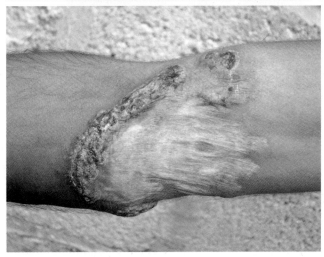

(A) Cercarial dermatitis

(B) Chronic Chagas' disease

(C) Disseminated cutaneous leishmaniasis

(D) Scabies

(E) Tungiasis

72 A young child who lives in a rural community in the Appalachia and who has been ill for 10 days presents with abdominal pain, anorexia, steatorrhea, and watery diarrhea. There is no indication of blood in the stool, but a fecal smear stained with trichrome reveals an abundance of cystlike structures like the one shown in the image. What is the agent responsible for the clinical manifestations?

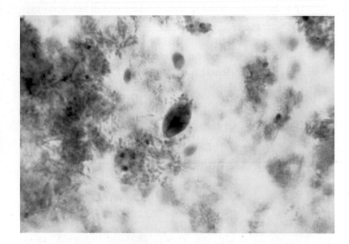

(A) *Cryptosporidium parvum*
(B) *Entamoeba histolytica*
(C) Enterotoxigenic *Escherichia coli*
(D) *Giardia lamblia*
(E) Rotavirus

73 In August, a previously healthy 12-year-old girl, who enjoys swimming in farm ponds in central Florida, is evaluated for meningitis. Gram stain of the CSF demonstrates no bacteria or yeast; however, there are indications of a PMN leukocytosis. A wet mount shows motile cells that resemble WBCs. Intravenous ceftriaxone therapy is initiated, but within 24 hours she slips into a coma. CT shows brain swelling or edema. Unfortunately, she is unresponsive to anticonvulsant drugs and dies the following day. Based on the available information, which diagnosis is the most plausible?

(A) Bacterial meningitis
(B) Cryptococcal meningitis
(C) Disseminated coccidioidomycosis
(D) Neurocysticercosis
(E) Primary amebic meningoencephalitis

74 In the summer, CDC investigates a series of outbreaks of cryptosporidiosis in upstate New York. The cluster of cases occurs in separate suburban communities, which are all upscale and feature a complete range of city services (e.g., sewage, water, and trash collection). Which of the following is the most plausible source of transmission for these outbreaks?

(A) Bird–mosquito–human route
(B) Drinking water contaminated with manure
(C) Fecal-oral person-to-person route
(D) Inhalation of dust seeding with bird droppings
(E) Parasite-infected meat (e.g., beef, mutton)

75 An HIV-positive student is considering part-time work to help with living expenses. Of the following jobs, which would be the most suitable, especially when considering the potential for contracting cryptosporidiosis?

(A) Assistant at an animal hospital
(B) Child day care worker
(C) Life guard at a public pool
(D) Pet store attendant
(E) Print shop worker

ANSWERS

1 **The answer is A: Creatine kinase serum level.** The most reliable diagnosis is trichinellosis (trichinosis), specifically *Trichina nativa*—a close relative of the pig species *Trichinella spiralis*. Infected patients are usually positive for creatine kinase, probably because *Trichina* larvae invade striated muscle cells inducing myositis. Creatinine clearance pertains to the renal function (i.e., filtering capacity), which is not relevant to this particular case. At this point in the disease process, seroconversion has not occurred, and, therefore, ELISA results would be inconclusive. Larvae are almost never recovered in a fecal preparation or visualized in a stained blood slide.

2 **The answer is B: Albendazole plus a corticosteroid.** Albendazole therapy is most effective in a patient who is experiencing the intestinal phase of the disease. Usually, this patient will have significant relief within a few weeks following completion of the anthelminthic drug. Patients with encapsulated disease could possibly experience residual myalgia, at least until the larvae are calcified. Corticosteroid will help the person cope with the adverse hypersensitivity reactions that invariably occur when the larvae are killed.

3 **The answer is C: Nurse cell.** Even though limited clinical information was given, the apparent diagnosis for these patients is trichinellosis (trichinosis) or a *Trichinella spiralis* infection. Certain groups of people who come to the United States are not always aware of the dangers of eating raw pork that has been raised in the family farm setting—especially one that allows the pigs to wander freely in the yard. Of course it is illegal to feed uncooked refuse to pigs, but on a small farm, these animals may acquire the infection by feeding on rat carcasses. Rats often harbor trichina larvae in this way. More to the question: When the larval stage of *T. spiralis* penetrates a striated muscle fiber, it promotes the development of a protective collagenous capsule often called the nurse cell. Referencing the correct name of a parasite stage will avoid frustrating moments with the pathologist in the hospital setting. The cysticercus is a tapeworm stage (e.g., *Taenia solium*); an onchocercoma is a fibrous growth common to an *Onchocerca volvulus* infection, and metacercaria is the infective stage for certain flukes.

4 **The answer is A: *Balantidium coli*.** This ciliated protozoan is associated with individuals who raise pigs or who work in slaughterhouses. Infections are often self-limiting, but if treatment is required, tetracycline is the preferred drug for adult patients. The protozoan is characterized with a macronucleus in both the trophozoite and cyst. In fact the macronucleus is the key factor with this question. *Cryptosporidium* produces an oocyst; *Entamoeba dispar* and *E. coli* are

nonpathogenic species and are merely indicators of fecal contamination; and, the nucleus of *Entamoeba histolytica* cannot be mistaken for a macronucleus.

5 **The answer is C: Enterobiasis.** Pinworms sometimes are seen in tissue sections from the appendix. Whether the parasite is able to induce appendicitis or is merely incidental to the medical condition is open to debate. What is real, however, is the fact that pinworm infections in children are often underappreciated. The parasite is capable of producing minute ulcerations in the intestinal mucosa, and heavy infections have been associated to perianal pain and pruritus. The worms usually amass in the ileocecal region but also have the potential to wander throughout the entire gastrointestinal tract. The female will eventually deposit thousands of eggs on the perianal folds. Infectivity of the eggs may be as rapid as 6 hours, and the newly hatched juveniles may then migrate into the reproductive canal of a young girl. Infections are treatable with pyrantel pamoate, albendazole, or mebendazole. Since the eggs are viable for about a week, treatment should definitely be repeated in order to prevent a recurrence of symptomatic disease. With regards to the incorrect answers, cross sections of helminths may be misidentified as protozoans (e.g., *Entamoeba histolytica*, *Giardia lamblia*) by the unprepared student. Note that there are no nuclei or other internal structures common to protozoans. Hookworms do not commonly involve the appendix, and *Ascaris lumbricoides* is a huge worm when compared to the human pinworm.

6 **The answer is D: *Taenia solium*.** This is a microscopic view of the scolex or holdfast organ of the ribbon stage of a taeniid tapeworm like *T. solium*. It routinely infects the small intestine. The suckers and crown of hooks are characteristic. *E. granulosis* (echinococcosis) is also a taeniid; however, it occurs as hydatid sand or protoscolices (shown in the image) within a liver or pulmonary cyst. *Ascaris* and *Toxacara* are roundworms, and *Fasciola* is a fluke. Roundworms and fluke do not possess scolices.

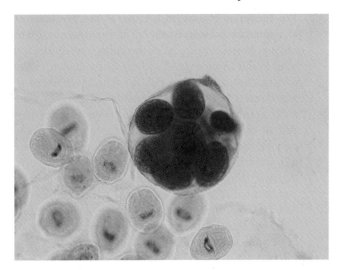

7 **The answer is C: *Hymenolepis nana*.** The presumed viral illness is more than likely responsible for the clinical manifestation. It is unlikely that *H. nana* is causing the problem in so many children in this situation. Even so, abdominal pain is sometimes a complaint in infected young children; however, symptoms may be negligible or absent altogether. Regardless, *H. nana* is the most commonly diagnosed intestinal tapeworm infection in the United States and likely the world. It is related in part to the direct life cycle (i.e., egg is the infective stage). This is especially true with younger patients who live in institutions. The parasite thrives in habitats where sanitation and personal cleanliness are wanting. The delicate membrane that surrounds the egg and the scolex armed with a crown of hooks are identifying features of this species of *Hymenolepis*. *T. saginata* is the beef tapeworm, which is much larger than *H. nana*. Transmission of this parasite occurs when the person eats insufficiently cooked beef. The hookworm *Ancylostoma* is a geohelminth and not likely transmitted in an institution such as a homeless shelter. *Enterobius* and *Strongyloides* are parasites which in theory could involve institutionalized children, but they are roundworms. Consequently, their eggs and morphology should not be confused with *Hymenolepis*.

8 **The answer is D: Praziquantel.** The anthelminthic praziquantel is effective for treating intestinal tapeworm infections. Niclosamide is also effective.

9 **The answer is D: Uphold good hygiene practices.** To a limited degree, all the answers are at least technically correct because feces could theoretically contaminate food and drink. Also, certain insects serve as intermediate hosts on occasion and inadvertently eating the insect would result in an infection. Considering issues of prevalence, however, it is far more likely for exposure to come about as a result of hand-to-mouth transmission (i.e., fecal-contaminated fingers) of the infective egg.

10 **The answer is C: Guarded because of the development of secondary echinococcosis.** The microscopic granule is a protoscolex, part of the collection of hydatid sand found in the cyst. If spillage of the hydatid fluid occurs, the patient is at risk for the development of additional cysts (i.e., dissemination of disease). The most appropriate intervention is extended albendazole or mebendazole therapy. Additional surgery may also be indicated. Amebic abscesses in the liver are not watery, and cryptosporidiosis does not involve the liver. Visceral larva migrans is a larval nematode condition that is more associated with granulomas. Anisakiasis occurs as a result of eating raw marine fish but cysts, if formed at all, would be tiny in comparison to echinococcosis and probably not fluid filled.

11 **The answer is D: Echinococcosis.** *Echinococcus granulosus* is a tiny tapeworm of dogs, especially sheepdogs that have been fed sheep viscera. The dog harbors the ribbon stage in the small intestine, tapeworm eggs are passed in the excrement and contaminate pasture, the sheep inadvertently eats the egg, and the juvenile or metacestode stage (hydatid cyst) develops in the liver or lungs of the sheep. Echinococcus or the development of the hydatid cyst also can occur in humans. Dipylidiasis is a dog flea tapeworm that has minor medical importance; diphyllobothriasis is transmitted to people via raw fish; cysticercosis occurs with the pork tapeworm; and, taeniasis refers to intestinal infections with the tapeworms *Taenia solium* and *T. saginatus*.

12 **The answer is D: Ingesting dog excrement.** Echinococcosis or hydatid disease is transmitted to people via oral exposure to the egg stage in excrement from dogs. Sheep droppings are not involved in the life cycle. Proper hand washing is imperative after working with dogs, especially before eating a meal. The person does not become infected by eating sheep livers or mutton or by handling sheep.

13 **The answer is B: Stop feeding raw sheep livers to dogs.** Simply stated, if the dog is denied access to the sheep offal, the life cycle is broken.

14 **The answer is B: Consumption of insufficiently cooked sirloin.** Based on the number of uterine branches stained by the India ink, the correct identification is *Taenia saginata* or commonly referred to as the beef tapeworm (i.e., a steer or cow serves as the intermediate host). The bladderworm or *Cysticercus*—a juvenile tapeworm of sorts—is the infective stage for people, and the vehicle for transmission is insufficiently cooked beef. The parasite may only produce vague abdominal discomfort, and the patient becomes aware of an infection when proglottids are noticed in the undergarments or after a bowel movement. *T. saginata* rarely is transmitted in the United States, but endemicity is high in Asia, Africa, and Latin America.

15 **The answer is D: Praziquantel.** Praziquantel therapy has a high degree of efficacy. Chloroquine is an antimalarial drug; ivermectin is used in filarial worm infections; metronidazole is used for anaerobic bacterial infections as well as in some protozoal infections, and piperazine is used for infections with the nematodes *Ascaris vermicularis* and *Enterobius vermicularis*. Niclosamide is also used for *Taenia* infections.

16 **The answer is A: *Diphyllobothrium latum*.** This cestode, sometimes called the broad fish tapeworm, has the tendency to absorb large quantities of vitamin B_{12}

from the intestinal tract of the human host—thus producing a tapeworm pernicious anemia. The species is common in parts of Finland, but similar species occur elsewhere in northern boreal regions and other areas of the world. Freshwater fish carry infective juvenile tapeworms, but cooking the fish will inactivate these encysted juveniles. The egg—noted in the stool concentration—features an anopercular knob, and the scolex is adorned with bothria (shown in the image) and not suckers or hooks. These are considered reliable markers in the identification of the species in the clinical laboratory.

17 **The answer is D: *Taenia solium*.** The diagnosis is cysticercosis. The condition is a result of cysticerci or bladderworms (sometimes referred to as juvenile tapeworms) infecting the tissue of the patient. Almost any tissue can be infected, but intraocular cysticercosis and neurocysticercosis pose grave challenges for the patient. Other serious infections involve cardiac and parenchymal brain tissue. Seizures are regularly reported in the CNS patient. Direct visualization of the juvenile parasites in biopsy or excised tissue can be done. The immunoblot assay is the test of choice to confirm the diagnosis of neurocysticercosis suggested by CT and MRI findings. Although the cystic form of the parasite is sensitive to the taeniacidal drugs like albendazole, the dead and dying worms may promote adverse inflammatory reactions. To minimize this situation, coadministration of an antiseizure medication and a corticosteroid is generally recommended.

18 **The answer is E: Ingestion of fecal-contaminated salad vegetables.** This is an imported case of cysticercosis. The daughter presumably acquired the infection from a household contact—her father being the likely candidate. *Taenia solium* eggs are infectious immediately when they are passed in feces. Further environmental development is unnecessary. Therefore, contaminated salad or possibly other uncooked vegetables is the most probable means of transmission. Since the child did not harbor the adult tapeworm, autoinfection will not occur. Although fairly common in Latin America, *T. solium* has a low-degree of endemicity in the United States. The disease is most prevalent in countries that are challenged with issues of poor hygiene and sanitation. Cysticercosis takes approximately 1 year to develop, which would discount the possibility of polluted drinking water and the recent eating of raw pork. Cysticercosis should not be viewed as merely a medical curiosity but an important and potentially life-threatening parasitic disease.

19 **The answer is C: Cutaneous larva migrans.** Sometimes referred to as creeping eruptions, this is solely a dermal disease in people. The person becomes infected when the filariform larva, which is found in moist soil or sand, penetrates bare skin. Individuals who go barefoot in a tropical setting are prime targets. The linear or serpiginous lesion is primarily an inflammatory response to the microscopic larval worm wandering through the skin. *Ancylostoma braziliense*, a hookworm that infects dogs and cats, is believed to be the most frequently encountered species, and the human is an unsuitable host for this particular hookworm species. Recommended therapy includes topical thiabendazole, albendazole, or ivermectin. Cercarial dermatitis or swimmer's itch is produced by an avian schistosome and the rash is widespread and produces pruritic papules. Chiggers and the *Demodex* mites both are capable of producing dermatitis, but the rash will usually not appear serpiginous. *Dracunculus medinensis*, a nematode that can cause skin lesions, is not found in the United States.

20 **The answer is E: Anisakiasis.** *Anisakis* and similar marine worms may be transmitted to humans in raw fish dishes like sushi. These are clearly nematodes in the photograph. *Diphyllobothrium* is a cestode. *Clonorchis*, *Paragonimus*, and *Schistosoma* are flukes.

21 **The answer is B: Submit to a thorough screening for common sexually transmitted infections.** *Phthirus pubis*, affectionately referred to as the crab louse (see photograph), is associated with sexual activity, and promiscuous behavior is a major risk factor. The possibility of being simultaneously infected with additional sexually transmitted organisms must be considered. The pubic region is the customary location for crabs, but other areas of the body may also be infested. As stated, the transmission of lice is through direct person-to-person contact, which would discount normal restroom and hot tub use. Antibacterial gels are not reliable when attempting to control ectoparasites. Clothing stored for extended periods poses no risk, since lice that might be attached to the fiber will die within a few days.

22 **The answer is E: Pediculosis capitis.** Lice infestations continue to be a major medical problem internationally and within the United States. In developing countries *Pediculus humanus capitis* (head louse) are of concern for people who live under crowded conditions. In the United States, families may also experience issues of social embarrassment and the frustration of dealing with a zero nit policy at the school level—a policy that is ruthlessly enforced by a school nurse who often has difficulty distinguishing between hair casts and viable nits. The photograph shows a clear-cut heavy infestation of nits and lice. This fact alone eliminates all other consideration with regard to the question. Itchy scalp is a usual complaint for pediculosis, but rashes are also possible. Definite diagnosis of pediculosis is even more straightforward when the nits or captured lice are observed under magnification.

23 **The answer is D: *Toxocara canis*.** Although several nematode species have been linked to ocular parasitic infections in humans, *T. canis* is the most common cause of ocular toxocariasis or ocular larva migrans—a variety of visceral larva migrans. Children who suffer from pica, especially geophagy, are the ones at most risk. Dogs and cats naturally harbor the parasitic worm. Embryonated eggs are infective to children, even though the human is an unsuitable host for parasite maturation. Retinal involvement is simply a matter of chance as the worm has the potential to migrate to any visceral organ. Unfortunately, due to the inflammatory response, visually distinguishing the condition *in situ* from a retinoblastoma is difficult. Enucleation and subsequent histopathogenic examination might be required for an accurate diagnosis. *Trichuris trichiura* matures in the intestinal tract; *A. caninum* is an agent of cutaneous larva migrans; and, *O. volvulus* and *L. loa* are tropical filarial worms that are transmitted by an arthropod vector.

24 **The answer is C: Paragonimiasis.** The causative agent is the Asian lung fluke, *Paragonimus westermani*, which is endemic to countries like Korea, Japan, and China. Although arguably minutia that is not required to answer the question, a distinctive diagnostic feature of the egg is its flattened operculum (see micrograph). More importantly, the matter of sputum-associated eggs is really the key to making the correct diagnosis. With the help of ciliated epithelium, fluke eggs work their way up to the pharynx. Swallowing these eggs is the means by which the eggs reach the intestinal track and are then excreted during a bowel movement. The bronchopneumonialike manifestations often persist for years, long after the person has left eastern Asia. People who have the tendency to consume raw crabs are most at risk for acquiring paragonimiasis. A similar lung fluke is found in certain areas of the United States.

25 **The answer is B: *Clonorchis sinensis*.** Clonorchiasis, a liver–bile duct parasitic disease, is endemic to Taiwan and many other regions of Southeast Asia. Millions of people harbor this parasite. Although not the intent of this question, there may be a more-than-causal connection between cholangiocarcinoma and *Clonorchis*. The important point here is the fact that this is a liver fluke. The cross section of the parasite in the histological section clearly demonstrates the presence of twin intestinal caeca, a reliable morphological marker for flukes. *Ascaris* is a huge worm in comparison and appears round in cross section; *Fasciola* is also large

and the fluke is more endemic to North America; both the adult and juvenile stages of *T. solium* do not customarily involve the bile ducts; and, *E. histolytica* would present as a liver abscess.

26 **The answer is C: Eating metacercariae in raw or partially cooked fish.** The image is of *Metagonimus yokogawai*, an intestinal fluke that infects millions in eastern Asia. What is important here, however, is the type of parasite—not the specific identification—and then obviously the mode of transmission. The metacercaria is the infective stage, and insufficiently cooked freshwater fish is the vehicle for transmission to people. The liver fluke, *Clonorchis sinensis*, also is transmitted via freshwater fish. Regarding flukes, a person cannot become infected by ingesting eggs, cercariae, or miracidia. The cysticercus is a tapeworm stage.

27 **The answer is A: Africa.** The endemicity of schistosomiasis haematobia (a blood fluke disease) is mostly confined to the African continent and some countries in the Middle East. It has not been successfully exported to the point that it is able to establish in other regions of the world. The terminal spine on the eggs is diagnostic for this fluke disease. The principle risk factor for contracting schistosomiasis is to come in contact with a cercariae-infested freshwater source like a canal, stream, or lake.

28 **The answer is E: *Schistosoma mansoni*.** Of the five schistosomes that are evolutionarily capable of infecting humans, *S. mansoni* is the species that routinely involves the liver as egg granulomas. Hepatomegaly and splenomegaly are a direct result of the encapsulated eggs. Hematochezia oftentimes occurs in chronically infected individuals, and the ova are shed in the feces. The adult fluke of *S. mansoni* normally resides in the inferior mesenteric vein of the intestines. The prominent lateral spine (most obvious in the single egg photograph in this case) is diagnostic of *S. mansoni*. *S. haematobium* and *S. intercalatum* feature prominent terminal spines, whereas *S. japonicum* and *S. mekongi* are characterized with tiny lateral spines.

29 **The answer is C: Praziquantel.** *Schistosoma mansoni* is endemic to tropical areas of South America. The characteristic egg allows for an easy identification. Furthermore, an ELISA offered by CDC has a high degree of sensitivity and specificity for *S. mansoni* infections. Even though his symptoms are mild—as they often are—a no-nonsense approach with regard to therapy is indicated. Praziquantel is an effective drug for all schistosome species.

30 **The answer is E: Schistosomiasis.** The micrograph is of the cercarial stage or the infective stage of schistosomiasis, a fluke disease that involves veins near the intestinal tracks or bladder. Chlorine treatment and heating the water will kill this stage—highly unlikely with this scenario. Cercariae emerge from snails and remain viable in the water for more than 24 h. Even a brief exposure like wading in the water is ample time for the cercaria to penetrate intact skin. This water source appears to be regularly contaminated with human waste, and drinking from it would also pose a risk for acquiring other microbial diseases.

31 **The answer is E: *Wuchereria bancrofti.*** Hydroceles are perhaps the most common presentation of *W. bancrofti*, a filarial worm that is endemic to Brazil. The diagnostic microfilaria is described as being sheathed but is often not visible in Giemsa-stained material. Chyluria is an associated sign. Scrotal elephantiasis is successfully managed through surgery. The other nematodes listed are not associated with this presentation.

32 **The answer is C: *Onchocerca volvulus.*** In many regions of Africa, *O. volvulus* is a leading cause of blindness; however, the helminth has migrated into areas of Central America and Ecuador. *L. loa* affects people of West Africa and parts of the Sudan; *W. bancrofti* is more commonly associated with elephantoid manifestations; *D. medinensis* has a completely different presentation and is currently confined to specific regions of Africa. Occasionally, cases are diagnosed in people immigrating into the United States. Juveniles of *T. canis*, an important agent of visceral larva migrans, provokes retinal granulomatous reactions.

33 **The answer is B: Drinking contaminated lake or stream water.** The children are infected with the Protozoan *Giardia lamblia*. Airborne transmission of dust most closely fits the clinical picture of certain fungal diseases (e.g., cryptosporidiosis, histoplasmosis). Urinating while wading in a stream is somewhat nonsensical since this is clearly an intestinal infection. Although it is theoretically possible for a patient to be introduced to *Giardia* through poor hygiene habits or via contaminated food, a preponderance of the cases occurs by ingesting the cystic stage in water. The micrograph is of the trophozoite (indicating that at least this sample was taken from a patient with significant diarrhea) and the cystic form of *Giardia lamblia*.

34 **The answer is E: *Trichuris trichiura.*** In all probability, this is a case of pseudoappendicitis. Along with several types of bacteria (e.g., *Yersinia*, *Campylobacter*, and *Salmonella*), many parasitic roundworms (e.g., agents of anisakiasis, *Enterobius*, and *Trichuris*) have been implicated in pseudoappendicitis. The bacillary band, short muscle fibers, and the stichosome esophagus are reliable morphological attributes consistent

with *T. trichiura*. However, from the medical student's perspective, the point of the question is not so much worm morphology but rather if the appendix is able to sustain the growth of a parasite. Whipworms normally reside in the large intestine, hookworms (*Necator* and *Ancylostoma*) in the small intestine, *B. malayi* in the lymphatics, and *D. medinensis* in the skin. The vermiform appendix is considered large intestine by histologists and theoretically would support the physiological needs of a whipworm but not the other choices. In view of the clinical presentation, an appendectomy seems reasonable; however, healthcare professionals should recognize the possibility of parasites mimicking appendicitis, especially when dealing with patients who have recently lived in the tropical areas of the world. The clinical importance of *T. trichiura* should not be underestimated.

35 **The answer is B: Heavy parasite burden covering the epithelial surface of the duodenum.** *Giardia* is not a tissue invader. It does not lyse epithelial cells, and therefore, blood in a stool sample cannot be attributed to giardiasis. Iron-deficiency anemias are signs of hookworm disease or diphyllobothriasis. Intestinal blockage is most often a result of ascariasis. The ventral adhesive disc of *Giardia* allows the parasite to firmly attach to the epithelial lining of the small intestine. Oftentimes, the parasitic burden is so great that this surface is nearly completely covered with protozoans, thus mechanically interfering with the digestive process. Steatorrhea and stools with mucus are reliable signs of a heavy infection.

36 **The answer is A: Amebiasis.** Trophozoites that have engulfed red blood cells and quadrinucleate cysts are strongly suggestive of amebic dysentery or a case of *Entamoeba histolytica*. Untreated infections may lead to intestinal perforation (due to cysteine proteinases and other tissue-damaging enzymes), peritonitis, or a liver abscess. To complicate matters, nonpathogenic amebae, like *E. dyspar*, are difficult to distinguish from *E. histolytica*—except that that nonpathogenic species do not ingest erythrocytes. Parasite antigen detection by ELISA is more sensitive and specific than examination of stool smears.

37 **The answer is C: Prescribe albendazole for trichuriasis.** In this case, the detection of bipolar eggs in the stool and abdominal symptoms are highly suggestive of a *Trichuris trichiura* or a human whipworm infection. Even though the worm embeds in the mucosa of the large intestine, only patients with heavy worm burdens are treated. Such is apparently the case here.

38 **The answer is B: Enterobiasis.** *Enterobius vermicularis*, the causative agent of enterobiasis or human pinworm disease, is a common childhood parasitic infection in the United States, especially in middle-class families. The child becomes infected by ingesting embryonated eggs indoors, usually in a home or school setting. The human pinworm does not infect household pets; therefore, dogs and cats are not involved in the life cycle. Controversy still exists; however, as to the parasite's medical importance, but most microbiologists consider infections to be underrated. Treatment is almost always recommended.

39 **The answer is E: *Plasmodium falciparum.*** The double ring trophozoites seen in the red blood cells, and the lack of erythrocytic Schüffner's dots are consistent with *P. falciparum.* This is the most severe form of malaria and rapid diagnosis is critical. This type of malaria is wide spread in Africa and young children are extremely vulnerable to the disease largely because they are immunologically naive. Frequently, the manifestations of fever are experienced by children with a falciparum infection. Complications of this infection include renal failure and cerebral malaria. *Babesia* is a related organism that typically causes mild disease, and is transmitted by ticks in the northeastern United States. *Brugia* is a helminth parasite associated with elephantiasis. *Cryptosporidium* is an intestinal protozoan associated with severe diarrhea in the immune compromised and *L. tropica* is an intracellular protozoan causing skin ulcers.

40 **The answer is C: Atovaquone plus proguanil (Malarone).** Chloroquine is not recommended for falciparum malaria treatment in many areas of the world due to resistance of this organism to the drug. Resistant strains of *Plasmodium falciparum* express an energy-dependent efflux pump which prevents accumulation of chloroquine in the parasite cell body. Malarone is one of the several agents that can be used for the treatment of chloroquine-resistant *P. falciparum.* Other treatment regimens include quinine sulfate plus either doxycycline, tetracycline, or clindamycin, or mefloquine. Carbapenems are β-lactam antibiotics; amphotericin is an antifungal drug and foscarnet is an antiviral drug used for the treatment of infections with cytomegalovirus.

41 **The answer is A: The child was infected with a different strain of the same organism.** A person may be infected with a different strain of malaria if they move to another geographic area. This accounts for why the child was reinfected a year later. Falciparum malaria is nonrelapsing. Vivax malaria, because of the hypnozoite stage latent in the liver, may relapse for up to 5 years. Recrudescence, due to a subclinical infection, has been reported for *P. malariae.* Complement deficiencies are linked to recurring meningococcal infections.

42 **The answer is A: West African man.** Most people who are indigenous to West Africa are resistant to *P. vivax* infections because they lack the Duffy glycoprotein receptor for the merozoite stage on the erythrocyte. This receptor ordinarily serves as the receptor for interleukin-8. Lacking the receptor gives the person protection against vivax malaria. Other forms of genetically determined resistance to malaria—specifically, *P. falciparum*—include sickle cell trait, thalassemia, and deficiency of glucose-6-phosphate dehydrogenase.

43 **The answer is E: Vivax malaria.** Based on the clinical picture, the most reasonable diagnosis is a *Plasmodium vivax* infection. The intraerythrocytic trophozoite and Schüffner's dots are irrefutable evidence. Geographically, *P. vivax* is the most prevalent form of malaria in Latin America and possibly the world. *P. ovale* is an African parasite. Due to its small size, *Babesia* might be mistaken for *P. falciparum* but never *P. vivax.* Leishmaniasis and Chagas' disease are not characteristically intraerythrocytic.

44 **The answer is A: Bite of an infected mosquito.** In general, all species of malaria are transmitted via the bite of an anopheline mosquito.

45 **The answer is A: To treat the exoerythrocytic stages and reduce the chance of relapse.** Chloroquine by itself is considered incomplete therapy. *Plasmodium vivax,* due to the hypnozoite stage in the liver, will relapse every few months for 3 to 5 years. Primaquine targets this stage of the parasite. Although *P. vivax,* if left untreated, can lead to organ damage, cerebral malaria, and renal manifestations (blackwater fever) are typically associated with *P. falciparum.*

46 **The answer is D: Spontaneous resolution within several months to a few years.** The two infected erythrocytes are much enlarged and densely stippled (i.e., Schüffner's dots), characteristics consistent with *Plasmodium vivax.* This form of malaria does not usually result in mortality. Although vivax malaria commonly relapses—usually for up to 3 years—it eventually totally resolves, even without therapy. Kidney failure, severe anemia, cerebral manifestation, and capillary obstruction are traits more common with falciparum malaria.

47 **The answer is E: Scabies.** Eggs of *Sarcoptes scabiei* var. *hominis* are commonly recovered from skin scrapings and are diagnostic for the condition. The presence of eggs indicates that the infestation is of human origin and not zoonotic. The variety that is associated with dogs produces only transitory infestation in people. The location of the lesions and the shape of the egg are reliable attributes of scabies. Body and pubic lice do burrow and the *Demodex* mite most commonly involves the pore around the nares of the face. Chiggers are not active during the winter months.

48 **The answer is C: Ingesting soil contaminated with embryonated eggs.** The thick shell of the egg stage identifies the disease as ascariasis or an infection of *Ascaris lumbricoides*. The parasitic helminth is often described as a geohelminth (i.e., to be infective to people, the egg must first develop or embryonate in soil). Ingestion of the contaminated soil results in an infection. The egg stage is remarkably resistant to the environmental pressures and remains viable for years in the soil. Drinking polluted water is the vehicle of transmission for protozoans like the diarrheogenic organisms of *Giardia* and *Entamoeba*. Meat is the vehicle for a taeniid tapeworm infection, wading in water best describes the means of acquiring schistosomiasis, and barefoot exposure pertains to the transmission of hookworms.

49 **The answer is D: Fluke eggs.** Certain parasites like the Asian liver fluke (e.g., *Clonorchis sinensis*) are associated with neoplastic disease. The patient emigrated from an endemic region of the world, which further supports the physician's supposition. *Schistosoma haematobium*, although not a response to this question, is a blood fluke that inhabits the veins around the bladder and is also believed to promote neoplastic disease, squamous cell carcinoma of the bladder in this case.

50 **The answer is D: Fecal-oral taeniid eggs.** Ingesting the eggs of the pork tapeworm (*Taenia solium*) in fecal-contaminated food items is the likely means for transmission of cysticercosis. Because of the shape, the cysticercus is sometimes referred to as bladderworm (a type of metacestode) and is the stage responsible for the pathogenesis of neurocysticercosis. To minimize the possibility of an autoinfection, it is critical that the infection be aggressively managed. *Ascaris* is a geohelminth and must first embryonate in soil to be infective, *Cyclospora* and *Toxoplasma* produce protozoan infections, and raw beef is the vehicle for transmission of another tapeworm that is not believed to be associated with neurocysticercosis.

51 **The answer is B: Food or water contaminated with tapeworm eggs.** The tapeworm egg is the infective stage for echinococcosis or hydatid disease and sheepdogs are the usual source of the infection in people. The finding of protoscolices within the liver is proof of hydatid disease. Cysticerci in raw pork has reference to the intestinal form of the pork tapeworm, anisakiasis and diphyllobothriasis are associated with raw fish, and contaminated fruit like raspberries is a vehicle for transmission for *Cyclospora*.

52 **The answer is D: Prolapse of the rectum.** Oftentimes light infections of the human whipworm (*Trichuris trichiura*) are only treated palliatively; however, a child who is symptomatic and who harbors heavy parasite burdens should be aggressively managed. Failure to treat with an anthelminthic could theoretically result in rectal prolapse. Hypochromic anemia is a possibility, but pernicious anemia (the choice here) refers to the broadfish tapeworm, *Diphyllobothrium latum*. The human whipworm is small and resides in the large intestine, which would eliminate choice C. Intestinal obstruction anywhere in the intestinal tract would be highly unlikely. The juvenile worms have no pulmonary phase like *Ascaris* and hookworms. Again, the adult worm resides in the large intestine and occasionally the appendix.

53 **The answer is C: Operculated eggs with an anopercular knob.** Scandinavian countries are endemic for this species of tapeworm. Characteristically, the eggs are operculated and adorned with a prominent anopercular boss. Responses B, D, and E are descriptive of nematode infections (*Ascaris*, *Enterobius*, and *Strongyloides*, respectively). With regard to response C, although segments of *Diphyllobothrium latum* may be seen in a stool sample, it is unlikely that the medical technologist in the laboratory would find a scolex. Regardless, the scolex of *D. latum* is unarmed (lacks hooks).

54 **The answer is B: Raw fish.** *Diphyllobothrium latum* and similar species are transmitted to people when raw or insufficiently cooked fish is consumed. The plerocercoid or the infective stage resides in the flesh of freshwater fish like trout and salmon. Although human sewage may play a role in the perpetuation of the life cycle, a person cannot become infected by ingesting the tapeworm eggs in drinking water.

55 **The answer is C: *Cyclospora*.** Imported raspberries from Central America have also been linked to cluster cases of cyclosporiasis in the United States. More than likely the use of contaminated river water to wash the berries or to apply fungicide and insecticide prior to shipping is a contributing factor. Cyclosporan oocysts are noticeably larger than those of *Cryptosporidium*. Although both *Cyclospora* and *Cryptosporidium* have oocysts that are acid-fast, the sensitivity to the antimicrobial TMP–SMZ is the distinguishing attribute.

56 **The answer is B: Hookworm.** The consumption and the oozing of blood from the intestinal site where the worm attaches explains the iron-deficiency anemia. Heavy infections of *Trichuris trichiura* or the human whipworm (not a choice in this question) has also been linked to anemia. *Diphyllobothrium latum* or the broad fish tapeworm has been noted to produce a type of pernicious or megaloblastic anemia.

57   The answer is A: Ability to produce cytotoxins. *E. histolytica* is a tissue-invading parasite as evidenced by extraintestinal abscesses. Cytotoxins, cysteine proteases, phospholipases, and other virulence factors that relate to tissue invasion separate this protozoan from look-alike nonpathogenic amebae.

58   The answer is D: Strongyloidiasis. The identification of a *Strongyloides stercoralis* infection is determined in part because of the presence of rhabditiform larvae in a fecal sample. On the other hand, the laboratory diagnosis of hookworms, *Ascaris*, *Enterobius*, and *Trichuria* are based on the recovery of parasite eggs in the feces. Once in a while, however, a pinworm egg will hatch on the perianeum and a larva may be seen in a stool sample. The presence of pinworm larvae in a stool sample, which has been properly stored and processed, is a very rare occurrence. A key word in the stem, therefore, is "abundance" and indicates the presence of numerous larvae in the stool. *Strongyloides* is a common parasite in children who reside in developing nations, especially children who are confined to an orphanage. A pulmonary phase of the *Strongyloides* life cycle has been linked with pneumonitis and also asthmalike manifestations. Enteritis is also a possibility. More than not, intestinal involvement will produce a benign infection. From time to time, this nematode is identified from patients in the United States.

59   The answer is B: Mite ova and scybala. A simple skin scraping in mineral oil from patients who have signs of scabies will demonstrate whole or fragmented parts of the female mite, mite eggs, and mite fecal debris (i.e., scybala). The microfilariae are diagnostic for filariasis (i.e., elephantiasis), nurse cells are found in the skeletal muscle of a patient with trichinosis, nits are louse eggs cemented to hair shafts, and mesocercariae refers to a tissue-migrating fluke.

60   The answer is A: Ascariasis with biliary involvement. More than 1 billion people worldwide are infected with *Ascaris lumbricoides*. Children are more likely candidates than adults to be infected. The worms commonly reside in the small intestine, but migration into the biliary tract is fairly common. Based on the exquisite radiating pain in this case, biliary involvement should be ruled out, probably though radiographic findings. It is not unusual for a child to spit up a worm upon being treated. Children in Latin America will harbor multiple worms—sometimes hundreds—and intestinal obstruction is a potential complicating factor. Usually, however, abdominal symptoms are vague with nothing more than a loss of appetite and occasional episodes of diarrhea.

61   The answer is C: Ingestion of contaminated soil or water. *Ascaris lumbricoides* is a geohelminth, meaning that the eggs that are passed in the stool must first embryonate in the soil or the environment. The parasite is not commonly transmitted person-to-person via feces. Consequently, the embryonated egg—not the unembryonated egg in fresh feces (choice A)—is the infective stage. Ingesting food and drink contaminated with these embryonated eggs would be the most likely way for humans to become infected. Lack of proper hand washing before eating only compounds the problem. Choice C has reference to hookworm disease, D refers to schistosomiasis, and E hemorrhagic *Escherichia coli*.

62   The answer is A: Babesiosis. The intraerythrocytic parasites are similar to falciparum on casual glance; however, clinical presentation and the fact that the patient has not traveled to areas which are known to be endemic to malaria strongly point to babesiosis as the correct diagnosis. *Babesia microti*, the causative agent, is fairly common in this area of New York (also Massachusetts). It is transmitted to people via a deer tick. At this point in time, clindamycin plus quinine is considered the best possible treatment.

63   The answer is A: Acute Chagas' disease. Chagas' disease is endemic to many countries in Central and South America. The acute phase is defined when motile trypanosomes are detected in the anticoagulated blood or the buffy coat (layer of white blood cells and platelets just above the erythrocyte zone). The trypomastigote stage, often C-shaped (see micrograph), is readily visualized in a fixed Giemsa-stained blood smear. The clinical manifestations in this case clearly pertain to the acute phase of the disease. Sleeping sickness is endemic to Africa and not South America, blackwater fever is linked to falciparum malaria. Malaria is an intraerythrocytic life cycle, and leishmaniasis is characterized with amastigotes and not tryptomastigotes.

64   The answer is C: He inoculated himself by rubbing infected reduviid feces into the bite site. The reduviid bug, *Triatoma infestans*, is responsible for transmitting most of the infections of Chagas' disease. The parasite (*Trypanosoma cruzi*) is passed in the feces of the bug, a process described as posterior station. A pseudocyst or a pocket of amastigotes, is clearly depicted in the micrograph and is characteristic of *T. cruzi* infection. Cardiac disease, including sudden death, is connected with chronic Chagas' disease. *Toxoplasma* is associated with litter boxes of cats. Tickborne diseases include Rocky Mountain spotted fever, Lyme disease, and babesiosis. Malaria is transmitted by anopheline mosquitoes, and sand fly species are vectors for leishmaniasis.

65 **The answer is A: A liver abscess.** The causative agent is *Entamoeba histolytica*. This is the most common extraintestinal manifestation. Amebic liver abscess develops as a result of a hematogenous spread (i.e., hepatoportal to the liver) and may grow to the size of a grapefruit. In the majority of the patients, leukocytosis occurs. The micrograph depicts a trophozoite.

66 **The answer is E: Trichomoniasis.** Motility is a key factor in identifying trophozoites of *Trichomonas vaginalis* in a wet mount. The preparation should be fresh, however. No clue cells in the micrograph would eliminate the possibility of bacterial vaginosis. Also, the lack of specificity of a stain to distinguish *Neisseria gonorrhoeae* from normal reproductive tract flora, no budding yeast cells eliminating a vaginal candidiasis, and identifying *Chlamydia trachomatis* from a saline prep or Gram stain is open to question.

67 **The answer is C: Epidemic typhus.** Of the choices, epidemic typhus is the only louseborne disease. The rickettsial organism is transmitted to people via louse defecations and then infects the endothelial cells of the capillaries, producing fever, vasculitis, and rash. It is a potentially fatal disease that is most likely to occur as a result of marked decline in personal hygiene (i.e., inability to bathe during poverty or wartime conditions).

68 **The answer is B: Hookworm disease.** Distinctive clues with this case include the geographic location, socioeconomic conditions, the anemia, and most importantly the fragile nature of the egg. *Ancylostoma* and *Necator* hookworms are transmitted when the filariform larvae penetrate bare skin. Parasite eggs are passed in the stool and, under austere sanitary conditions, will contaminate soil. The warm moist soil of the South favors development of the infective stage or the filariform larva. Protein deficiency and mental dullness are clinical manifestations of severe disease.

69 **The answer is C: Glycoprotein switching.** The diagnosis is African sleeping sickness—caused by the acute form of *Trypanosoma brucei rhodesiense*. The trypomastigote stage, seen in the micrograph, is able to hide from host defenses by regularly changing or switching its glycoprotein surface molecules. Cysteine proteinases, phospholipases, and lectin are virulence factors of the diarrheogenic ameba, *Entamoeba histolytica*. Schistosome blood flukes disguise themselves with a coating of host blood product (i.e., host antigenic mimicry). The occurrence of African sleeping sickness in the United States is extremely rare, but arguably, the real significance of this disease gives insight into a critical microbial mechanism that leads to successful invasion of the human host.

70 **The answer is D: Soldiers protecting themselves from the bites of sand flies.** Cutaneous leishmaniasis is the obvious diagnosis—based on the clinical presentation and the fact that New World leishmaniasis is endemic to tropical environments in Latin America. Direct microscopic or visualization of the amastigote diagnostic stage or the immunochromatographic procedure, which detects antibodies to *Leishmania* antigen K39, would be more conclusive, however. Both dermotropic and viscerotropic leishmaniasis are endemic to the Middle East. As a result of the Iraq and Afghanistan wars, hundreds of laboratory-confirmed cases have been reported in GIs. Without question, this parasitic disease has military importance. Avoiding contact with water alludes to schistosomiasis, a disease that is not that common in Central America. There is no evidence of a louse (i.e., nits cemented to clothing fibers) or tick infestation. Targeting anopheline mosquito larva in water would have no relevance since the sandfly is the only reported vector and does not breed in water.

71 **The answer is C: Disseminated cutaneous leishmaniasis.** The patient appears to be infected with one of the New World *Leishmania* organisms, probably *L. braziliensis* or *L. mexicana*. The sand fly is the vector. The insect bite will progressively evolve into a cutaneous ulcer. If untreated, the ulcer will spontaneously heal—after several weeks. Because the parasite attacks the reticuloendothelial system, it has the potential to reappear with a vengeance (i.e., as disseminated disease). Such is the case with this patient. T cell cytotoxicity is a major virulence component of all forms of leishmaniasis. Cercarial dermatitis is a schistosome disease, an accidental parasite of no real consequence. Tungiasis, although caused by a tropical parasite (specifically a flea that embeds in tissue), usually involves only the ankle or foot. The scabies mite will most often manifest as small, circumscribed, pruritic eruptions.

72 **The answer is D: *Giardia lamblia*.** Mature cysts of *G. lamblia* feature four nuclei; however, two of the nuclei are often not visible because of the limited depth of field of the micrograph (shown in the image). The axonemes and the hyaline cyst wall make the diagnosis irrefutable. The clinical presentation, especially the watery diarrhea without blood, is consistent with a giardiasis diagnosis. More than likely the child consumed water that was contaminated with *Giardia* cysts, a definite possibility in a rural setting.

73 **The answer is E: Primary amebic meningoencephalitis.** The fumigant course of the disease and the lack of bacterial and fungal elements in the Gram stain are most consistent with amebic meningoencephalitis. Neurocysticercosis (*Taenia solium*) is a tapeworm disease and is statistically more likely to occur in a patient who emigrated from developing countries in Latin America, Asia, and Africa. *Naegleria fowleri*, the etiologic agent in this particular case, is transmitted during the summer months in warm ponds or streams. The ameba in reality is a free-living freshwater species that inadvertently invades the nasal passageways of swimmers. It craws up the olfactory nerve, a pathway of sorts that leads to the central nervous system. A number of tissue-damaging virulence determinants (e.g., cysteine protease, phospholipase A) have been identified, which account for the severe hemorrhagic meningoencephalitis seen in fatal infections. Mortality rates are especially high, largely because the disease is rare and progresses rapidly. A correct diagnosis may easily be unrecognized and made at autopsy. Motile trophozoites (directional movement) can be observed in a wet mount preparation of centrifuged CSF. Effective therapy includes amphotericin B.

74 **The answer is B: Drinking water contaminated with manure.** Due of the circumstances of this outbreak, *Cryptosporidium parvum* is the likely culprit. The parasite normally involves livestock, and flooded stockyards contaminating drinking water supplies probably account for the large-scale epidemics. Cryptosporidiosis, because it is refractory to treatment, is especially serious in AIDS patients.

75 **The answer is E: Print shop worker.** The infective stage of cryptosporidiosis is the oocyst, and it could be transmitted to the patient via human or animal feces. Changing diapers and working with excrement from animals are risk factors. It is not uncommon for a child to have an accident in a public pool, and, unfortunately, the oocysts are resistant to normal levels of chlorine. The only job listed that would pose no risk for ingesting oocysts would be to work in a print shop.

Chapter 5

Infectious Diseases

QUESTIONS

1 An 18-year-old woman preparing to enter college is required to be up-to-date on vaccinations. In addition to required childhood vaccinations, students entering college are often required to be vaccinated against which organism?
(A) *Chlamydia trachomatis*
(B) Hepatitis C virus
(C) Human papillomavirus
(D) *Neisseria meningitidis*
(E) *Treponema pallidum*

2 A 24-year-old previously healthy man presents with cough and dyspnea of 5 days duration. A chest radiograph reveals bilateral infiltrates and the man is treated empirically for walking pneumonia as an out patient. Which antibiotic is he most likely given?
(A) Azithromycin
(B) Clindamycin
(C) Fluconazole
(D) Imipenem
(E) Linezolid

3 A 54-year-old man is being treated with anticancer drugs, which have reduced the production of white blood cells from his bone marrow. He develops an infection with an organism that does not cause disease in immunologically healthy individuals. What description best fits this infection?
(A) Asymptomatic
(B) Chronic
(C) Latent
(D) Opportunistic
(E) Persistent

4 A resident in his first week of outpatient clinic work prescribes erythromycin for the treatment of a UTI, presumably a simple case *Escherichia coli*. The attending countermands his order and suggests the resident consider TMP–SMZ. Why are the antimicrobial choices proposed by the attending more appropriate?

(A) Bacterial glycocalyx impedes the absorption of erythromycin
(B) Erythromycin is likely to be inactivated by transpeptidases
(C) Macrolides are principally secreted in the feces
(D) Macrolides promote *Candida* overgrowth in women
(E) Oral macrolides are linked to Stevens–Johnson syndrome

The next two questions are linked.

5 Two weeks after visiting a construction site in Ohio that was a former poultry farm, a 56-year-old Florida man with chronic myelogenous leukemia presents with fever of 39°C and difficulty breathing. The illness began with flulike symptoms and progressed to nonproductive cough and dyspnea. A chest radiograph reveals diffuse pulmonary infiltrates and mediastinal lymphadenopathy. Results of a needle biopsy of lung tissue stained with methamine silver are shown in the accompanying photograph. What is the etiology of this man's disease?

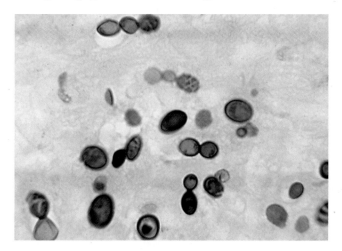

(A) *Histoplasma capsulatum*
(B) *Nocardia asteroides*
(C) *Pneumocystis jiroveci*
(D) *Streptococcus pneumoniae*
(E) *Toxoplasma gondii*

6 How did the infection in the above case most likely occur?
- (A) Colonization of skin with the organism
- (B) Contact with an AIDS patient with similar symptoms
- (C) Inhalation of spores from soil
- (D) Ingestion of contaminated water
- (E) Through intravenous drug use

7 A 19-year-old college student had emergency surgery for a ruptured appendix. Prior to surgery, the patient was placed on IV antibiotics. Which of the following is most likely to cause sepsis in this situation and must therefore be covered by the prescribed antibiotics?
- (A) Aerobic Gram-negative rods, Gram-positive cocci, and anaerobes
- (B) Aerobic Gram-positive rods and Gram-negative cocci
- (C) Anaerobic Gram-positive rods and *Pseudomonas aeruginosa*
- (D) Anaerobic Gram-positive cocci and methicillin-resistant *Staphylococcus aureus* (MRSA)
- (E) *Staphylococcus*, *Streptococcus*, and anaerobic Gram-positive rods

8 A 25-year-old woman presented with a painful, swollen, red, warm left ankle and a temperature of 38°C. She reports no history of trauma to the ankle. Skin lesions, as shown in the photograph, are also found. Analysis of the synovial fluid revealed an elevated white blood cell count with a predominance of neutrophils. Organisms isolated on chocolate agar from the synovial fluid are shown in the photograph. What is the most likely cause of this patient's current condition?

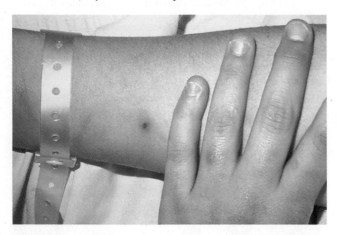

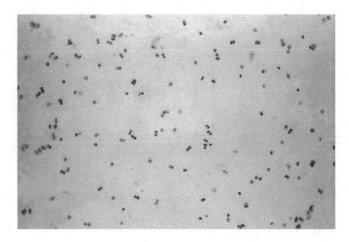

- (A) *Borrelia burgdorferi*
- (B) *Neisseria gonorrhoeae*
- (C) *Salmonella* sp.
- (D) *Staphylococcus aureus*
- (E) *Yersinia enterocolitica*

9 A 3-year-old boy presented to the emergency department with a 2-day history of coldlike illness and a 1-day history of difficulty breathing and an unusual, barklike cough. Physical exam revealed a fever of 38°C, tachypnea, tachycardia, and stridor. A chest radiograph revealed narrowing of the upper airways (a steeple sign). A clinical diagnosis of croup was made. What is the most likely etiologic agent in the above case?
- (A) *Haemophilus influenzae*
- (B) *Moraxella catarrhalis*
- (C) *Mycoplasma pneumoniae*
- (D) Parainfluenza virus
- (E) Respiratory syncytial virus

10 A 19-year-old woman presented with a 3-day history of fever, sore throat, malaise, and headache. Physical exam revealed a temperature of 39°C, cervical lymphadenopathy, and a whitish tonsillar exudate. Of the following, which is the most likely cause?
- (A) *Haemophilus influenzae*
- (B) *Moraxella catarrhalis*
- (C) *Neisseria gonorrhoeae*
- (D) *Streptococcus pyogenes*
- (E) Viral

11 A 21-year-old college student was hospitalized with meningitis due to *Neisseria meningitidis*. Room mates of the patient can be protected from the disease by chemoprophylaxis. Which drug is most commonly used for this purpose?
- (A) Amoxicillin
- (B) Ciprofloxacin
- (C) Doxycycline
- (D) Isoniazid
- (E) TMP–SMZ

12 A 7-year-old girl was hospitalized for severe dehydration. Of note, she recently traveled with her mother to the Caribbean for a 1-week vacation. Within a few days of her return, she became febrile and had episodes of cramping diarrhea. Her abdominal distress worsened to the point that she now had little desire to eat or drink. Microscopic examination of fresh stool revealed abundant fecal leukocytes. Which of the following diagnoses is most consistent with her clinical presentation?
(A) Adenovirus gastroenteritis
(B) *Campylobacter* enterocolitis
(C) Cholera
(D) Giardiasis
(E) Rotavirus gastroenteritis

13 A 15-year-old boy with acne is being treated with a topical antimicrobial. Which organism is associated with this disease and with which antimicrobial is he most likely being treated?
(A) *Malassezia furfur*/Ketoconazole
(B) *Propionibacterium* sp./Clindamycin
(C) *Staphylococcus aureus*/Cloxacillin
(D) *Streptococcus pyogenes*/Penicillin
(E) *Trichosporon* sp./Clotrimazole

14 A neonate is delivered 3 weeks prematurely. Because she was uninsured, the mother did not receive adequate prenatal care; however, she reported no illness during pregnancy. The infant has no signs of illness at birth; however, develops meningitis soon afterward. The causative organism, which would have been screened for during pregnancy had she received prenatal care was isolated from the vagina of the mother as well as from the cerebral spinal fluid of the neonate. Which of the following organisms is the likely cause?
(A) Cytomegalovirus
(B) Herpes simplex type 2
(C) *Listeria monocytogenes*
(D) *Streptococcus agalactiae*
(E) *Toxoplasma gondii*

15 A 42-year-old man with HIV, presenting for his regular checkup, is found to have a CD4 cell count of 180/cmm. He is given a prescription for TMP–SMZ for the prevention of which opportunistic pathogen?
(A) *Cryptococcus neoformans*
(B) *Cryptosporidium parvum*
(C) *Histoplasma capsulatum*
(D) *Mycobacterium avium* complex
(E) *Pneumocystis jiroveci*

16 A 43-year-old man presents with fever of 104 °F, progressively worsening headache, diffuse abdominal pain, constipation, anorexia, and malaise of 5 days duration. Physical exam revealed hepatosplenomegaly, but no icterus. A rash, described as rose spots, was seen on the trunk. His history is significant for having returned from a mission trip to Haiti 1 week ago. What is the most likely microbial cause of this man's condition?
(A) *Entamoeba histolytica*
(B) *Giardia lamblia*
(C) Hepatitis A virus
(D) *Salmonella typhi*
(E) *Vibrio cholerae*

The next two questions are linked.

17 A 67-year-old hospitalized woman was treated for 7 days with clindamycin and cefuroxime for a postsurgical infection when she developed profuse, watery diarrhea, cramping abdominal pain, and fever. An enzyme immunoassay of the stool revealed the presence of a bacterial enterotoxin. How should this woman be treated?
(A) Continue clindamycin and cefuroxime
(B) Amoxicillin plus clavulanate
(C) Ceftriaxone
(D) Ciprofloxacin
(E) Metronidazole

18 Which virulence factor of the etiologic agent in the above case contributes to its ability to cause nosocomial infections?
(A) Intracellular growth
(B) Lipopolysaccharide
(C) Shiga toxin production
(D) Spore formation
(E) Type III secretion system

The next three questions are linked.

19 A 42-year-old man who recently immigrated to Los Angeles, California from Cambodia presents with a 2-week history of fever, night sweats, a 15-pound weight loss, and cough productive of bloody sputum. Granulomatous lesions can be visualized on a chest radiograph. What is the most likely organism causing this infection?
(A) *Histoplasma capsulatum*
(B) *Echinococcus granulosus*
(C) *Mycobacterium tuberculosis*
(D) *Streptococcus pneumoniae*
(E) *Salmonella typhi*

20 Sputum from the patient in the above case showed acid-fast bacilli. A nucleic acid amplification test confirmed the diagnosis. What is the appropriate initial therapy for this patient?
(A) Isoniazid
(B) Drug combination of isoniazid and rifampin
(C) Drug combination of isoniazid, ciprofloxacin, and amikacin
(D) Drug combination of isoniazid, rifampin, pyrazinamide, and ethambutol
(E) Drug combination of isoniazid, streptomycin, pyrazinamide, ciprofloxacin, and amikacin

21 Virulence factors of the organism in the above question enable it to:
(A) Adhere tightly to respiratory epithelial cells
(B) Alter cAMP levels in respiratory epithelial cells
(C) Induce immune suppression through infection of T cells
(D) Lyse secretory IgA
(E) Survive intracellularly within macrophages

The next three questions are linked.

22 A 57-year-old man complains of worsening abdominal pain for the past 2 months, which he describes as heartburn. He notes that the pain improves temporarily with food, or by taking antacids. Definitive diagnosis includes serology to detect antibodies to which organism?
(A) Adenovirus
(B) *Cryptosporidium parvum*
(C) Enteroaggregative *Escherichia coli*
(D) *Helicobacter pylori*
(E) *Proteus vulgaris*

23 What treatment regimen is recommended for the man in the above case?
(A) Bismuth and ampicillin
(B) Metronidazole
(C) Proton pump inhibitors
(D) Proton pump inhibitor plus amoxicillin and clarithromycin
(E) Tetracycline plus metronidazole

24 How is successful treatment of the condition in the above case best determined?
(A) Resolution of symptoms
(B) Endoscopy
(C) Urea breath test
(D) Hemoccult test
(E) Stool culture

25 A 15-year-old home schooled boy presented with a 3-day history of low-grade fever and malaise, followed by significant swelling and tenderness in the submaxillary area bilaterally and unilateral, painful, testicular edema. His history is significant for a lack of most childhood vaccines due to parental concerns of vaccine-related autism. Two weeks previously, he had attended summer camp with other home schooled children from various countries. Other teenaged boys attending the summer camp developed similar symptoms and some also developed meningitis. The etiologic agent was isolated from respiratory secretions and urine. What is the most likely etiologic agent?
(A) *Haemophilus influenzae* b
(B) Mumps virus
(C) *Neisseria meningitidis*
(D) Respiratory syncytial virus
(E) *Streptococcus pneumoniae*

26 A 67-year-old hemodialysis patient with a history of frequent hospitalizations presents with a fever and signs of severe sepsis. Her history is significant for treatment of *Clostridium difficile* colitis 3 months previously. *Enterococcus faecium* was isolated from the blood. Which antibiotic would most likely be effective in this patient?
(A) Ampicillin
(B) Gentamicin
(C) Linezolid
(D) TMP–SMZ
(E) Vancomycin

27 A 58-year-old man developed tinnitus and vertigo after being treated for *Escherichia coli* septicemia while hospitalized for colon cancer surgery. Which antibiotic was he most likely given?
(A) Azithromycin
(B) Clindamycin
(C) Gentamicin
(D) Levofloxacin
(E) Linezolid

28 A 43-year-old AIDS patient with a CD4 cell count of 15/cmm develops toxoplasmosis. Which of the following describe his likely symptoms?
(A) Abdominal pain, anorexia, nausea, vomiting
(B) Fever, malaise, nonproductive cough, dyspnea
(C) Fever, weight loss, night sweats
(D) Fever, headache, confusion, motor weakness
(E) Profuse, watery diarrhea occasionally streaked with blood

29 A 32-year-old prison inmate presented with fever of 38.5 °C, unexplained weight loss of 12 pounds, and a cough of 3 weeks duration. The cough was productive of bloody sputum. A sputum Gram stain failed to reveal any predominant organisms. An acid-fast stain of the sputum is shown in the figure. Chest radiographs showed cavitary lesions in the right upper lobe; however, an intradermal skin test showed a 5 mm area of induration after 72 h. In addition to the organism causing the respiratory symptoms, for which other organism should he be tested?

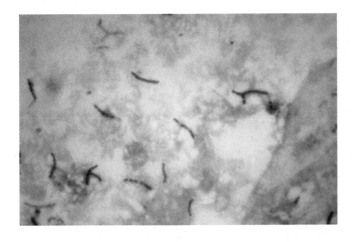

(A) *Aspergillus fumigatus*
(B) *Histoplasma capsulatum*
(C) Human immunodeficiency virus
(D) *Klebsiella pneumoniae*
(E) *Streptococcus pneumoniae*

The next two questions are linked.

30 While removing trash and brush from a canal in Florida, a man is pierced with a thorn in one of his fingers. At the time of the injury, the wound seemed insignificant. After a few days, however, it becomes inflamed and swollen (shown). Eventually, the wound becomes so painful that he is compelled to seek medical assistance. The physician astutely observes that with minimal pressure applied, greenish, sweet-smelling pus freely oozes from the lesion. Considering the clinical picture, which of the following etiologies is most likely?

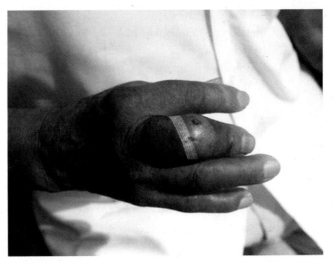

(A) *Actinomyces* sp.
(B) *Leptospira interrogans*
(C) MRSA
(D) *Pseudomonas aeruginosa*
(E) *Sporothrix schenckii*

31 Which of the following antimicrobial regimens is most suitable for treating the man in the above case?
(A) Amoxicillin–clavulanate
(B) Amphotericin B
(C) Piperacillin plus an aminoglycoside
(D) Doxycycline
(E) Vancomycin

32 An outbreak of watery diarrhea occurring in a Chicago center housing young children awaiting foster care is investigated by the health department. The stool is positive for fecal leukocytes but is not heme-positive. The etiologic agent is isolated on MacConkey agar. Which of the following is the most likely etiologic agent?
(A) *Bacillus cereus*
(B) *Escherichia coli* O157:H7
(C) Enterotoxigenic *E. coli*
(D) *Salmonella typhi*
(E) *Shigella sonnei*

33 A 12-year-old boy in central Africa presents to a medical mission with a noticeable mass on the left side of his face at the jaw line. His bottom teeth on the left side are loosened and cervical lymph nodes are enlarged. His parents report that the swelling appeared about 2 weeks ago and has grown very rapidly in size. A biopsy of the mass subsequently reveals cells of fairly uniform size and shape, with round to oval nuclei containing multiple nucleoli. Many mitotic figures are seen suggesting that the mass is a cancer. With which microorganism is this cancer causally associated?

(A) *Actinomyces israelii*
(B) *Blastomyces dermatitidis*
(C) Epstein–Barr virus
(D) *Plasmodium falciparum*
(E) *Trypanosoma brucei*

34 A 47-year-old AIDS patient with a CD4 cell count of 95/cmm presents with an insidious onset of severe headache and fever for the past 3 weeks. In the past few days, he had become mildly confused and developed diplopia. Papilledema is seen on physical exam. Ring-enhancing lesions are seen on MRI. Cerebral spinal fluid (CSF) showed 150 mononuclear cells/cmm, mild elevation of protein, and decreased glucose. An India ink stain of the CSF was negative; however, capsular polysaccharide antigens, found in the CSF, allowed for a definitive diagnosis. What is the etiology of this man's infection?
(A) *Cryptococcus neoformans*
(B) *Haemophilus influenzae* b
(C) *Listeria monocytogenes*
(D) *Mycobacterium tuberculosis*
(E) *Neisseria meningitidis*

The next two questions are linked.

35 A 45-year-old obese patient is hospitalized with fever, cough, and dyspnea. Her history is significant for severe asthma that requires frequent treatment with oral prednisone. A chest radiograph reveals cavitary lesions. Growth of the organism on buffered charcoal yeast extract (BCYE) agar is slow and characterized by the formation of aerial hyphae. Gram stain of the cultured organism is shown in the photograph. What is the etiology of this woman's disease?

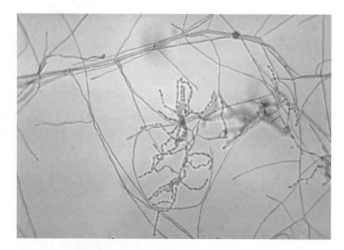

(A) *Coccidioides immitis*
(B) *Histoplasma capsulatum*
(C) *Legionella pneumophila*
(D) *Mycobacterium tuberculosis*
(E) *Nocardia asteroides*

36 How did the patient in the above question become infected?
(A) Ingestion of cysts in undercooked meat
(B) Inhalation of arthroconidia from soil
(C) Inhalation of microconidia from soil
(D) Inhalation of the bacterium in soil
(E) Person-to-person by inhalation of respiratory droplets

37 A 47-year-old man presents with fever, vomiting, and severe headache. His history is positive for a recent upper respiratory tract infection. Physical exam reveals stiff neck. Kernig and Brudzinski signs are positive. What is the most likely clinical diagnosis?
(A) Brain abscess
(B) Encephalitis
(C) Meningitis
(D) Myelitis
(E) Sinusitis

38 A 14-year-old girl with leukemia had been neutropenic for 5 weeks when she developed fever, cough, shortness of breath, pleuritic chest pain, and hemoptysis. The causative organism is seen in a lung biopsy stained with methenamine silver. With which antimicrobial should she be treated?

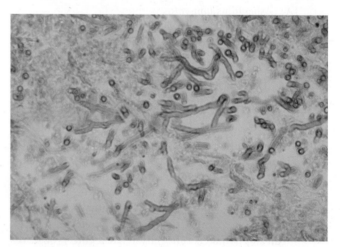

(A) Ciprofloxacin
(B) Imipenem–cilastatin
(C) Piperacillin–tazobactam
(D) Rifampin
(E) Voriconazole

39 A Down syndrome child, who lives in an institution, was seen because of crusted lesions on his hands (shown, first image). A skin scraping of the lesions is shown in the second image. How should this condition be treated?

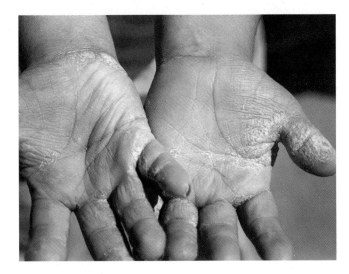

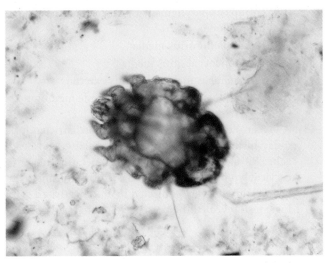

(A) Albendazole
(B) Griseofulvin
(C) Metronidazole
(D) Permethrin
(E) Praziquantel

40 A college student who has a summer job clearing brush from hiking trails in Utah has an abrupt onset of fever and chills. He seeks medical help after a day of illness, when he becomes keenly aware of a painful lymph node in his groin area near an ulcerated and infected tick bite. After evaluation and subsequent consultation with an infectious disease specialist, streptomycin therapy is recommended. What is the most likely diagnosis?
(A) Endemic typhus
(B) Human granulocytotropic anaplasmosis
(C) Human monocytic ehrlichiosis
(D) Lyme disease
(E) Ulceroglandular tularemia

41 A 67-year-old homeless, alcoholic male presented with fever, headache, malaise, anorexia, weight loss, and night sweats of 2 weeks duration. Physical exam revealed abnormalities in extraocular movements and papillary response, indicating cranial nerve dysfunction. A chest radiograph revealed numerous small nodules up to 1 mm in diameter. Examination of cerebral spinal fluid (CSF) revealed decreased glucose, moderately elevated protein, and a lymphocytic pleocytosis. What is the expected description of organisms that would most likely be seen in stained CSF?
(A) Acid-fast bacilli
(B) Gram-positive rods
(C) Gram-negative rods
(D) Gram-negative diplococci
(E) Gram-positive diplococci

42 A 20-year-old woman presented in July with a rubeolalike rash on the extremities, chills, fever, myalgia, and malaise 5 days after returning from a hiking trip in North Carolina. A history of tick bites is noted and Rocky Mountain spotted fever is suspected. How would a definitive diagnosis most likely be made?
(A) Culture of the organism on blood agar
(B) Gram stain
(C) Indirect immunofluorescence testing
(D) Radioimmunoassay
(E) Weil–Felix test

The next two questions are linked.

43 A 45-year-old day care provider presents in August with a fever of 38°C, headache, photophobia, and neck stiffness. A clinical diagnosis of meningitis is made. Based on the epidemiology of meningitis in the United States, what is the most likely cause of her disease?
(A) *Cryptococcus neoformans*
(B) *Haemophilus influenzae*
(C) *Neisseria meningitidis*
(D) *Streptococcus pneumoniae*
(E) Viral

44 If infected with the most common cause, what would a cerebral spinal fluid analysis from the above patient most likely show?
(A) Lymphocytes, decreased glucose, elevated protein
(B) Lymphocytes, normal glucose, elevated protein
(C) Neutrophils and lymphocytes, normal glucose, normal protein
(D) Neutrophils, elevated glucose, normal protein
(E) Neutrophils, low glucose, elevated protein

45 A masters-level zoology student, who is researching the behavior of rats in urban St Louis, Missouri, develops a febrile illness, marked with headaches, conjunctival hemorrhages, and signs consistent with renal failure. He is hospitalized for 2 weeks before the etiologic agent is found in blood, CSF, and urine samples. Confirmatory serologic tests are positive. What is the most likely etiological agent?

(A) Arenavirus

(B) *Babesia microti*

(C) Hantavirus

(D) *Leptospira interrogans*

(E) *Toxoplasma gondii*

46 In early July, a 45-year-old man from rural eastern Tennessee is taken to the emergency department with a high fever and episodes of delirium which appear to be connected to the high fever. History reveals that he has been sick for more than 10 days—his condition began about a week following a fishing trip. Positive tick exposure is verified; the hospital laboratory reports a WBC count of 3.1 (th/μL); and, the illness responds favorably to doxycycline treatment. Later, a reference laboratory confirms the suspected diagnosis with a type-specific antibody titer of 1:256 and granulocytic morulae. Which of the following is most the compatible diagnosis?

(A) Babesiosis

(B) Brucellosis

(C) Endemic typhus

(D) Ehrlichiosis

(E) Lyme disease

47 An elderly woman, with uncontrolled diabetes, has a yellowish-green discharge that chronically drains from her left ear canal (shown). The external canal is inflamed and the tympanic membrane appears to be ruptured. The attending physician empirically diagnoses the condition and orders a combination antibiotic regimen of an IV aminoglycoside and a third-generation cephalosporin. She initially responds, but when treatment is suspended, she relapses. Of the following, which is the most likely diagnosis?

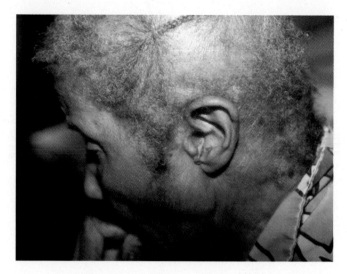

(A) Group A pharyngitis with Eustachian tube involvement

(B) *Haemophilus* otitis media

(C) Pneumococcal otitis media

(D) *Pseudomonas* malignant otitis externa

(E) Staphylococcal abscessed tympanic membrane

48 A 9-year-old boy was brought to his pediatrician for a 3-day history of fever, sore throat, malaise, and headache. Physical exam revealed a temperature of 39°C, cervical lymphadenopathy, and a whitish tonsillar exudate. A throat swab, subjected to an office-based serologic test, revealed the presence of which pathogen?

(A) Adenovirus

(B) Enterovirus

(C) *Haemophilus influenzae*

(D) *Moraxella catarrhalis*

(E) *Streptococcus pyogenes*

The next two questions are linked.

49 A 78-year-old man was hospitalized and placed on a respirator following a stroke. After 10 days of hospitalization, he developed a fever. Lung infiltrates were seen on chest radiographs. Sputum and blood cultures were obtained and he was placed on empiric antimicrobials. Which of the following is a suitable empiric antimicrobial regimen?

(A) Amphotericin B

(B) Azithromycin

(C) Levofloxacin plus vancomycin

(D) Penicillin V

(E) Piperacillin plus tazobactam

50 Sputum and blood cultures obtained from the patient in the above case and cultured on nutrient agar grew Gram-negative, oxidase-positive bacilli that produced pyocyanin and pyoverdin pigments, as shown in the accompanying photograph. With which organism did the patient become infected?

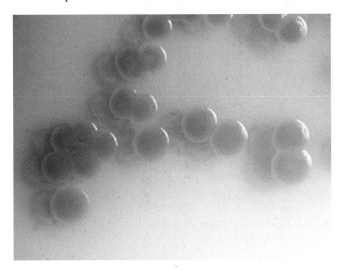

(A) *Klebsiella pneumoniae*
(B) *Aspergillus flavus*
(C) *Legionella pneumophila*
(D) *Pseudomonas aeruginosa*
(E) *Pneumocystis jiroveci*

51 A 47-year-old man has a serious skin infection due to aerobic, Gram-positive bacteria. He is unable to receive β-lactam antibiotics due to a history of penicillin allergy. Which of the following antibiotics could he be given?
(A) Ampicillin
(B) Aztreonam
(C) Cefazolin
(D) Clindamycin
(E) Meropenem

52 A 67-year-old man developed an insidious onset of fever, chills, and night sweats. Over the course of a week or so he became increasingly weak and short of breath. A heart murmur was heard on auscultation. Blood tests revealed an elevated erythrocyte sedimentation rate. Valvular vegetations were seen on transesophageal echocardiography. Which of the following diseases and etiologies fit this clinical picture?
(A) Acute endocarditis—*Staphylococcus aureus*
(B) Atherosclerosis—*Chlamydophila pneumoniae*
(C) Dilated cardiomyopathy—*Coxsackievirus*
(D) Myocarditis—*Borrelia burgdorferi*
(E) Subacute endocarditis—Viridans group streptococci

53 A 2-month-old infant presents with violent coughing spells often ending with vomiting for the past 2 days. The parents report that she had been well until 2 weeks ago when she had coldlike symptoms including a fever, profuse runny nose, sneezing, and poor appetite. History reveals a chronic cough in the father and recent respiratory illness in two older siblings. Vaccination history is unknown. No retractions, wheezing, rales, or stridor were noted on physical exam; however, the patient did appear mildly dehydrated. Chest radiographs were normal. A CBC revealed a white blood cell count of 20,000 with 70% lymphocytes. Which of the following diseases is most likely?
(A) Bronchiolitis
(B) Croup
(C) Epiglottitis
(D) Pertussis
(E) Pneumonia

54 A 16-year-old girl presents with fever, exudative pharyngitis, profound fatigue, and cervical lymphadenopathy of 2-days duration. Palpation revealed mild splenomegaly. A blood test revealed 10% atypical lymphocytes and lymphocytosis, and a heterophil antibody test was positive. How should this patient be treated?
(A) Acyclovir
(B) Amphotericin
(C) Corticosteroids
(D) Penicillin
(E) Symptomatically

The next two questions are linked.

55 An infant is born with very low birth weight, microcephaly, petechial rash, hepatosplenomegaly, and chorioretinitis. *In utero* infection with which organism could account for these problems?
(A) *Chlamydia trachomatis*
(B) Cytomegalovirus
(C) Group B *Streptococcus*
(D) Rubella virus
(E) *Toxoplasma gondii*

56 How can the infant in the above question be treated?
(A) Erythromycin
(B) Ganciclovir
(C) MMR vaccine
(D) Penicillin
(E) Pyrimethamine and sulfadiazine

57 A previously healthy 24-year-old male who is an avid spelunker presents with non-productive cough, dyspnea, chest tightness, and fever 2 weeks after visiting caves in the Ozark Mountains in Arkansas. Chest radiographs are shown in the accompanying photograph. Blood and sputum cultures are obtained, and he is treated empirically with azithromycin for community-acquired pneumonia. Standard cultures are negative for bacteria; however, the etiologic agent is cultured from sputum on brain–heart infusion agar with antibiotics and cycloheximide. How does this finding change the treatment regimen?

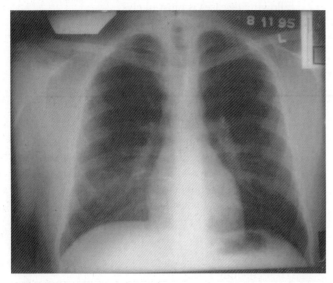

(A) Change to amphotericin B to cover for *Coccidioides immitis*

(B) Change to doxycycline to cover *Chlamydia psittaci*

(C) Change to itraconazole to cover for *Histoplasma capsulatum*

(D) Change to penicillin to cover *Mycoplasma pneumoniae*

(E) Increase the dose of azithromycin to cover drug-resistant *Legionella pneumophila*

The next two questions are linked.

58 A 73-year-old man presents with a painful vesicular rash on the left side of his face including within the ear canal, left ear pain, facial weakness, and altered sensations on the affected side of his face, as well as vertigo. The photograph shows the patient 1 week after the onset of the rash. What is the most likely diagnosis?

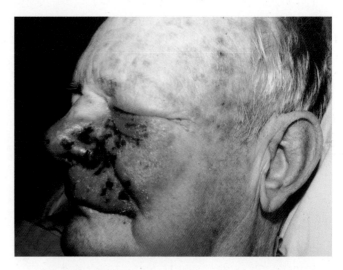

(A) Brown recluse spider bite

(B) Erysipelas

(C) Ramsey Hunt syndrome

(D) Superficial pyoderma

(E) Tabes dorsalis

59 Which of the following is the most likely complication of infection that the man in the above case may experience?

(A) Encephalitis

(B) Optic neuritis

(C) Parkinson disease

(D) Postherpetic neuralgia

(E) Temporal arteritis

60 A 25-year-old woman developed fever, chest pain, and arrhythmia 1 week after experiencing a flulike illness. A variety of tests lead to the diagnosis of myocarditis of microbial origin. What is the most likely etiology?

(A) *Borrelia burgdorferi*

(B) *Corynebacterium diphtheriae*

(C) Coxsackievirus B

(D) Influenza virus

(E) *Trypanosoma cruzi*

61 The Atlanta health department investigates an outbreak of watery, nonbloody diarrhea which occurred in a day care center and affected 25 children 8 to 24 months of age and 3 adult day care providers. The organism shown in the image is found in the stool samples from most of the affected individuals. What is the appropriate treatment?

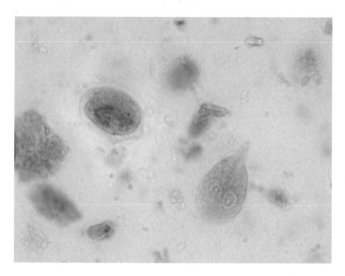

(A) Amoxicillin

(B) Amoxicillin–clavulanate

(C) Erythromycin

(D) Metronidazole

(E) Trimethoprim–sulfamethoxazole

62 A 68-year-old man undergoes heart valve replacement due to chronic valvular stenosis. His physician explains to him that his valve problem probably stemmed from repeated episodes of which childhood disease?

(A) Chickenpox

(B) Diphtheria

(C) Measles

(D) Rotavirus

(E) Strep throat

63 A 60-year-old man was diagnosed clinically with subacute infective endocarditis. Routine blood cultures failed to grow any organisms and the infection was initially described as culture-negative. However, after 14 days of culture, organisms that are part of the normal mouth flora and an uncommon cause of endocarditis were isolated from the blood. A Gram stain of the organisms is shown in the accompanying photograph. With which group of organisms is he most likely infected?

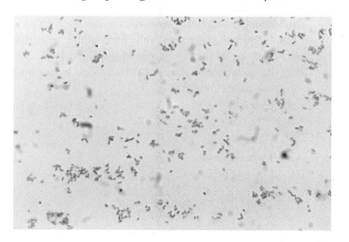

(A) Coagulase-negative staphylococci

(B) Coagulase-positive staphylococci

(C) Enterococci

(D) HACEK group

(E) Viridans group streptococci

64 A 2-year-old girl presents to the emergency department with a 2-h history of difficulty breathing. She appears toxic and acutely distressed, has a low-grade fever, and is drooling. She requires intubation and a course of ceftriaxone. What is the most likely diagnosis?

(A) Bronchiolitis

(B) Croup

(C) Diphtheria

(D) Epiglottitis

(E) Pertussis

65 A 3-month-old child presents to the emergency department in March with low-grade fever, tachypnea, dyspnea, wheezing, and cyanosis. A chest radiograph reveals hyperinflation. What is the most likely microbial cause of this child's symptoms?

(A) Adenovirus

(B) *Chlamydophila pneumoniae*

(C) Influenza virus

(D) *Mycoplasma pneumoniae*

(E) Respiratory syncytial virus

66 A 27-year-old female is diagnosed with acute retroviral syndrome and is placed under the management of infectious disease specialists. Which of the following, if it occurred in this patient, would indicate that she has progressed from HIV infection to AIDS?

(A) CD4 cell count 50% of normal

(B) Invasive cervical carcinoma

(C) Shingles

(D) Thrush

(E) Viral load >100,000/cmm

The next two questions are linked.

67 A 6-month-old child presents to the emergency department in January with a severe bout of watery, nonbloody diarrhea without dehydration. What is the most likely cause and treatment?

(A) *Escherichia coli* K1/
    trimethoprim–sulfamethoxazole

(B) Enteroinvasive *E. coli*/ampicillin

(C) *Giardia lamblia*/metronidazole

(D) Rotavirus/oral rehydration therapy

(E) *Shigella dysenteriae*/ampicillin

68 How could this infection best be avoided?
(A) Avoidance of crowded conditions such as day care
(B) Breast feeding
(C) Cleaning environmental surfaces with chlorine-containing disinfectants
(D) Hand washing
(E) Vaccination

69 A 48-year-old obese alcoholic man who is being treated for pulmonary tuberculosis presents with severe pain in his right big toe of 1 day's duration. Physical exam reveals an exquisitely tender, swollen, and erythematous right hallux. Acute gouty arthritis is suspected and upon testing, a serum uric acid level is found to be elevated. Which antituberculosis agent could have precipitated these symptoms?
(A) Ethambutol
(B) Isoniazid
(C) Pyrazinamide
(D) Rifampin
(E) Streptomycin

70 A 54-year-old neutropenic man undergoing cancer chemotherapy presents with difficult and painful swallowing. Endoscopy of the esophagus reveals multiple raised 2 mm diameter white plaques with no ulceration. Which organism is the most likely cause?
(A) *Candida albicans*
(B) Cytomegalovirus
(C) Enterovirus
(D) *Helicobacter pylori*
(E) Herpes simplex virus

71 Hand washing and good community sanitation would have the greatest effect on reducing the transmission of which of the following infectious diseases?
(A) Influenza
(B) Malaria
(C) Poliomyelitis
(D) Schistosomiasis
(E) Tuberculosis

72 A 20-year-old British woman died in September of 2005 after 2 months of progressive neurologic deterioration. Her symptoms began with depression and behavioral changes and she was initially diagnosed with an anxiety disorder. However, soon she began developing progressive ataxia and incontinence. Autopsy findings of her brain are shown in the accompanying photograph. She was one of over 100 patients to develop this disease in Great Britain since 1995. What is the origin of the disease that caused the death of this woman?

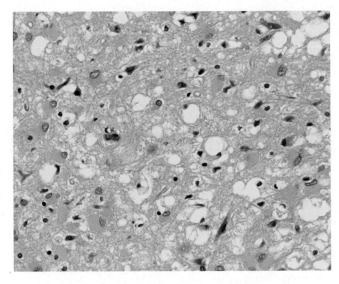

(A) Bovine tuberculosis
(B) Chronic wasting disease of deer and elk
(C) Creutzfeldt–Jacob disease
(D) Kuru in African monkeys
(E) Scrapie-infected sheep

73 A 43-year-old AIDS patient with a CD4 cell count of less than 50/μL was brought by a friend to the emergency department after suffering a seizure. The friend reported that the patient had been lethargic, confused, and forgetful for the past week. Physical exam revealed a confused, afebrile man with focal neurological signs. A ring enhancing lesion was seen on CT and MRI of the brain. Cytology of the CSF showed malignant appearing lymphocytes. A PCR of the cerebral spinal fluid revealed viral DNA. Which virus is most likely involved in the etiology of this man's neurological signs?
(A) Cytomegalovirus
(B) Epstein–Barr virus
(C) Herpes simplex virus type 1
(D) JC virus
(E) St Louis encephalitis virus

74 A 23-year-old woman had been treated for 2 weeks with antibiotics for a persistent cough. Shortly after finishing her antibiotic regimen, she develops a thick, white vaginal discharge and perivaginal pruritus. Examination of the discharge did not show clue cells, but did demonstrate pseudohyphae. What is the most appropriate treatment?
(A) Cidofovir
(B) Clindamycin
(C) Clotrimazole
(D) Metronidazole
(E) Ofloxacin

The next three questions are linked.

75 A 33-year-old pregnant woman in her 34th week of gestation presents with a mucopurulent vaginal discharge. No growth from the discharge is obtained on Thayer-Martin agar. A direct immunofluorescent stain of the discharge reveals elementary bodies. With which organism is she infected?

(A) *Chlamydia trachomatis*
(B) Herpes simplex virus
(C) *Neisseria gonorrhoeae*
(D) *Treponema pallidum*
(E) *Trichomonas vaginalis*

76 What is the preferred method of diagnosis of this infection?

(A) Antigen detection from cervical swabs
(B) Cell culture
(C) Cytology (Pap smear)
(D) Nucleic acid amplification
(E) Serology

77 If the woman in the above case is not treated appropriately, for what disease would her infant be at risk?

(A) Conjunctivitis
(B) Hydrops fetalis
(C) Late onset deafness
(D) Meningitis
(E) Patent ductus arteriosus

78 A 65-year-old man, a South American immigrant, presents with biventricular heart failure with peripheral edema, hepatosplenomegaly, and pulmonary congestion. Global heart enlargement is seen on chest radiography. Electrocardiography reveals right bundle-branch block and left anterior fascicular block. Serum collected from the patient and run on ELISA detects antibodies to an agent transmitted by the bite of reduviid bugs. What is the etiology of this man's disease?

(A) *Borrelia burgdorferi*
(B) *Cardiobacterium hominis*
(C) *Coxiella burnetii*
(D) *Rickettsia akari*
(E) *Trypanosoma cruzi*

79 A 3-week-old female infant is brought to the emergency room following a seizure. Physical exam reveals fever and a vesicular rash on the infant's extremities and trunk. The rash did not affect the palms of the hands or soles of the feet. Her mother, a 17-year-old single parent, claims the infant was well until about 3 days ago. She denies any illness during pregnancy or exposure of the infant to anyone with similar symptoms. Nevertheless, the physician suspects a perinatal infection and orders diagnostic tests. Which of the following tests would most likely be positive as related to the cause of this infant's disease?

(A) Herpes simplex virus isolation from the skin lesions
(B) Infant IgM for toxoplasmosis
(C) Maternal IgM for cytomegalovirus
(D) Maternal VDRL
(E) Nucleic acid amplification tests for *Neisseria gonorrhoeae*

80 A 43-year-old man presents with an acute onset of diarrhea, upper right quadrant abdominal pain, and fatigue. Physical exam reveals hepatomegaly, yellow sclera, and dark urine. About 1 month ago, he returned from the Gulf coast of Texas where he had consumed raw oysters. What is the most likely microbial etiology of this man's disease?

(A) *Diphyllobothrium latum*
(B) Hepatitis A virus
(C) *Vibrio cholerae*
(D) Yellow fever virus
(E) *Yersinia enterocolitica*

81 A 6-year-old boy develops an acute onset of malaise, anorexia, hematuria, decreased urine output, and periorbital edema. Physical exam reveals hypertension. Hematology reveals a mild normocytic, normochromic anemia and a normal white blood cell and platelet count. His history is significant for an infection from which he recovered 2 weeks previously. What was the most likely type of infection he experienced which subsequently led to his current condition?

(A) Acute toxoplasmosis
(B) Gastroenteritis
(C) Leptospirosis
(D) Pyoderma
(E) Urinary tract infection

82 An 8-month-old child presents with fever of 37.8°C, cough, and runny nose of 2 days duration. On examination, she is not fussy, and does not appear to be in pain. Her chest is clear to auscultation and tympanic membranes are reddened and slightly bulging. Which is the most likely etiologic diagnosis and recommended treatment option?

(A) *Moraxella catarrhalis*—amoxicillin–clavulanate
(B) Nontypeable *Haemophilus influenzae*—ampicillin–sulbactam
(C) Respiratory syncytial virus—ribavirin
(D) Rhinovirus—symptomatic treatment
(E) *Streptococcus pneumoniae*—amoxicillin

83 A 72-year-old man dies following a stroke. An autopsy reveals the cause of the stroke as shown in the accompanying photograph of the aorta. Which pathogen may play a role in the pathogenesis of the lesions seen in the photograph?

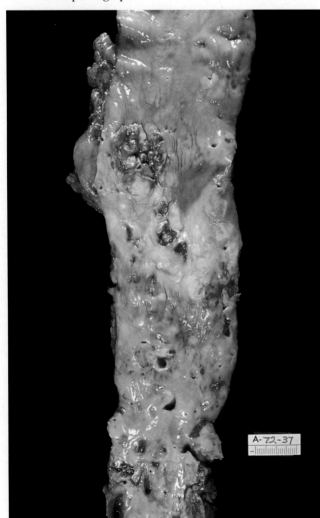

(A) *Candida albicans*
(B) *Chlamydophila pneumoniae*
(C) Group A *Streptococcus*
(D) Measles virus
(E) Viridans group streptococci

84 An 8-year-old child has an exacerbation of asthma symptoms concurrent with an upper respiratory infection (low fever, nasal discharge, and sore throat). Which of the following organisms is most likely involved in causing the exacerbation?

(A) Adenovirus
(B) Group A *Streptococcus*
(C) *Haemophilus influenzae*
(D) Influenza virus
(E) Rhinovirus

85 A 25-year-old army recruit develops a vaccine-associated skin lesion as shown in the accompanying photograph. The lesion began as a papule at the inoculation site 5 days after vaccination, and progressed to a pustular lesion before forming a scab. Against which bioterrorism agent does this vaccine protect?

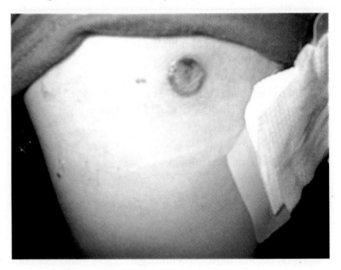

(A) Arenavirus
(B) *Bacillus anthracis*
(C) *Clostridium botulinum*
(D) Smallpox virus
(E) *Yersinia pestis*

86 A previously healthy 35-year-old male develops an acute onset of fever, chills, myalgia, and headache which rapidly progressed over 36 h to a severe respiratory illness. He is hospitalized in the intensive care unit and despite appropriate supportive care, dies 24 h later from acute respiratory distress. He is diagnosed postmortem with hantavirus pulmonary syndrome. How might he have acquired this infection?

(A) Cleaning out a rodent-infested warehouse
(B) Exploring caves inhabited by infected bats
(C) Exposure to mosquito bites
(D) Hiking in tick-infested woods
(E) Swimming in a contaminated farm pond

87 An outbreak of a gastrointestinal illness occurs on a cruise ship. The affected passengers experienced 36 h of vomiting and watery diarrhea. The ship returns early from the cruise, is cleaned thoroughly with chlorine-containing products and reboarded with new passengers. Despite the efforts to clean the ship, the second group of passengers endures a similar outbreak. What is the most likely microbial etiology of these outbreaks?

(A) *Cryptosporidium parvum*
(B) Enterotoxigenic *Escherichia coli*
(C) *Giardia lamblia*
(D) Norovirus
(E) *Shigella sonnei*

88 A 27-year-old female in her 36th week of pregnancy has routine vaginal and rectal swabs taken for screening of a pathogen which she may carry asymptomatically and which is associated with neonatal sepsis, pneumonia, and meningitis. For which pathogen is she being screened?

(A) Group B *Streptococcus*
(B) Herpes simplex virus type 2
(C) *Neisseria gonorrhoeae*
(D) *Toxoplasma gondii*
(E) *Treponema pallidum*

89 An outbreak of food poisoning occurs after a catered lunch attended by 112 people. Thirty percent of the individuals who ate the lunch developed nausea and vomiting 3 h after consumption of the food. A health department investigation linked the outbreak to contamination of chicken fried rice with a spore-forming organism. What is the cause of this outbreak?

(A) *Bacillus cereus*
(B) *Clostridium perfringens*
(C) *Cryptosporidium parvum*
(D) *Staphylococcus aureus*
(E) *Sporothrix schenckii*

90 A 20-year-old female presents to a sexually transmitted disease clinic with a thin grayish-white vaginal discharge, the odor of which she describes as "fishy smelling." Vaginal exam reveals a discharge adherent to the vaginal wall with no underlying erythema. The discharge has a pH of 5. Microscopic examination of the discharge reveals clue cells. What is the most likely cause of this discharge?

(A) *Candida albicans*
(B) *Chlamydia trachomatis*
(C) *Gardnerella vaginalis*
(D) *Neisseria gonorrhoeae*
(E) *Trichomonas vaginalis*

91 An increase in cases of childhood paralysis in an African country followed the cessation of a crucial vaccination program. The vaccine in question protected children against which infectious disease?

(A) Malaria
(B) Measles
(C) Meningitis
(D) Polio
(E) Schistosomiasis

92 A previously healthy 19-year-old male is brought by frantic parents to the emergency department after suffering a seizure. Hours prior to the seizure, he complained of headache and fever. His parents report that he also seemed to be acting odd, and seemed confused prior to the seizure. Following the results of an MRI, the patient is diagnosed clinically with encephalitis and treated empirically with an antimicrobial drug pending results of further tests. Which drug is recommended in this situation?

(A) Acyclovir
(B) Amphotericin B
(C) Cefotaxime
(D) Pyrimethamine
(E) Vancomycin

93 A 55-year-old diabetic male presents to urgent care with a fever of 39 °C, swelling, erythema, and pain in his left calf as shown in the accompanying photograph. A few weeks previously, the patient fell, hitting his left anterior shin, resulting in a bruise but no bleeding. What empiric antibiotic therapy is appropriate for this man?

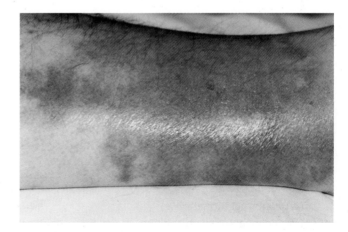

(A) Ampicillin
(B) Dicloxacillin
(C) Doxycycline
(D) Gentamicin
(E) Itraconazole

The next three questions are linked.

94 A 23-year-old newly diagnosed HIV-infected male has a CD4 cell count of 150/cmm and a viral load of 10,000 copies per mL. He is placed on an antiretroviral drug regimen that includes efavirenz, atazanavir + ritonavir and abacavir/lamivudine. What is the mechanism of action of the drugs atazanavir and ritonavir?

(A) Block entry of HIV into the cell by inhibiting conformational change in gp41

(B) Block budding from the cell by preventing cleavage of sialic acid residues

(C) Block the formation of the provirus by inhibiting reverse transcription

(D) Prevent incorporation of the provirus into host cell chromosomes

(E) Prevent maturation of the virus by blocking formation of essential structural and nonstructural proteins

95 Which drug being taken by the patient in the above question is a non-nucleoside reverse transcriptase inhibitor?

(A) Abacavir

(B) Atazanavir

(C) Efavirenz

(D) Lamivudine

(E) Ritonavir

96 After several months on the drug regimen, the individual in the above case develops a buffalo hump, central obesity, and dyslipidemia. Which of the following drugs could account for these findings?

(A) Abacavir/lamivudine

(B) Atazanavir + ritonavir

(C) Efavirenz

(D) Lamivudine alone

97 A 4-year-old child was hospitalized for suspected bacterial meningitis. Antigens of the infectious agent were detected in the cerebral spinal fluid and an etiologic diagnosis was made. Which laboratory test allowed for the detection of bacterial antigens?

(A) Gram stain

(B) Indirect immunofluorescence

(C) India ink stain

(D) Latex agglutination

(E) Polymerase chain reaction

The next two questions are linked.

98 A 45-year-old neutropenic cancer patient presents with fever, dyspnea, and hemoptysis. Imaging studies reveal cavitary lung lesions and are strongly suggestive of angioinvasive disease. Elevated galactomannan levels are found in serum and bronchoalveolar lavage (BAL) fluid. What is the etiology of this man's disease?

(A) *Aspergillus fumigatus*

(B) *Candida glabrata*

(C) *Klebsiella pneumoniae*

(D) *Mycobacterium tuberculosis*

(E) *Nocardia asteroides*

99 Which of the following antimicrobial agent is most appropriate in this case?

(A) Azithromycin

(B) Isoniazid

(C) Penicillin G

(D) Pentamidine

(E) Voriconazole

100 A 12-year-old Jordanian boy presents with migrating arthritis and a new onset of a heart murmur. He has had similar episodes of arthritis during his childhood, each one occurring about 3 weeks after recovery from an episode of pharyngitis. The boy was evaluated and a diagnosis was made on the basis of the Jones criteria. What is the diagnosis?

(A) Acute rheumatic fever

(B) Kala azar

(C) Lyme disease

(D) Reactive arthritis

(E) Viral arthritis

101 A 56-year-old Indian woman with a chronic cough, night sweats, and weight loss for 4 months goes to a pharmacy for a medication. In addition to a cough suppressant, the medicine she can buy over-the-counter in her country contains isoniazid. Her symptoms initially improve dramatically, but return in a few weeks and her illness continues to progress. What is the most likely diagnosis?

(A) Asthmatic reaction to the medication

(B) *Chronic* bronchitis

(C) *Mycoplasma* pneumonia

(D) Pneumococcal pneumonia

(E) Tuberculosis

ANSWERS

1 **The answer is D: *Neisseria meningitidis.*** Infection with this agent is most common in children; however, young adults in crowded conditions such as college dormitories are also at high risk. Many colleges and universities require or strongly recommend vaccination for their incoming students. The only other agent listed for which a vaccine is available is human papillomavirus.

2 **The answer is A: Azithromycin.** Macrolides, such as azithromycin, are recommended for outpatient treatment of pneumonia in adults who have not previously received antibiotics for the condition. The most likely causes of mild pneumonia that can be treated in an outpatient setting are *Mycoplasma pneumoniae* and *Chlamydia (Chlamydophila) pneumoniae*, both of which are susceptible to macrolides. Doxycycline can also be used in this setting. Clindamycin is often used to treat anaerobic infections; fluconazole is an antifungal drug; imipenem is a carbapenem available only in intravenous formulation and used for seriously ill patients; and linezolid is an oxazolidine useful for treatment of methicillin-resistant *Staphylococcus aureus* and vancomycin-resistant enterococci.

3 **The answer is D: Opportunistic.** Opportunistic agents are typically of low virulence in immune competent individuals, causing disease only when a person becomes compromised. Opportunistic pathogens include certain members of all groups of microorganisms including bacteria, fungi, viruses, and parasites.

4 **The answer is C: Macrolides are principally secreted in the feces.** The macrolide group (e.g., erythromycin, clarithromycin, and azithromycin) is concentrated in the liver and biliary excretion is the reason why the drug does not give good coverage for UTI enteric and staph organisms. Only minute quantities are secreted in the urine. Stevens–Johnson syndrome, a rare hypersensitivity reaction, may be drug related but is not the reason for the change in the choice of antibiotic. TMP–SMZ is appropriate but the attending could have also ordered a fluoroquinolone or an aminopenicillin. All are concentrated in the urine and have good activity against most bacterial UTI agents. The glycocalyx, β-lactamases (transpeptidases), and candidiasis are not significant factors.

5 **The answer is A: *Histoplasma capsulatum.*** This is a case of acute pulmonary histoplasmosis. The photograph shows the yeast form of this dimorphic fungus. The patient was at increased risk of severe disease due to his age and leukemia. *H. capsulatum* is a soil fungus

endemic in the Mississippi and Ohio River valleys and is found in soils enriched with bird droppings. The patient, a man from Florida (outside of the endemic area), was exposed to large amounts of fungal spores by visiting a construction site on a former poultry farm. Most individuals living in areas endemic for *H. capsulatum* show serologic evidence of infection. Infection of the immune competent may be asymptomatic, or can result in a flulike illness, although more serious pulmonary disease can result if the infecting dose is unusually high and if the patient is very young, elderly, or immune compromised. In an immune competent individual, the fungus is walled off by a strong cell-mediated immune response; however, the organism may remain viable for several decades within lung granulomas. Immune suppression resulting, for example, from HIV infection, cancer, or transplantation, allows the organism to escape from the granuloma and spread throughout the body, causing disseminated histoplasmosis. The clinical description, including persistent fever, weight loss, hepatosplenomegaly, and skin lesions are frequent manifestations of disseminated histoplasmosis. Yeast forms of the fungus can be visualized in tissue using periodic acid Schiff stain or silver stains, both of which stain the carbohydrates of the fungal cell wall. Diagnosis of disseminated histoplasmosis can also be made by antigen detection in the urine. While all of the organisms listed with the exception of *T. gondii* cause respiratory illness, they can be ruled out on the basis of the chest radiograph and photograph. *N. asteroides* occurs in immune compromised individuals such as this patient; however, it is a Gram-positive filamentous rod that causes a slowly developing, necrotic form of pulmonary disease. *P. jiroveci* is an opportunistic fungus causing pulmonary disease in the immune compromised, particularly AIDS patients with CD4 cell counts of less than 200/cmm. *S. pneumoniae*, a Gram-positive diplococcus, is the most common cause of community-acquired pneumonia.

6 **The answer is C: Inhalation of spores from soil.** *Histoplasma capsulatum* is a soil fungus. It does not colonize the skin, is not transmitted person-to-person or through ingestion of contaminated food or water, or by IV drug use.

7 **The answer is A: Aerobic Gram-negative rods, Gram-positive cocci, and anaerobes.** Of the commensal organisms in the gut, including the appendix, the most likely ones to cause disease are members of the Enterobacteriaceae family of aerobic, Gram-negative rods (e.g., *Escherichia coli*), enterococci, and anaerobes such as *Bacteroides* sp.

8 **The answer is B: *Neisseria gonorrhoeae.*** This is a case of disseminated gonorrhea. One of the manifestations of this disease is arthritis. Pustular skin lesions are commonly found. While all of the organisms listed are causal agents of arthritis, *N. gonorrhoeae* is the only Gram-negative diplococcus on the list. In addition, *N. gonorrhoeae* is the most common cause of septic arthritis in sexually active young adults.

9 **The answer is D: Parainfluenza virus.** Although all the organisms listed can cause respiratory disease, croup is generally a viral illness. While respiratory syncytial virus can also cause croup, about 80% of cases are caused by parainfluenza virus.

10 **The answer is E: Viral.** All of the organisms listed can cause febrile pharyngitis; however, viral causes are more common, in both children and adults, than are bacterial causes. It is not possible to distinguish between viral and bacterial causes of pharyngitis based on clinical manifestations. This is an important point to keep in mind, as unnecessary use of antibiotics to treat viral infections is common.

11 **The answer is B: Ciprofloxacin.** A single dose of 500 mg of ciprofloxacin is the preferred regimen for prophylaxis of adults against *Neisseria meningitidis*. Rifampin can also be used. Children can be protected using a single dose of ceftriaxone as fluoroquinolones are usually contraindicated in children.

12 **The answer is B: *Campylobacter* enterocolitis.** An important clue to this diagnosis is the presence of fecal leukocytes. Of the agents listed, only *Campylobacter* is inflammatory—although sometimes it is not. Most of the cases of *Campylobacter* are self-limiting and resolve spontaneously without antimicrobial intervention. Other microbial agents of inflammatory diarrhea include *Entamoeba histolytica*, some virulent strains of *Escherichia coli*, *Shigella*, and *Salmonella*. In the above case, additional laboratory evaluation is probably warranted. Campylobacteriosis is one of the many causes of traveler's diarrhea; however, the disease is also endemic in the United States.

13 **The answer is B: *Propionibacterium* sp./Clindamycin.** The anaerobic, Gram-positive rod, *P. acnes*, is associated with the common form of acne. Several nonmicrobial factors are also involved in the pathogenesis. The presence of this organism in sebaceous follicles stimulates an inflammatory response. The infiltration of neutrophils leads to pus formation in the follicles. Treatment with topical clindamycin or with oral doxycycline or minocycline is commonly prescribed. The other organisms listed cause various skin diseases; however, they are not associated with acne. *M. furfur* and various species of *Trichosporon* cause cutaneous fungal infections. *S. aureus* and *S. pyogenes* can cause a variety of skin infections ranging in severity from impetigo to cellulitis and necrotizing fasciitis (*S. pyogenes*).

14 **The answer is D: *Streptococcus agalactiae*.** This organism, also known as Group B *Streptococcus* (GBS), is the most common cause of meningitis and septicemia in neonates. All the organisms listed can cause neonatal disease and can be transmitted from mother to infant without a maternal illness during pregnancy; however, GBS is the only one on the list for which routine screening is carried out during pregnancy. GBS colonizes the intestinal tract and can spread to the vagina. The presence of GBS in the vagina can be asymptomatic or can lead to disease in the woman, including amnionitis and endometritis. GBS is also an important cause of urinary tract infections in pregnant women. Neonates can be exposed to the bacterium *in utero*, or during or after birth. *In utero* exposure can lead to premature birth and subsequent early-onset disease. Shortly after birth, infants with early-onset disease manifest with signs of sepsis, meningitis, or pneumonia.

15 **The answer is E: *Pneumocystis jiroveci*.** All of the organisms listed are opportunistic infections that may occur in AIDS patients. Prophylaxis for *P. jiroveci* is recommended to begin when CD4 cell levels decline to less than 200/cmm. No chemoprophylaxis is recommended to prevent infections with *C. neoformans* due to its relative infrequency. Nitazoxanide is approved for treatment of *C. parvum*; however, no drug has been recommended for prophylaxis. Persons with AIDS and CD4 cell counts of <150/cmm and who live in areas hyperendemic for *H. capsulatum* can be protected from disease with prophylactic itraconazole. Azithromycin or clarithromycin can be used in AIDS patients with CD4 cell counts of <50/cmm to prevent infections due to *M. avium* complex.

16 **The answer is D: *Salmonella typhi*.** The signs and symptoms of this case are consistent with typhoid fever. Of the signs and symptoms presented in this case, the high fever and rose spots are the two most important clues for *S. typhi* infection. The rose spots, which are bacterial emboli, are often considered classic signs of typhoid fever; however, they may be difficult to detect. Infection with *E. histolytica* typically presents as bloody diarrhea usually without fever. Symptomatic infection with *G. lamblia* presents as watery, foul-smelling diarrhea and cramps. Symptoms of hepatitis A virus infection include abdominal pain, anorexia, and malaise, and hepatomegaly can often be found. However, high fever is not associated with this disease. A watery diarrhea, described as rice-water stools, is the typical presentation of infection with *V. cholerae*.

17 **The answer is E: Metronidazole.** This is a case of antibiotic-associated colitis, an important nosocomial infection caused by *Clostridium difficile*. This condition can develop rapidly following the initiation of antibiotic therapy. Although many antibiotics have been implicated, clindamycin and cephalosporins are among the most common antibiotics that can lead to *C. difficile* overgrowth. Diagnosis of this condition can be made by the detection of toxins produced by the bacteria and involved in the pathogenesis. Toxin A is an enterotoxin that increases permeability of the intestinal wall by disrupting intercellular tight junctions. Toxin B leads to disruption of intestinal cell cytoskeletons by causing actin within the cell to depolymerize. Metronidazole and vancomycin are used for the treatment of *C. difficile* colitis.

18 **The answer is D: Spore formation.** *Clostridium* spp. are anaerobic, spore-forming Gram-positive rods. Spores are highly resistant to environmental conditions, commonly contaminating areas within hospitals and causing infections in patients being treated with antibiotics. *C. difficile* does not grow intracellularly. It is a Gram-positive organism and thus lacks lipopolysaccharide. Shiga toxin is produced by *Shigella dysenteriae* and enterohemorrhagic *Escherichia coli*. Type III secretion systems are typically found in Gram-negative organisms.

19 **The answer is C: *Mycobacterium tuberculosis*.** The history, signs, and symptoms of this case are consistent with tuberculosis. This infection is more common among immigrants from Southeast Asia. California is one of several states from which most of the diagnoses of TB are reported. None of the other infections present in the manner described in this case. Although a cause of lung granulomas, *H. capsulatum* is not endemic to California, or to Southeast Asia. *E. granulosus* is associated with sheep-raising areas. Pulmonary infections due to *S. pneumoniae* typically have an abrupt onset. Rust-colored sputum may be produced; however, granulomas are not found. *S. typhi* presents with fever and abdominal complaints.

20 **The answer is D: Drug combination of isoniazid, rifampin, pyrazinamide, and ethambutol.** Current treatment guidelines recommend these four drugs for the first 2 months of therapy for TB. A reduction in the number of drugs after 2 months is dependent on finding no cavitation of chest radiographs and no acid-fast bacilli on sputum stain. The rationale for a four drug combination is to cover for drug-resistant organisms as well as to prevent the development of drug resistance.

21 **The answer is E: Survive intracellularly within macrophages.** A major aspect of the virulence of *Mycobacterium tuberculosis* is its ability to infect and grow within macrophages by preventing fusion of the lysosomes with the phagosome. *M. tuberculosis* does not demonstrate the other activities listed in the question.

22 **The answer is D: *Helicobacter pylori*.** This bacterial organism is involved in the pathogenesis of peptic ulcer disease, which can manifest as heartburn. A serologic test is available for diagnosis and has high sensitivity and specificity. None of the other organisms listed are associated with peptic ulcer disease. Adenoviruses cause respiratory disease or diarrhea. *C. parvum* is a sporozoite parasite associated with diarrhea. Enteroaggregative *E. coli* is a pathogenic strain of *E. coli* that causes diarrhea. *P. vulgaris* is associated with urinary tract infections that lead to struvite stone formation.

23 **The answer is D: Proton pump inhibitor plus amoxicillin and clarithromycin.** The case is descriptive of peptic ulcer disease, associated with *Helicobacter pylori* infection. This condition can be diagnosed by several means. The urease breath test is sensitive and specific for *H. pylori*; however, it requires expensive equipment. Alternatively, a stool antigen test is now available for patients without blood in their stools. In addition, enzyme immunoassay can detect anti-*H. pylori* IgG in patient's serum. Triple therapy is recommended to promote healing of the ulcer and eradicate *H. pylori* from the stomach. First-line regimens include a proton pump inhibitor as well as clarithromycin plus amoxicillin or metronidazole.

24 **The answer is C: Urea breath test.** This test is the most sensitive method to detect the eradication of *Helicobacter pylori*.

25 **The answer is B: Mumps virus.** This case is descriptive of mumps in a postpubertal male. Mumps has an incubation period of 2 weeks. Symptomatic infections in postpubertal males manifest not only as parotitis (tenderness in the submaxillary area), but can also result in orchitis. Meningitis is also a potential outcome of infection. Mumps infections have been markedly reduced in the United States due to vaccination; however, occasional outbreaks do occur in unvaccinated or under-vaccinated individuals. None of the other organisms cause this constellation of symptoms. While *H. influenzae* b, *N. meningitidis*, and *S. pneumoniae* cause meningitis and are preventable by vaccination, they are not associated with parotitis or orchitis. Respiratory syncytial virus (RSV) is the primary cause of pneumonia and bronchiolitis in infants, and an important cause of colds in older children. It is not associated with parotitis or orchitis. There is no vaccine available for RSV.

26 **The answer is C: Linezolid.**   *Enterococcus* is one of the most frequently isolated pathogens from patients on long-term hemodialysis. Enterococci, particularly *E. faecium*, are resistant to a broad range of antibiotics. Ampicillin resistance can result from altered penicillin-binding proteins or through the secretion of β-lactamases. Aminoglycoside resistance is mediated through the acquisition of genes coding for aminoglycoside-modifying enzymes. These genes are found on plasmids or transposons and are transferable to other bacteria. Vancomycin resistance, more common in *E. faecium* than in *E. faecalis*, can be induced during therapy with oral vancomycin, a potential treatment for *C. difficile*-associated colitis. TMP–SMZ shows activity when tested *in vitro* against Enterococci; however, in vivo, the bacteria can absorb folic acid from the environment. Linezolid, as well as the streptogramins (quinupristin and dalfopristin) can be used for highly resistant enterococcal infections.

27 **The answer is C: Gentamicin.**   Tinnitus and vertigo as well as nephrotoxicity are potential side effects of aminoglycosides including gentamicin. These antibiotics are often given for Gram-negative infections, and patients should be monitored for the development of toxicity while on these drugs. Azithromycin is a macrolide antibiotic that is well tolerated, but is not used for most Gram-negative infections. Clindamycin is useful for infections with some strains of *Staphylococcus* and *Streptococcus*, as well as many anaerobic infections. It is not used for Gram-negative infections. A major caution with clindamycin use is the development of *Clostridium difficile* colitis. It can also cause diarrhea and rash. Levofloxacin is a fluoroquinolone antibiotic. Fluoroquinolones are used for a wide variety of bacterial infections, particularly with Gram-negatives and atypical bacteria. A major toxicity of this group of antibiotics that limits their use especially in children and pregnant women is cartilage damage. Linezolid is an oxazolidine antibiotic used for Gram-positive infections, particularly MRSA. It is generally well tolerated.

28 **The answer is D: Fever, headache, confusion, motor weakness.**   Toxoplasmosis is a neurologic disease in AIDS patients and other severely immune compromised patients. Neurological disease in this patient population typically represents reactivation

of an old infection. Individuals become infected with *Toxoplasma gondii* either through ingestion of oocysts shed in cat feces, or ingestion of cysts in undercooked meat. Serologic evidence suggests that about 15% of adults in the United States harbor the parasite. Most infections are asymptomatic, although some people experience a mononucleosislike illness. The organism replicates as tachyzoites in muscle and brain tissue. Eventually, cysts containing bradyzoites are formed in these tissues and the organism can remain viable for years without causing harm to the infected individual. Reactivation of the parasite can occur in infected persons who become severely immune suppressed due to AIDS or organ transplantation. The parasite can also cause serious congenital neurological disease if a woman becomes infected during pregnancy.

29 **The answer is C: Human immunodeficiency virus.**   While the bacteria and fungus listed cause pulmonary disease, the clinical manifestations and acid-fast sputum results are consistent with pulmonary TB. In immune competent individuals without identifiable risk factors for TB, an area of induration of ≥15 mm is considered positive. In contrast, a ≥10 mm area of induration is considered positive for at-risk individuals including immigrants from endemic countries, intravenous drug abusers, or children. Persons infected with HIV or who have other causes of severe immune suppression are considered to have a positive TB skin test if they develop an area of induration of ≥5 mm in diameter. Thus, the patient in this case, with a positive sputum and symptoms of pulmonary TB who developed a 5 mm area of induration may be infected with HIV. In addition, the patient is in a well-documented risk group for both infections. The CDC recommends HIV screening for all TB patients.

30 **The answer is D: *Pseudomonas aeruginosa*.**   This organism, ubiquitous in water and soil, is the only one listed that produces greenish, sweet-smelling pus. Although *S. schenckii* is associated with rose thorns, it characteristically causes ulcerative lesions at the initial site with secondary nodules along the draining lymphatics.

31 **The answer is C: Piperacillin plus an aminoglycoside.**   Piperacillin is in the class of penicillins sometimes referred to as "anti-pseudomonal penicillins." Synergy with an aminoglycoside is not uncommon. The other antimicrobials listed are not effective against *Pseudomonas*.

32 **The answer is E: *Shigella sonnei*.**   *Shigella*, like all of the Enterobacteriaceae can be isolated from stool on MacConkey agar. *Shigella* sp. is the cause of bacillary dysentery. There are four species, *S. sonnei*, *S. flexneri*,

S. boydii, and *S. dysenteriae.* All species infect the large intestine. While *S. flexneri, S. boydii,* and *S. dysenteriae* are found in developing countries, *S. sonnei* occurs in developed countries. Clinical manifestations of *S. sonnei* infection are the mildest, usually resulting in watery diarrhea. Fecal examination reveals the presence of neutrophils, indicating an invasive process; however blood in the stool is rare with *S. sonnei.* In contrast, infection with *S. dysenteriae* is most severe, resulting in fever, tenesmus, abdominal cramps, and frequent mucoid and bloody stools. Infection with *S. flexneri,* the most common *Shigella* sp. in developing countries and *S. boydii,* an uncommon cause of infection, results in symptoms similar to *S. dysenteriae.* Infection with enterotoxigenic *E. coli* presents as watery diarrhea; however, this organism is found in developing countries and is a common cause of traveler's diarrhea. Infection with *E. coli* O157:H7 results in bloody diarrhea. Infection with *S. typhi* does not occur in the United States, and does not present with watery diarrhea. Watery diarrhea can result from food poisoning due to *B. cereus;* however, fecal leukocytes would not be found and this organism is not isolated on MacConkey agar.

33 **The answer is C: Epstein–Barr virus.** The mass described is Burkitt lymphoma. This B-cell lymphoma occurs on the face or jaw of children in malaria-endemic areas of Africa. The virus induces a translocation of the *c-myc* oncogene from chromosome 8 to chromosome 14 near the promoter for the immunoglobulin heavy chain genes. Relocation of *c-myc* to this transcriptionally active area allows for the aberrant expression of the oncogene protein, and subsequent transformation of the cell. Additional evidence of the role of EBV in tumorigenesis is provided by the finding of EBV DNA and Epstein–Barr nuclear antigen-1 in tumor cells.

34 **The answer is A: *Cryptococcus neoformans.*** This is a typical presentation of *C. neoformans*-induced meningitis. It occurs most commonly in T-cell immune suppressed individuals such as those with AIDS. Its onset is typically insidious rather than sudden, and it can wax and wane in severity delaying time of diagnosis by several weeks. The most common presenting symptom is headache, although changes in mental status such as confusion may occur as well, especially as the disease progresses. Papilledema is a common sign of meningeal inflammation. Stiff neck is another common indicator if meningitis is often absent in patients with *C. neoformans* meningitis. The CSF analysis is typical of nonbacterial meningitis (mononuclear pleocytosis, mildly increased protein, and moderately decreased glucose). India ink staining of the CSF shows encapsulated budding yeasts in 25% to 50% of patients; thus a negative India ink smear

should not be considered conclusive. Tests to detect polysaccharide capsular antigens are positive in about 90% of patients. Alternatively, diagnosis can be made by culture of the organism on routine fungal medias. *Haemophilus* and *Listeria* are ruled out as possibilities, even though *Haemophilus* has a polysaccharide capsule, because both would elicit a neutrophilic pleocytosis. *M. tuberculosis* can present with meningitis and can cause mononuclear pleocytosis; however it lacks a polysaccharide capsule and is not diagnosed by antigen detection in the CSF. Instead, an acid-fast stain of centrifuged CSF may detect the organism. More typically, cultures and/or PCR provide diagnosis of *M. tuberculosis* meningeal infections.

35 **The answer is E: *Nocardia asteroides.*** Several clues in the case point to this organism. The patient had a chronic pulmonary disease and was immune suppressed due to frequent exposure to oral prednisone. Most patients with nocardiasis are immune suppressed (secondary to cancer, transplantation, diabetes, AIDS, or corticosteroid use) or have a chronic pulmonary disease. Pulmonary nocardiasis may show cavitations, as does tuberculosis and less commonly chronic histoplasmosis or coccidioidomycosis; however, other radiographic patterns also occur. *Nocardia* stains weakly Gram-positive and is partially acid fast (does not uniformly pick up the acid-fast stain). It has a beaded appearance in stained specimens as shown in the picture. Growth of the organism is slow, and rapidly growing commensal organisms in sputum can prevent detectable growth of *Nocardia.* Thus, if this organism is suspected, the laboratory should be advised to culture on a selective media such as BCYE, a medium used for the isolation of *Legionella.* The filamentous appearance of *Nocardia* in stained specimens and the formation of aerial hyphae in culture resemble fungi. *Histoplasma,* however, does not appear as filaments in sputum. Rather, yeast forms can be seen in sputum stained with giemsa or periodic acid-Schiff. Although pulmonary disease can result from infection with *Coccidioides immitis,* it appears in sputum as endosporulating spherules. Culture of *Histoplasma* and *Coccidioides* is normally done on mycologic media such as brain–heart infusion (BHI) agar or Sabouraud dextrose and BHI (SABHI) agar.

36 **The answer is D: Inhalation of the bacterium in soil.** *Nocardia* is a ubiquitous organism found in soil and water. It is not transmitted person-to-person. Arthroconidia and microconidia are the infectious forms of *Coccidioides* and *Histoplasma,* respectively. None of the organisms listed in the above form tissue cysts.

37 **The answer is C: Meningitis.** The classic signs of meningitis are headache, fever and stiff neck or nuchal rigidity. Muscle spasms in the back of the neck occur secondary to meningeal irritation and lead to nuchal rigidity in many patients. Vomiting is a frequent symptom in meningitis and may occur as a consequence of elevated intracerebral pressure and/or brainstem irritation Kernig and Brudzinski signs are maneuvers commonly used to make a clinical diagnosis of meningitis; however, they are not uniformly positive in patients with this disease.

38 The answer is E: Voriconazole. The photograph depicts the fungus, *Aspergillus*. *Aspergillus* and *Candida* are the most common fungal infections in neutropenic cancer patients. The only antifungal drug listed is voriconazole, which is the drug of choice for invasive aspergillosis.

39 The answer is D: Permethrin. This is a case of crusted scabies. This condition most commonly affects individuals with immunodeficiency disorders. The second micrograph depicts a sexually adult female mite, which readily burrows into the epidermis. The crusted lesions teem with hordes of mites, thus allowing the clinician to make an accurate diagnosis with a modicum of effort. Five percentage of permethrin is one of the treatment options. Both albendazole and praziquantel are typically used to treat helminth infections. Griseofulvin is an antifungal drug and metronidazole is most commonly used to treat infections with anaerobic bacteria.

40 The answer is E: Ulceroglandular tularemia. This is the most common form of tularemia diagnosed in the United States. Tularemia, caused by *Francisella tularensis*, is endemic to the Midwest and some Western States. This patient most likely acquired the disease through the tick bite, although deer flies can also transmit the infection. Infection can also result from contact with the tissues of infected animals such as rabbits. After seroconversion, an immunodiagnosis is possible, but sufficient time probably has not passed in this case. *F. tularensis* has an extremely low infective dose, and, therefore, a high potent for accidental transmission in the hospital laboratory. Isolation and identification of the Gram-negative coccobacillus requires a facility rated for a biosafety level three category. In this case, diagnosis and treatment based on the clinical presentation is appropriate. Streptomycin therapy is considered the standard of care. Other aminoglycosides may also prove to be efficacious, however. For Lyme disease, erythema migrans at the bite site would be more likely. Endemic typhus is a fleaborne rickettsial disease that is produces a rash. Human granulocytotropic anaplasmosis and human monocytic ehrlichiosis are not commonly found in Utah.

41 The answer is A: Acid-fast bacilli. The case described is of miliary tuberculosis with meningitis. This form of tuberculosis is characterized by dissemination of the organism throughout the body. Miliary TB is most common in the very young or elderly, the immune suppressed, as well as those with chronic conditions such as alcoholics, cancer patients, or patients with connective tissue disorders. Its onset is insidious, and patients present as described in the case. The majority of patients with miliary tuberculosis show evidence of nodules resembling millet seeds in the lung. Meningeal involvement frequently leads to dysfunction of cranial nerves III, IV, and VI, manifested as abnormal eye movements and papillary responses. The CSF findings in tuberculosis meningitis are consistent with those described in the case. In contrast, CSF findings in acute bacterial meningitis include neutrophilic pleocytosis, very low glucose, and elevated protein.

42 The answer is C: Indirect immunofluorescence testing. The Weil–Felix test, used in the past for the diagnosis of rickettsial infections, is based on the cross reaction of antibodies to *Rickettsia* and *Proteus*. This test is nonspecific and insensitive and is no longer used. Instead, diagnosis is confirmed most commonly by detecting antibodies to the organism in the patient's serum. This can be done by indirect immunofluorescence, latex agglutination, or enzyme immunoassay. Culture of the organism from the blood can be done, but is limited to reference laboratories. Rickettsial organisms do not grow on bacteriologic agars, but instead must be cultivated in cells. The organisms do not pick up a Gram stain, although they will pick up Giemsa or Gimenez stains.

43 The answer is E: Viral. Viruses are the most common cause of meningitis. Viral infection of the meninges is known as aseptic meningitis. This disease is less severe than bacterial meningitis. Whereas viral meningitis may not require hospitalization, bacterial meningitis is a medical emergency requiring prompt clinical diagnosis and administration of empiric antibiotics. To avoid unnecessary hospitalization and administration of antibiotics, it is essential to be able to distinguish between septic (bacterial) and aseptic meningitis. CSF findings help make this distinction. Enteroviruses, specifically coxsackieviruses and echoviruses cause the greatest number of cases of aseptic meningitis. These viruses are common infections of children and adults with close contact with children. They show a seasonal occurrence, with most cases occurring in the summer and early fall. *S. pneumoniae* and *N. meningitidis* are important cause of meningitis in both children and adults. Vaccination has decreased the occurrence of these two causes of meningitis. *C. neoformans* is a cause of meningitis in immune suppressed individuals.

44 **The answer is B: Lymphocytes, normal glucose, elevated protein.** These are typical CSF findings for persons with viral meningitis. Bacterial meningitis typically results in CSF findings of neutrophils, low glucose and elevated protein while the CSF in fungal or tuberculosis meningitis typically shows lymphocytes, decreased glucose and elevated protein.

45 **The answer is D: *Leptospira interrogans*.** The most plausible diagnosis is Weil disease, caused by *L. interrogans*. Leptospirosis is a zoonotic disease transmitted to people by rodents (including synanthropic rats of the inner city). Individuals who handle these animals or other types of wild animals are the most likely candidates to contract the infection, especially if mucous membranes or broken skin is contaminated with positive urine. *Leptospira* organisms can be identified from the patient's urine or tissue via darkfield microscopy or direct fluorescent-antibody staining, although these techniques are insensitive. Culture of the organism on specialized medium may take 2 weeks or longer. The finding of antibodies in the patient's serum to the organism is the preferred method of diagnosis. Like syphilitic spirochetes, leptospires are sensitive to β-lactam and tetracycline antibiotics. *B. microti*, arenaviruses, and hantaviruses are zoonotic infections with rodent hosts. Babesiosis does not present as described in the case, and the organism is restricted to the coastal regions of the northeast United States. Lymphocytic choriomeningitis virus, an Arenavirus, most commonly causes a self-limiting flulike illness, although meningitis can also occur. Other arenaviruses are found in South America or Africa. Hantavirus in the United States is associated with rapidly progressive respiratory distress. *T. gondii* infection is most commonly associated with contact with oocysts in cat feces, or transplacental transmission. If infected as an adult, it is often asymptomatic, or may result in a mononucleosislike syndrome.

46 **The answer is D: Ehrlichiosis.** The case is most descriptive of human monocytic ehrlichiosis (*Ehrlichia chaffeensis*), an emerging disease that attacks the hematopoietic system. It has been reported from the Eastern and Midwestern United States. A primary risk factor is contact with ticks (e.g., *Dermacentor variabilis*, *Amblyomma americanum*), especially during the warm-weather months when tick infestations are most likely. In most cases, an empirical diagnosis is not feasible; however, a history of a tick bite in an endemic area, a CBC that is remarkable for leucopenia and possibly thrombocytopenia, monocytes with morulae (characteristic clusters of the cocci within a cytoplasmic vacuole), and an indirect fluorescent antibody test of greater than 1:128 is sufficient evidence for a firm diagnosis. Middle-aged individuals are more likely to present with symptoms. Headaches, myalgia, malaise, and gastrointestinal disturbances further characterize the disease. Ehrlichiosis can be fatal, especially in the elderly. The drug of choice is doxycycline, and treatment should be initiated early for favorable prognosis, definitely before laboratory confirmatory results are available.

47 **The answer is D: *Pseudomonas* malignant otitis externa.** This disease occurs in immune compromised individuals, particularly those with diabetes. It is an invasive infection of the external ear which can spread to involve nearby cartilage and bone. Malignant otitis externa is most commonly caused by *Pseudomonas*. An aminoglycoside in synergy with a third-generation cephalosporin is commonly used to treat pseudomonal infections. The other diseases listed do not fit the clinical picture described in the case, nor would this combination of antibiotics be typical for treatment.

48 **The answer is E: *Streptococcus pyogenes*.** All of the organisms listed can cause febrile pharyngitis; however, *S. pyogenes* is the most common bacterial cause. It is the only pharyngitis pathogen for which in-office serologic tests are available.

49 **The answer is C: Levofloxacin plus vancomycin.** The man in the case developed nosocomial pneumonia, the most common causes of which are Gram-negative rods and *Staphylococcus aureus*. Gram-negative rods that may be involved in nosocomial pneumonia include the Enterobacteriaceae (*Escherichia coli*, *Klebsiella*, *Serratia*, and *Enterobacter*), *Pseudomonas aeruginosa*, and *Legionella pneumophila*. *S. aureus* strains include both methicillin-sensitive *S. aureus* (MSSA) and methicillin-resistant *S. aureus* (MRSA). Empiric antimicrobials must provide coverage for these organisms. Levofloxacin provides coverage for the Gram-negative rods as well as MSSA. Vancomycin provides coverage for MRSA. None of the other antimicrobial regimens listed provide coverage for all the organisms involved in nosocomial pneumonia.

50 **The answer is D: *Pseudomonas aeruginosa*.** While all of the organisms listed can cause pneumonia, only *P. aeruginosa* and *L. pneumophila* are common causes of nosocomial pneumonia. Further, only *P. aeruginosa* fits the characteristics of the organism described. *A. flavus* and *P. jiroveci* are fungi. *K. pneumoniae*, a Gram-negative rod is not noted for pigment production, and is more typically grown on MacConkey agar. *L. pneumophila* does not easily pick up a Gram stain, does not grow on nutrient agar, and does not produce pigments.

51 **The answer is D: Clindamycin.** Penicillin is a β-lactam antibiotic. Serious allergies to penicillin dictate avoidance of other β-lactams due to the possibility of immunologic cross-reactivity with the breakdown products of penicillin, penicilloyl, and penicillanic acid. Clindamycin is the only antibiotic listed that is not a β-lactam. Although aztreonam lacks the side chain responsible for β-lactam allergies, and can be used safely in penicillin-allergic patients, it does not bind to the penicillin-binding proteins of Gram-positive organisms, and thus cannot be used in this case.

52 **The answer is E: Subacute endocarditis—Viridans group streptococci.** This case is descriptive of subacute endocarditis and the most common cause of this condition is Viridans group streptococci. Acute endocarditis shares much of the same findings; however, the onset is rapid. It most often occurs in injection drug users. The other diseases listed do not have this classic presentation.

53 **The answer is D: Pertussis.** Aspects of the case which are consistent with a diagnosis of pertussis include the violent cough spells that end with vomiting, the preceding catarrhal phase of the disease, the lack of vaccination history, and the respiratory illness in other family members. Also consistent with a diagnosis of pertussis is the lymphocytosis, and the mild dehydration, presumably stemming from poor feeding as well as vomiting. The characteristic whoop of pertussis may not be heard in an infant younger than 6 months of age. *Bordetella pertussis* is transmitted person-to-person. Vaccination is recommended for all infants; however immunity wanes over time and older children and adults are considered reservoirs of the disease. Pneumonia or bronchiolitis in an infant of this age would be associated with RSV infection. Wheezing and rales would be an expected finding by auscultation. Chest radiographs in RSV infection typically show hyperinflation and diffuse infiltrates in both lung fields. Stridor is typically heard in infants with croup, and chest radiographs often show a steeple sign secondary to edema in the subglottic area. Cough is rare in epiglottis, and in this disease, an enlarged epiglottis would be seen on neck radiographs.

54 **The answer is E: Symptomatically.** The case is descriptive of infectious mononucleosis due to Epstein–Barr virus infection. There is no antimicrobial treatment available for this infection and it is generally treated symptomatically to reduce fever and pain. Acyclovir is used to treat herpes simplex virus and varicella-zoster virus. Amphotericin is used to treat serious fugal infections. Corticosteroids are not used in uncomplicated cases of infectious mononucleosis such as the one described here. They may be required in cases involving hematologic complications such as hemolytic anemia or thrombocytopenia or if enlarged tonsils or cervical lymph nodes threaten closure of the airways. Penicillin is an antibiotic that can be used for streptococcal pharyngitis; however, although some of the symptoms are similar (exudative pharyngitis, cervical lymphadenopathy, and fever), it is not the patient's diagnosis.

55 **The answer is B: Cytomegalovirus.** All of the organisms listed cause perinatal infections. The incidence of congenital cytomegalovirus (CMV) in the United States is 1,000/100,000 births. Congenital CMV results when a pregnant woman has a primary infection or reactivation of a latent CMV infection. Infants born to mothers who experience primary infections during pregnancy are far more likely to present as described in this case. Manifestations of congenital CMV at birth include low birth weight, petechiae, hepatosplenomegaly, jaundice, microcephaly, deafness, and chorioretinitis. Most congenitally infected infants, however, are born to mothers with reactivated CMV and are more likely to be asymptomatic at birth. Late manifestations of congenital CMV can occur in asymptomatic and symptomatic infants and include sensorineural hearing loss which can develop months to years after birth. Routine screening for CMV during pregnancy is currently not done. Pregnant women should be advised to take extra precautions during pregnancy to avoid exposure to CMV in saliva and urine of young children. *C. trachomatis* is acquired by infants during birth and most commonly results in eye infections characterized by purulent ocular discharge (ophthalmia neonatorum) developing about 1 week after birth. Pneumonia can also occur about 2 to 3 weeks after birth. Acquisition of Group B *Streptococcus* by infants also occurs during birth, with manifestations developing after about 1 week. Bacteremia, shock, and pneumonia are most common; meningitis, septic arthritis, and osteomyelitis can also occur. Congenital rubella can result in a variety of manifestations depending on the age of the fetus at the time of infection. Some of these manifestations are present at birth, including low birth weight, a rash described as "blueberry muffin rash," microcephaly, and hepatosplenomegaly. The classic triad of congenital rubella virus infection is deafness, patent ductus arteriosus, and cataracts. Late onset manifestations, particularly deafness, but also mental retardation, intellectual impairment, and language disorders can occur. Congenital infection with *T. gondii* has the worst outcome if the mother acquires a primary infection during the first trimester. Congenitally infected infants are born with intracranial calcifications, hydrocephalus, microcephaly, and chorioretinitis and suffer from encephalitis and seizures.

56 **The answer is B: Ganciclovir.** This antiviral is recommended for individuals, including neonates, with symptomatic CMV infections. Infants with symptomatic congenital CMV treated with ganciclovir have been reported to show improved outcomes, particularly in the rate of deafness. Erythromycin is used to treat infants infected with *Chlamydia trachomatis*. Penicillin is used to treat infants with group B streptococcal infections. Pyrimethamine and sulfadiazine are used to treat immunocompromised adults and congenitally infected infants with toxoplasmosis. No specific antimicrobial treatment is available for infants with congenital rubella syndrome (CRS). The wide-spread use of the measles, mumps, and rubella (MMR) vaccine in children has dramatically reduced the incidence of CRS in the United States.

57 **The answer is C: Change to itraconazole to cover for *Histoplasma capsulatum*.** The history suggests the patient became infected while spelunking in the Ozark Mountains. Outbreaks of histoplasmosis have occurred from exposures to soils from caves rich in bat guano or soil rich in bird droppings such as chicken coops or decaying buildings. Transmission occurs by inhalation of macroconidia found in abundance in such soils. The hilar lymphadenopathy and patchy infiltrates seen on the chest radiograph are supportive of acute pulmonary histoplasmosis. The negative culture results on standard bacteriologic media rule out typical bacterial causes of community-acquired pneumonia such as *Streptococcus pneumoniae*. The growth of the organism on brain–heart infusion agar with antibiotics and cycloheximide supports the diagnosis of fungal pneumonia while the finding of *Histoplasma* antigens in the urine confirms the diagnosis. The drug of choice for acute pulmonary histoplasmosis is itraconazole. Although *Coccidioides immitis* can cause similar pulmonary symptoms, this endemic fungus is found in the deserts of the southwestern United States. None of the bacterial species listed grow on standard bacteriologic media. *Chlamydia psittaci* can cause pneumonia; however, *Chlamydia* spp. are intracellular organisms and must be grown on cultured cells, not agar. *Mycoplasma* can also cause similar symptoms, but is not generally diagnosed by culture results due to its fastidious nature and slow growth. In addition, penicillin is not used to treat *Mycoplasma* infections. This organism lacks a cell wall; thus penicillin, a cell wall inhibitor, is of no use against this agent. *Legionella* is cultured on buffered-charcoal yeast extract agar and a standard dose of azithromycin is the drug of choice

58 **The answer is C: Ramsey Hunt syndrome.** This syndrome is seen when herpes zoster (shingles) involves the geniculate ganglion of the seventh cranial nerve. The classic signs of this condition include the rash of shingles with lesions occurring in and around the ear canal on the affected side, vertigo and facial paralysis on the affected side. None of the other choices present in the manner described in this case. Brown recluse spider bites result in a necrotic and ulcerative skin lesion which enlarges over time at the site of the bite. Erysipelas is an infection of the superficial layers of the skin most commonly due to Group A *Streptococcus* (GAS). Impetigo is a superficial pyoderma, caused by GAS or *Staphylococcus aureus*. Tabes dorsalis is a form of progressive ataxia associated with neurosyphilis.

59 **The answer is D: Postherpetic neuralgia.** Postherpetic neuralgia (PHN) is one of the most common complications of shingles, regardless of where on the body the rash occurs. The risk of PHN following shingles is high in patients over the age of 70. Complications of Ramsey Hunt syndrome are not as common, but include persistent facial weakness and hearing loss. Encephalitis is very rare in patients with shingles. Eye involvement in herpes zoster typically involves structures of the eye itself (eyelids, conjunctiva, sclera, cornea, or anterior chamber), not the optic nerve. Parkinson disease and temporal arteritis are not complications of herpes zoster.

60 **The answer is C: Coxsackievirus B.** All of the organisms listed can cause myocarditis; however, the most common cause of infection-induced myocarditis is Coxsackievirus B.

61 **The answer is D: Metronidazole.** The photograph shows trophozoites of *Giardia lamblia*, an important cause of watery diarrhea in daycare and other institutional settings. The drug of choice for this infection is metronidazole, although tinidazole, furazolidone, or quinacrine can also be used.

62 **The answer is E: Strep throat.** Chronic rheumatic heart disease, which results from repeat episodes of rheumatic fever, is a cause of chronic valvular stenosis. Rheumatic fever results from pharyngeal infection with certain strains of group A *Streptococcus*. None of the other childhood infectious diseases listed are associated with valvular stenosis.

63 **The answer is D: HACEK group.** HACEK refers to the following Gram-negative bacilli which are part of the normal flora of the oral cavity: *Haemophilus aphrophilus* or other *Haemophilus* sp. (*H. parainfluenzae* and *H. paraphrophilus*), *Actinobacillus actinomycetemcomitans*, *Cardiobacterium hominis*, *Eikenella corrodens*, and *Kingella kingae*. They are slow growing bacteria requiring as much as 2 weeks before being detectable in blood cultures. The HACEK group cause 5% to 10% of cases of infective endocarditis, and should be suspected in all cases of culture-negative endocarditis. HACEK group endocarditis is seen in patients with poor dental hygiene or who have a history of recent dental procedures. The photograph shows Gram-negative bacilli. The other organisms listed are important causes of culture-positive endocarditis, and are all Gram-positive cocci. Coagulase-negative staphylococci are especially important causes of prosthetic valve endocarditis. *Staphylococcus aureus* is coagulase-positive and is overall the most common cause of endocarditis. This species is especially important as a cause of infective endocarditis in injection drug users. Enterococci are the third most common cause of endocarditis, and occur particularly in patients with intestinal disease. Viridans group streptococci are the most common cause of native valve endocarditis.

64 **The answer is D: Epiglottitis.** Epiglottitis is a serious childhood condition with both infectious and noninfectious causes. Life-threatening airway obstruction makes this disease a medical emergency which may require intubation. Infectious causes of epiglottitis include *Staphylococcus aureus*, *Streptococcus pneumoniae*, *Haemophilus influenzae*, Group A *Streptococcus*, and even some respiratory viruses. Prior to widespread use of the vaccine, most cases of epiglottitis were caused by *H. influenzae* b. Recommended empiric therapy is ceftriaxone. The other respiratory conditions listed do not present in this alarming fashion and do not lead to intubation. Bronchiolitis and croup are common in young children and are most commonly viral in origin. Diphtheria can cause airway obstruction requiring mechanical ventilation. Typically, physical exam reveals a pseudomembrane covering the mucosa of the tonsils, uvula, and palate, and the patient is treated with antitoxin as well as erythromycin or penicillin. Patients with pertussis present with paroxysmal cough with intermittent gasps for air. Coughing fits can end with vomiting. Antibiotics are not effective at this stage of the infection, but can be used in the catarrhal phase to prevent the progress of the disease. Erythromycin or other macrolides are recommended for this purpose.

65 **The answer is E: Respiratory syncytial virus.** The case is descriptive of bronchiolitis, a lower respiratory tract infection. Lower respiratory infections in infants are most commonly viral in origin. All of the organisms listed can cause this condition; however, respiratory syncytial virus (RSV) is by far the most common cause. Infection of the epithelial cells of the small airways by RSV causes inflammation and edema, increasing the work of respiration. Infants present as in this case with rapid breathing, wheezing, and cyanosis. The chest radiographs show hyperinflation, and sometimes a diffuse infiltrate.

66 **The answer is B: Invasive cervical carcinoma.** This cancer is considered an AIDS defining condition. The other options listed are indicative of progression of disease, and/or poor control of virus replication but are not included in the case definition of AIDS.

67 **The answer is D: Rotavirus/Oral rehydration therapy.** Rotavirus is the most common cause of nonbloody, watery diarrhea worldwide. It causes an estimated 2.7 million infections in children less than 5 years of age in the United States, resulting in 410,000 office visits and at least 272,000 emergency department visits. An estimated 55,000 to 70,000 children are hospitalized each year with this infection in the United States. Most children can be treated symptomatically with oral rehydration. Despite the relative ease of treatment, this virus remains a major cause of mortality among young children in developing countries causing an estimated 600,000 childhood deaths each year. *E. coli* K1 is a cause of urinary tract infections. Trimethoprim–sulfamethoxazole is one of the recommended treatment regimens for this infection. Enteroinvasive *E. coli* is a rare cause of watery diarrhea, which can progress to dysentery. It is generally treated symptomatically. *G. lamblia* is an important cause of watery diarrhea in the United States and is treated with metronidazole. It is not nearly as common as rotavirus. *Shigella dysenteriae*, an important cause of bloody diarrhea in developing countries, rarely occurs in the United States. Most shigellosis in the United States is attributed to *S. sonnei* or *S. flexneri*. Ampicillin is no longer recommended for empiric treatment due to increasing rates of resistance.

68 **The answer is E: Vaccination.** All of the choices listed can reduce the likelihood of infection with rotavirus, but vaccination is the most effective. The agent is transmitted by a fecal-oral route and is very stable in the environment. Thus, infection following contact with contaminated surfaces as well as person-to-person transmission is possible. Infections are more likely in children attending daycare. Breast feeding helps protect infants from infection, delaying the age of first infection until the child is no longer being breast fed. Chlorine-containing disinfectants are important for reducing transmission of rotavirus, as is frequent hand washing. Vaccination is recommended for prevention of serious infection in infants. Two versions of the vaccine have been approved by the FDA. The RotaTeq vaccine, approved in 2006 is live, oral vaccine administered to children at 2, 4, and 6 months of age. The Rotarix vaccine, approved in 2008, is a live, attenuated vaccine administered orally in two doses to children beginning at 6 weeks of age.

69 **The answer is C: Pyrazinamide.** Hyperuricemia is the principle toxicity of this drug. High levels of uric acid in the blood can lead to gouty arthritis. Other risk factors for gout in this case are age (peak onset of gout in the 40s), gender (more common in males), obesity, and alcohol use. All of the drugs listed are considered first-line drugs for the treatment of tuberculosis. As treatment requires at least 26 weeks to complete, even less common toxicities can manifest, and physicians must be familiar with these. A major toxicity of ethambutol is optic neuritis. Isoniazid is associated with rash, fever, peripheral neuropathy, and hepatotoxicity. Drug interactions are of concern with rifampin as this drug induces the cytochrome P-450 system. Additionally, rifampin is associated with hepatotoxicity and can cause an orange–red discoloration of tears and urine. Streptomycin can cause ototoxicity leading to hearing loss and vertigo. It can also elevate creatinine levels.

70 **The answer is A: *Candida albicans*.** The case is descriptive of esophagitis. *Candida* is the most common infectious cause of esophagitis and is seen especially in cancer patients and AIDS patients. Cytomegalovirus and herpes simplex virus are also potential causes of esophagitis; however, ulcerations would be seen on endoscopy. The patient is at risk for *Candida* esophagitis due to his neutropenia. Candidal infections are controlled immunologically by phagocytes.

71 **The answer is C: Poliomyelitis.** Hand washing and good community sanitation together are most effective at reducing infections transmitted by a fecal-oral route. Community sanitation efforts involve improved disposal of human waste and provision of safe drinking water. Poliomyelitis is caused by polioviruses which are transmitted by a fecal-oral route. Even without vaccination, this disease can be reduced through improvements in community sanitation. Influenza and tuberculosis are transmitted by infectious aerosols. Hand washing is important to reduce transmission of influenza; however, reduction in cases relies on annual vaccination. Reduction in the transmission of tuberculosis relies on the identification and treatment of infected individuals. Malaria is a protozoan disease transmitted by mosquitoes. Eradication efforts are aimed at reducing vector mosquito populations and preventing mosquito bites with insecticide-impregnated bed nets. Schistosomiasis is associated with exposure to fresh water containing infected snails that serve as an intermediate host for the schistosome parasites. The cercarial form of this trematode parasite burrows through the skin of humans bathing or washing clothes in or engaging in agricultural activities while standing in fresh water. Schistosome eggs are shed in the feces or urine of infected humans, and the life cycle of the parasite continues if human waste contaminates fresh water rivers, streams, and irrigation ditches. Thus, improved community sanitation

is important for eradication of schistosomiasis. Hand washing will not reduce the incidence of this disease.

72 **The answer is E: Scrapie-infected sheep.** Scrapie, a neurological disease of sheep and goats, is caused by a proteinaceous infectious particle, or prion (PrP). These proteins are similar to a protein found in normal cells, particularly cells of the central nervous system. Abnormal prions, referred to as PrP^{Sc}, are associated with a group of diseases called spongiform encephalopathies so called because of the spongiform change seen in the brains of affected animals or humans. The large vacuoles seen in the photograph are the characteristic finding of spongiform encephalopathy. Infectious prions have no nucleic acid and replicate by binding to normal cellular prions causing refolding and polymerization of the normal proteins. Accumulation of this now abnormal version of the prion protein (PrP^{Sc}) causes cell death. British cattle became infected with the scrapie agent when rendering practices changed in the 1970s. This change in the processing of animal feed unwittingly allowed infectious prions from scrapie-infected sheep to be present in sheep byproducts used in cattle feed. Cattle infected with the scrapie prion developed a new disease that came to be known as mad cow disease. Tens of thousands of cases of this bovine disease occurred in Britain in the 1980s and 1990s. Many of the affected cattle entered the human food chain before efforts to control this new disease began. The first human case of spongiform encephalopathy derived from mad cow disease was diagnosed at postmortem in a young British man in 1995. Efforts to control the bovine disease and prevent further human cases lead to the culling of millions of cattle. Almost 200 human cases of what became known as variant Creutzfeldt–Jacob disease have occurred, primarily in Great Britain. Other spongiform encephalopathies believed to be due to infectious prions include chronic wasting disease of deer and elk, transmissible mink encephalopathy and feline spongiform encephalopathy. Creutzfeldt–Jacob disease is a rare human spongiform encephalopathy that occurs sporadically, and to a lesser extent, within families. The sporadic form is thought to be due to a spontaneous change in the normal prion protein into the disease-causing conformation. This altered conformational version binds to more normal prion protein, causing it too to change conformation and accumulate within the cell, ultimately leading to cell death. Thus, this disease is not due to an infectious prion, and did not give rise to variant Creutzfeldt–Jacob disease. Kuru was a human spongiform encephalopathy found in Papua New Guinea and transmitted by cannibalism. This disease has been eradicated with the outlawing of cannibalistic rituals. Bovine tuberculosis does not cause spongiform encephalopathy.

73 **The answer is B: Epstein–Barr virus.** Causes of ring-enhancing lesions in the brain of AIDS patients include EBV-associated lymphomas, toxoplasmosis, and cryptococcosis. The neurological disease described in this case is due to CNS lymphoma. The diagnosis of CNS lymphoma is aided by the finding of EBV DNA by PCR of the CSF. EBV is an oncogenic virus which is causally related to primary CNS lymphomas in AIDS patients. This disease arises in AIDS patients with CD4 counts of less than 100/µL. Its incidence has dropped dramatically since the introduction of highly active antiretroviral therapy. Cytomegalovirus causes encephalitis in AIDS patients, and the occurrence of herpes simplex encephalitis is not increased in patients with immune suppression. The diagnosis of CMV and HSV encephalitis is aided by the demonstration of viral DNA by PCR, and a lymphocytic pleocytosis can be seen; however, the cells are not malignant appearing. St Louis encephalitis virus causes encephalitis especially in the elderly, and is diagnosed by demonstration of antiviral IgM in the cerebral spinal fluid. JC virus is the cause of progressive multifocal leukoencephalopathy which often presents with focal neurologic signs including hemiparesis, ataxia, aphasia, or cortical blindness. Both JC virus and St Louis encephalitis virus are RNA viruses.

74 **The answer is C: Clotrimazole.** This case is descriptive of vaginal candidiasis. Antibiotics usage can kill normal bacterial flora in the vagina, allowing candidal organisms to grow unchecked. A thick white discharge and pruritis are characteristic of this condition. Of the antimicrobials listed, only clotrimazole is an antifungal. Cidofovir is an antiviral used for cytomegalovirus infections. Clindamycin is an antibiotic used for anaerobic infections, and can also be used for some infections with Gram-positive cocci. Metronidazole is also used for anaerobic bacterial infections, as well as infections with the protozoan parasites, Giardia lamblia and Trichomonas vaginalis. Vaginitis due to T. vaginalis is acquired sexually and not associated with antibiotic usage. In addition, it causes a thin grayish-white discharge. Ofloxacin is a respiratory fluoroquinolone.

75 **The answer is A: Chlamydia trachomatis.** This organism has a life cycle which includes two morphologically and metabolically distinct forms, the elementary body and the reticulate body. The elementary body is the metabolically inactive, infectious form of the organism that emerges from infected cells and is transmitted to other hosts. The reticulate form develops once the elementary body enters a cell within a phagosome. It is larger and metabolically active, replicating by binary fission. Genital discharges are also caused by N. gonorrhoeae, which grows on Thayer–Martin agar and T. vaginalis detected on microscopic examination of the discharge. A discharge may be present in primary genital herpes infections; however, genital herpes is characterized as an ulcerative disease. Primary infection with T. pallidum also leads to genital ulcers.

76 **The answer is D: Nucleic acid amplification.** This type of test is highly specific and is more sensitive and rapid than cell culture. Antigen detection is considerably less sensitive. Neither cytology nor serology is used to diagnose infections with this organism.

77 **The answer is A: Conjunctivitis.** Neonatal infection with Chlamydia trachomatis can result in purulent eye infections about 1 to 2 weeks after birth or pneumonia 2 to 3 weeks after birth. Hydrops fetalis is a potential outcome of in utero infection with parvovirus B-19. Late onset deafness can occur in congenital cytomegalovirus or congenital rubella virus infections. Meningitis can result from perinatal infections with a variety of bacteria, particularly Escherichia coli, Listeria monocytogenes and group B Streptococcus. Patent ductus arteriosus is a part of the classic triad of congenital rubella syndrome.

78 **The answer is E: Trypanosoma cruzi.** The case is descriptive of myocarditis in chronic Chagas disease. T. cruzi is a flagellated protozoan parasite transmitted by reduviid bugs and endemic to areas of South and central America. None of the other organisms listed are transmitted by this vector, although some are or can be vectorborne. With the exception of R. akari all can cause cardiac manifestations. B. burgdorferi, the causative agent of Lyme disease, is transmitted by ticks. Myocarditis can occur in patients with Lyme disease. C. hominis is a member of the HACEK group of Gram-negative bacilli found as mouth flora and cause culture-negative endocarditis. C. burnetii is the cause of Q fever, a disease characterized as a flulike illness which can progress to mild pneumonia. Human infection with this organism is usually acquired by inhalation of the organism in soil contaminated with livestock feces, birth fluids, or dried placental material; however, ticks transmit the organism among livestock. Chronic infections can lead to endocarditis. R. akari causes rickettsialpox, a mite-borne disease characterized by high fever, chills, myalgia, and a generalized rash. No cardiac disease occurs in rickettsialpox.

79 **The answer is A: Herpes simplex virus isolation from the skin lesions.** This case is descriptive of neonatal herpes. Infants are exposed to herpes virus during birth, and symptoms develop weeks later. The most serious neonatal disease results from women who have a primary infection around the time of delivery. In this instance, if lesions were present and detected by the physician, the infant would be delivered by caesarian section. Most commonly, the mother does not have lesions at the time of delivery, and not infrequently, persons with the virus are unaware of their infection status. No prenatal screening is done for genital herpes. Infants can present with infection of the skin, eyes, and mouth (SEM), encephalitis, or disseminated disease. The SEM form has low mortality and long-term morbidity; however, without prompt recognition and treatment, the virus can spread through the body involving the brain and other organs. This child has evidence of a skin infection that has spread to the brain. The mortality rate for neonatal herpes encephalitis is about 15%; however, the rate of long-term sequelae including seizure disorders and intellectual impairment is about 65%. Diagnosis of neonatal herpes is confirmed by virus isolation from skin lesions or other sites of viral involvement (eyes, throat, CSF). Polymerase chain reaction can also be used. The infant did not present with symptoms suggestive of the other perinatal infections listed. Congenital toxoplasmosis typically presents at or before birth with hydrocephalus, microcephaly, intracranial calcifications, and chorioretinitis. Seizures are also common in this disease. The mother may not have had symptoms of primary infection during her pregnancy. Cytomegalovirus is the most common congenital infection. Infected children may be born asymptomatically or symptoms such as petechial rash, microcephaly, low birth weight, and hepatosplenomegaly may be present at birth. Late-onset manifestations including sensorineural deafness and mental retardation are possible in both symptomatic and asymptomatic infants. A VDRL performed on the mother would indicate syphilis if positive. Manifestations of congenital syphilis shortly after birth include snuffles, maculopapular rash, and organ dysfunction seen as pneumonitis, DIC, nephritic syndrome, or hemolytic anemia. Asymptomatic gonorrhea infections are common in women. Infants infected with *N. gonorrhoeae* during birth usually present with purulent eye infections, although bacteremia, meningitis, and septic arthritis can also result.

80 **The answer is B: Hepatitis A virus.** This case is descriptive of hepatitis with evidence of icterus (yellow sclera, dark urine). Outbreaks of hepatitis A virus have been associated with consumption of raw shell fish, particularly from the Gulf of Mexico. Hepatitis A virus (HAV) is an enterovirus; thus it is highly stable in the environment and able to remain viable outside the body for long periods of time (weeks to months in the right conditions). Humans are the only hosts for HAV. Contamination of shellfish occurs when poorly treated or untreated sewage enters streams and rivers that ultimately empty into the Gulf. Infection results

in acute hepatitis, which manifests as described in this case. The incubation period is about 4 weeks. *D. latum* is the fish tapeworm. Infection is associated with the consumption of raw fresh water fish from northern lake regions and is usually asymptomatic. The parasite can compete with its host for vitamin B_{12}, leading to a deficiency of B_{12} in the host, and possible development of megaloblastic anemia. *V. cholerae* infections have resulted from the consumption of raw oysters. Copious watery diarrhea is the hallmark of this infection. Hepatitis results from infection with Yellow fever virus. This virus is found in central and South America as well as Africa where it is transmitted by the mosquitoes, most notably *Aedes aegypti*. Infection with *Yersinia enterocolitica* is associated with the consumption of raw milk, although infections have been associated with meat, fish, and even oysters. Infection causes fever, abdominal pain, and bloody diarrhea. This infection is more common in northern Europe than in the United States.

81 **The answer is D: Pyoderma.** This child is experiencing acute glomerulonephritis (AGN). Postinfectious glomerulonephritis is not common; however, *Streptococcus pyogenes* (also known as group A *Streptococcus*) is the most likely culprit when it does occur. Acute glomerulonephritis can follow 1 to 4 weeks after pharyngeal or skin infections with certain strains of *S. pyogenes*. These strains, referred to as nephritogenic, may have antigens that cross react with renal antigens. The finding of IgG and complement C3 in glomerular tissues suggests that a type III hypersensitivity response may play a role in pathogenesis. Diagnosis of acute poststreptococcal glomerulonephritis (APSGN) is made possible by the finding of antibodies to GAS antigens. Anti-DNase B antibodies can be found in pyoderma-associated APSGN, whereas antistreptolysin O antibodies are found in pharyngitis-associated APSGN. Acute toxoplasmosis is not associated with glomerulonephritis. Although the symptoms of renal disease associated with infection may suggest gastroenteritis caused by *E. coli* O157:H7, the hematology results suggest that this is not hemolytic uremic syndrome in which hemolytic anemia and thrombocytopenia are common. Leptospirosis is a rare disease with an incidence of about 0.03/100,000. Most cases of leptospirosis present as an acute febrile illness, although hepatic and renal involvement can occur in about 10%. Urinary tract infections are very uncommon in male children. Urinary symptoms of increased frequency and urgency occur concurrent with the infection, not after recovery.

82 **The answer is D: Rhinovirus—symptomatic treatment.** The case is descriptive of the common cold, the most frequent cause of which is rhinovirus. Acute otitis media (AOM) is a common complication of colds in young children and is often due to the virus. *Moraxella*, *Haemophilus*, and pneumococcus are the most important bacterial causes of AOM; however, they generally cause more severe symptoms. Treatment guidelines for AOM suggest in a case such as this one (no evidence of pain, low-grade fever) deferring the use of antibiotics to see if the child will improve without them. Infection with respiratory syncytial virus in a child of this age would be expected to elicit lower respiratory tract symptoms. Ribavirin is also not recommended for RSV infections except in the most severe cases.

83   **The answer is B: *Chlamydophila pneumoniae*.** The photograph shows atherosclerosis of the aorta. Rupture of atherosclerotic plaques lead to blood clots that can dislodge and travel to the brain to cause strokes. Atherosclerosis is an inflammatory disease and many factors, including endothelial cell infection, are suggested to play a role as inflammatory stimuli. The most frequently implicated pathogen is *C. pneumoniae*. This organism has been isolated from atheromas. Cytomegalovirus has also been implicated in the pathogenesis of this condition. No other organisms have been implicated as strongly as these two agents.

84   **The answer is E: Rhinovirus.** Respiratory pathogens, including all those listed in the question, are one of the most important causes of exacerbation of asthma symptoms. Of these, rhinovirus is the most frequently implicated. The child in this case is suffering from a cold and rhinoviruses are the most frequent causes of the common cold.

85   **The answer is D: Smallpox virus.** The vaccine reaction described occurs in immune competent individuals inoculated with vaccinia, the agent used for the smallpox vaccine. Vaccinia is a live virus which replicates locally at the site of inoculation, inducing the skin reaction. The vaccine virus can be spread to other sites on the body, or to susceptible individuals; thus the vaccination site should be covered with a bandage until the lesion is completely healed. The other agents listed are considered bioterrorism threats; however, the only other agent for which a vaccine is available is *B. anthracis*. Anthrax vaccine can cause a mild localized erythematous, indurated reaction at the site of inoculation.

86   **The answer is A: Cleaning out a rodent-infested warehouse.** Rodents are the natural hosts for hantaviruses. The virus is shed in rodent urine and feces and humans can be incidentally infected when they inhale viral particles while disturbing rodent habitat. The CDC recommends wearing masks while cleaning out

areas that may be contaminated with rodent waste. Hantaviruses are not transmitted in bat guano (as is rabies virus or the fungus *Histoplasma capsulatum*). Hantaviruses are not transmitted by ticks or mosquitoes, as are various arboviruses. While swimming in contaminated farm ponds can lead to infection with the free-living ameba, *Naegleria fowleri*, or the bacterium, *Leptospira interrogans*, this activity is not associated with the acquisition of hantaviruses.

87   **The answer is D: Norovirus.** This agent is a common cause of outbreaks of acute gastroenteritis, particularly in confined environments such as ships, military bases, and nursing homes. It can be transmitted person-to-person by a fecal-oral route. This virus is very stable in the environment and can be harbored by shellfish in areas contaminated with human sewage. It can even withstand heating and be transmitted in cooked shellfish. The virus is also highly resistant to chlorine and can thus be transmitted by contact with contaminated surfaces such as door knobs and stair railings. The other agents listed cause watery diarrhea; however, they are not as likely to cause back-to-back outbreaks such as the one described in the case.

88   **The answer is A: Group B *Streptococcus*.** The CDC recommends routine screening of all pregnant women for this organism between 35 and 37 weeks of gestation. Vaginal colonization with group B *Streptococcus* occurs in up to 30% of pregnant women and can cause serious neonatal disease if the infant is exposed to the organism during birth. The other organisms listed also cause congenital or perinatal infections. There is no routine testing recommended for herpes simplex virus type 2 or *T. gondii*. Screening for *N. gonorrhoeae* is recommended for pregnant women considered at high risk for infection. The most common outcome of neonatal infection with this agent is gonococcal ophthalmia neonatorum. Serological testing for syphilis (*T. pallidum*) is recommended for the first prenatal visit.

89   **The answer is A: *Bacillus cereus*.** This spore-forming bacterial species is associated with food poisoning. Spores of this organism are ubiquitous and contaminate a variety of foodstuffs. Under certain conditions of food preparation, the spores germinate and the organism grows, releasing toxins into the food. A heat-stable toxin induces vomiting by an unknown mechanism. A heat-labile enterotoxin has also been characterized. The action of this toxin is similar to that of enterotoxigenic *Escherichia coli* and *Vibrio cholerae*. It increases cyclic AMP concentrations in intestinal cells, which increases the secretion of sodium and other ions into the lumen of the intestine, resulting in watery diarrhea. Thus, the heat-stable toxin induces vomiting and the heat-labile toxin induces diarrhea. The conditions of food preparation determine which, if either, of these toxins is present in the food. *C. perfringens* is a spore-forming organism associated with food poisoning; however, it induces a diarrheal illness. The enterotoxin of *S. aureus* causes a vomiting illness within hours of consumption of contaminated food; however, this bacteria is not a spore-forming organism. *C. parvum* causes a diarrheal illness. Outbreaks have been associated with ingestion of contaminated water. *S. schenckii* is a fungus and is not associated with food poisoning.

90 **The answer is C: *Gardnerella vaginalis*.** All of the organisms listed can cause vaginal discharge. Many women with vaginal discharge seek medical care at sexually transmitted disease clinics; however, not all causes of vaginal discharge are transmitted in this manner. The case describes a woman with bacterial vaginosis as indicated by the finding of a pH higher than 4.5, clue cells, and the lack of additional symptoms such as vaginal pain or irritation. Clue cells are shed epithelial cells covered with adherent bacteria. Bacterial vaginosis is due to an overgrowth of normal vaginal flora. The discharge associated with candidal vaginitis is thick, white, and clumpy. It is usually accompanied by intense pruritus, and burning and pain on urination. *Trichomonas* vaginitis is characterized by a profuse, frothy discharge accompanied by pain and irritation. The cervix may be erythematous and demonstrate punctate hemorrhages (strawberry cervix). Mobile flagellated protozoans are seen on microscopic examination of the discharge. Both *N. gonorrhoeae* and *C. trachomatis* cause cervicitis. Pelvic exam in this case would reveal a thick puslike discharge coming from an erythematous, edematous cervix.

91 **The answer is D: Polio.** Global eradication of paralytic polio is a major endeavor of the World Health Organization. Many countries are no longer considered endemic for this virus due to a successful vaccination program. However, in endemic countries, wild-type polio virus still circulates in the population. Most infections are asymptomatic; thus, infected individuals are unaware that they are shedding the virus in their feces. Vaccination programs can be halted in times of civil unrest, economic crises, and even when the population has concerns over vaccine safety. When this occurs, as it has recently, increased numbers of paralytic disease cases can result.

92 **The answer is A: Acyclovir.** Viruses are the leading cause of acute encephalitis, and herpes simplex virus type 1 is the most common of these. Due to the mortality rate and high rate of sequelae from HSV-1

encephalitis, prompt empiric therapy with acyclovir is recommended for individuals presenting with signs and symptoms of acute encephalitis. Several viruses other than HSV can cause encephalitis in previously healthy individuals, but are not treatable with acyclovir. Cefotaxime and other third-generation cephalosporins can be used for treatment of meningitis, as well as other illnesses. Similarly, vancomycin can be used to treat meningitis due to highly penicillin-resistant *Streptococcus pneumoniae*. Although meningitis can present similarly to the patient in this case, he was diagnosed clinically with encephalitis. Pyrimethamine is a drug used to treat *Toxoplasma gondii* which can cause subacute encephalitis in immune compromised individuals. Amphotericin B is an antifungal drug.

93 **The answer is B: Dicloxacillin.** This patient has cellulitis, most commonly caused by *Streptococcus pyogenes* (Group A *Streptococcus*) or *Staphylococcus aureus*. Although GAS is susceptible to ampicillin, most *S. aureus* strains produce β-lactamases that render them resistant to penicillins and aminopenicillins. Thus, empiric treatment of cellulitis includes antibiotics that are not affected by staphylococcal β-lactamases including antistaphylococcal penicillins such as dicloxacillin, or first generation cephalosporins such as cephalexin. Doxycycline and gentamicin are not used for Gram-positive infections. (Aminoglycosides are sometimes used synergistically with a penicillin for Gram-positive infections.) Itraconazole is an antifungal drug.

94 **The answer is E: Prevent maturation of the virus by blocking formation of essential structural and nonstructural proteins.** This drug combination is a preferred regimen according to the 2008 treatment guidelines developed by the Department of Health and Human Services Panel on Antiretroviral Guidelines for Adults and Adolescents. The drugs atazanavir and ritonavir are both protease inhibitors. The HIV protease cleaves the polypeptide into individual structural proteins essential for the formation of infectious virions.

95 **The answer is C: Efavirenz.** The recommended regimen for a treatment of naïve HIV-infected patient is a combination of drugs consisting of either one nonnucleoside reverse transcriptase inhibitor (NNRTI) plus two nucleoside reverse transcriptase inhibitors (NRTI) or a protease inhibitor (PI) combination plus two NRTIs. It is important to know which drugs belong to those categories. Abacavir and lamivudine are NRTIs. Atazanavir and ritonavir are PIs.

96 **The answer is B: Atazanavir + ritonavir.** The patient has developed a problematic side-effect of many protease inhibitors. Atazanavir and ritonavir are both protease inhibitors. Abacavir and lamivudine are nucleoside reverse transcriptase (RT) inhibitors and efavirenz is a non-nucleoside reverse transcriptase inhibitor.

97 **The answer is D: Latex agglutination.** This test is used for the detection of *Streptococcus pneumoniae, Haemophilus influenza* b, *Neisseria meningitidis, and Cryptococcus neoformans* (a fungus) in cerebral spinal fluid. Latex agglutination is more sensitive than Gram stain of the CSF; however, it is not as sensitive as culture, and a negative test does not rule out an infectious cause of the patient's symptoms. Indirect immunofluorescence is usually used to detect specific antibodies in patient's serum. India ink stain can be used to detect the presence of *C. neoformans* in cerebral spinal fluid; however, this test is not as sensitive as latex agglutination. The polymerase chain reaction detects nucleic acid.

98 **The answer is A: *Aspergillus fumigatus*.** A prolonged deficiency of neutrophils may occur in cancer chemotherapy and predispose patients to fungal infections as well as other microbial diseases. Neutropenic patients are susceptible to *Candida* infections including *C. glabrata*. Pulmonary infections can result; however, they are not typically angioinvasive. Both *K. pneumoniae* and *M. tuberculosis* can present with hemoptysis and, along with *N. asteroides* can cause cavitary lung lesions. This case is descriptive of invasive aspergillosis. Fever, hemoptysis, and respiratory manifestations are classic manifestations of this disease. *A. fumigatus* is noted for its ability to invade blood vessels. Rapid diagnosis of invasive aspergillosis is possible by the detection of galactomannan, a polysaccharide component of the cell wall of *Aspergillus* that is released by the organism as it replicates. Serum and BAL samples are assayed for this substance by enzyme-linked immunoassay. The finding of galactomannan in serum and BAL fluid is diagnostic for invasive aspergillosis.

99 **The answer is E: Voriconazole.** Voriconazole, a newer azole, is the preferred drug, especially when compared to the renal toxicity issues associated with amphotericin B. Pentamidine has activity against *Pneumocystis*. Azithromycin, penicillin, and isoniazid are antibacterial agents.

100 **The answer is A: Acute rheumatic fever.** This disease is a sequela of pharyngeal infection with certain strains of group A streptococci. The Jones criteria were developed as an aid to the diagnosis of this acute rheumatic fever (ARF). Major criteria for diagnosis of ARF include carditis, polyarthritis, chorea, erythema marginatum, and subcutaneous nodules. The finding of two major or one major and two minor criteria allow the diagnosis of ARF. Kala azar is a form of leishmaniasis involving infection of multiple organs with *Leishmania donovani*. Lyme disease can present with migrating arthritis; however, it is not associated with pharyngitis. Reactive arthritis can result from certain enteric bacterial infections and is not seen in association with cardiac problems. Viral arthritis is usually not migratory and is not associated with pharyngitis and heart murmurs.

101 **The answer is E: Tuberculosis.** Isoniazid is used to treat infections with *Mycobacterium tuberculosis*. Resistance of *M. tuberculosis* to isoniazid is common and easily developed when infections are treated with only one drug. Thus, appropriate treatment of this infection begins with four drugs, isoniazid, ethambutol, pyrazinamide, and rifampin. Unfortunately, antimicrobials such as isoniazid can be purchased over-the-counter in many countries, setting the stage for the emergence of resistant organisms.

Chapter 6

Basic Immunology

QUESTIONS

Select the single best answer.

1 Which of the following cytokines supports proliferation and differentiation of developing lymphocytes in the primary lymphoid tissue?
(A) Interleukin-1
(B) Interleukin-4
(C) Interleukin-7
(D) Interleukin-12
(E) Interleukin-18

2 A workup on an ill child revealed low levels of complement C3 in her blood. Which one of the following presentations did this child most likely manifest?
(A) Chronic eczema
(B) Immune hemolytic anemia
(C) Incomplete recovery from viral infections
(D) Poor response to vaccination
(E) Recurrent infections with extracellular bacteria

3 Vaccination operates to generate a humoral immune response to the immunogen(s). Which one of the following represents the critical function of the resultant humoral response in protecting vaccinated patients from future infections by targeted pathogenic agents?
(A) Opsonization
(B) Extravasation
(C) Neutralization
(D) Complement activation
(E) Antibody-dependent cell cytoxicity (ADCC)

4 Positive selection in the thymus occurs when thymocytes express functional versions of which critical molecule?
(A) CD28
(B) Fc receptor
(C) MHC class I
(D) MHC class II
(E) T-cell receptor (TCR)

5 Which one of the following represents the major role of negative selection in the thymus?
(A) Elimination of self-reactive T cells
(B) Expansion of nonself-reactive T cells
(C) Maturation of professional antigen presenting cells such as dendritic cells
(D) Expression of T-cell receptors on mature T cells
(E) Differentiation of Th1 and Th2 CD4+ T cells

6 A blood sample from an individual with systemic lupus erythematosus was studied in a research project mapping T-cell receptor specificities. Many T cells were discovered to express receptors specific for autologous antigens. Failure of which process in the thymus leads to the large number of autoreactive T cells in the patient's blood?
(A) Affinity maturation
(B) Antigen processing
(C) Hematopoiesis
(D) Negative selection
(E) Receptor editing

7 Which cytokine is essential for T-cell proliferation and is also necessary for the production of CD25-positive regulatory T cells?
(A) IL-2
(B) IL-3
(C) IL-4
(D) IL-5
(E) IL-6

8 T helper cells interacting with antigen-presenting dendritic cells require signals generated by the molecular interactions of the T-cell receptor with the MHC–peptide complex. Additionally, costimulation is required to amplify the initial TCR signals provided through the T cell CD28 molecule interaction with which one of the following dendritic cell molecule(s)?

(A) CD4

(B) CD8

(C) CD45

(D) CD80/86

(E) CD152

9 T cells stimulated by peptide–MHC complexes, displayed on antigen presenting cells, in the absence of costimulation undergo which one of the following processes?

(A) Activation

(B) Anergy

(C) Apoptosis

(D) Differentiation

(E) Proliferation

10 Downregulation of T-cell activation is achieved by the binding of which molecule on the T cell with CD80/86 on the dendritic cell?

(A) CD4

(B) CD8

(C) CD45

(D) CD28

(E) CD152

11 Dendritic cells, macrophages, and what other cell types are considered "professional antigen presenting cells," capable of antigen presentation to T helper cells?

(A) B cells

(B) Basophils

(C) Eosinophils

(D) Mast cells

(E) Neutrophils

12 Antigens from which one of the following microbes would be presented on MHC class I molecules by macrophages?

(A) *Ascaris lumbricoides*

(B) *Candida albicans*

(C) *Haemophilus influenzae*

(D) Influenza virus

(E) *Streptococcus pneumoniae*

13 Activation of macrophages is best achieved by which cytokine?

(A) Interferon gamma (IFN-γ)

(B) Granulocyte monocyte colony-stimulating factor (GM-CSF)

(C) Interleukin-1

(D) Macrophage chemotactic protein (MCP)

(E) Transforming growth factor beta (TGF-β)

14 The intracellular signal initiated by antigen binding to the T-cell receptor is generated by which set of molecules expressed on the T cell membrane?

(A) CD3

(B) CD4

(C) CD28

(D) CD45

(E) CD152

15 The interaction of which molecule on the membrane of cells with its ligand signals apoptosis?

(A) B7 (CD80/86)

(B) CD40

(C) CTLA-4 (CD152)

(D) Fas (CD95)

(E) Fc receptor (CD16)

16 Which one of the following cells is the major source of tumor necrosis factor alpha (TNF-α), interleukin-1, and interleukin-12?

(A) B cells

(B) Macrophages

(C) Mast cells

(D) Th1 cells

(E) Th2 cells

17 Which cells are the source of interleukin-4, –5, –10, and –13?

(A) B cells

(B) Macrophages

(C) Mast cells

(D) Th1 cells

(E) Th2 cells

18 Which cells utilize reactive oxygen and nitrogen species and lysosomal enzymes to kill pathogens?

(A) Cytotoxic T cells

(B) Natural killer T (NKT) cells

(C) Macrophages

(D) Natural killer (NK) cells

(E) Th1 cells

19 If a person had a genetic defect affecting perforin production, which cells and immune function would be affected?

(A) Cytotoxic T cells and natural killer cells/cell killing

(B) Dendritic cells/antigen presentation

(C) Eosinophils and basophils/granule production

(D) Macrophages and neutrophils/phagocytosis

(E) Mast cells/fusion of granules to cell membrane

20 Which immune system cell is primarily responsible for the formation of granuloma in the lungs of tuberculosis patients?
(A) Cytotoxic T cells
(B) Dendritic cells
(C) Eosinophils
(D) Natural killer cells
(E) Th1 cells

21 Which one of the following cytokines plays the most important role in protection against intracellular growth (reactivation) of *Mycobacterium tuberculosis*?
(A) Interferon-γ
(B) Interleukin-2
(C) Interleukin-5
(D) Interleukin-10
(E) Tumor necrosis factor

22 A 14-year-old girl presented with an itchy, erythematous rash following exposure to poison ivy. Which term describes the role of poison ivy oils in this response?
(A) Allergen
(B) Carrier
(C) Cytokine
(D) Hapten
(E) Immunogen

23 Which type of hypersensitivity is associated with reactions to poison ivy oil?
(A) Type I
(B) Type II
(C) Type III
(D) Type IV

24 Which cell type is primarily responsible for the inflammation seen in poison ivy rash?
(A) B cells
(B) Cytotoxic T cells
(C) Eosinophils
(D) Natural killer cells
(E) Th1 cells

25 A 4-year-old child has atopic dermatitis due to severe allergies to dust, animal dander, and many kinds of pollens. Mediators released from which cell type are responsible for the clinical manifestations immediately following exposure to these substances?
(A) B cells
(B) Macrophages
(C) Mast cells
(D) Th1 cells
(E) Th2 cells

26 A 36-year-old woman with severe allergy to yellow jackets was stung multiple times at a soccer game. Within minutes she developed respiratory distress and became unconscious. Which mediator is primarily responsible for this reaction?
(A) Complement
(B) IgG
(C) Histamine
(D) TNF
(E) Norepinephrin

The next four questions are linked.

27 A person develops a viral infection and both T and B cells become activated to fight the infection. In which way is antigen recognition by B cells different from antigen recognition by T cells?
(A) B cells home to the paracortex of lymph nodes where they recognize the antigens trapped by helper T cells
(B) B cells recognize the antigens that have been processed and presented by follicular dendritic cells
(C) B cells undergo receptor editing to change receptors that fail to bind to an antigen
(D) B cells utilize membrane immunoglobulin molecules to bind to antigen in its natural state
(E) The antigen receptors on a single B cell have a broad specificity, and are able to recognize several chemically unrelated antigens

28 The person in the above question is experiencing a primary infection with the virus. B cells activated in a primary infection secrete which class of antibody first?
(A) IgA
(B) IgD
(C) IgE
(D) IgG
(E) IgM

29 The viral infection in the above question began in the respiratory tract. Which antibody class would best protect respiratory epithelial cells from viral infection?
(A) IgA
(B) IgD
(C) IgE
(D) IgG
(E) IgM

30 The virus in the above question spreads from the respiratory tract and causes viremia. Which antibody class would be most important in fighting the virus as it spreads through the body?

(A) IgA
(B) IgD
(C) IgE
(D) IgG
(E) IgM

31 In order for class switching from IgM to IgG to occur, B cells must receive two signals, one generated following binding to T helper cells and the other secreted by helper T cells. What are these two T helper cell-derived molecules?
(A) Antigen and IL-2
(B) CD40 ligand and interferon-γ
(C) CTLA-4 and IL-4
(D) B7 and IL-7
(E) CD20 and IL-13

32 What structural feature is uniquely found on IgA in breast milk and not found on serum IgM?
(A) Fab
(B) FcR
(C) Hinge region
(D) J chain
(E) Secretory piece

The next two questions are linked.

33 A 47-year-old woman developed toxic shock following an infection with a strain of *Staphylococcus aureus* that produced toxic shock syndrome toxin (TSST)-1. This toxin binds directly to MHC Class II molecules on macrophages and which molecule on T cells?
(A) CD3
(B) CD40 ligand
(C) Fas ligand
(D) The gamma chain of the IL-2 receptor
(E) The variable beta portion of the T-cell receptor

34 What response of T cells plays a role in the pathogenesis of shock following the binding of TSST-1 and similar molecules?
(A) Anergy
(B) Apoptosis
(C) Cell cytotoxicity
(D) Cytokine secretion
(E) Memory cell differentiation

35 Macrophages recognize microorganisms through the interaction of microbial substances with what type of receptors on macrophages?
(A) Antigen receptors
(B) Complement receptors
(C) Fc receptors
(D) Membrane immunoglobulin
(E) Pattern recognition receptors

36 Antigen receptors on T and B cells share which similar feature?
(A) Affinity maturation occurs following antigen recognition for both receptor types
(B) Interaction with MHC molecules is required for antigen recognition by both receptor types
(C) The constant regions of both receptor types are identical
(D) The specificity of both receptor types is determined following exposure of mature cells to antigen
(E) The variable portions of both receptor types are generated by random recombination of genes

37 Thymocytes interacting with self-peptides undergo negative selection. The self-peptides in this reaction act as:
(A) Allergens
(B) Tolerogens
(C) Haptens
(D) Immunogens
(E) Antigens

38 Persons with helminth infections mount immunologic responses that involve IgE and eosinophils. Which two cytokines are most important for these responses to occur?
(A) IL-1 and tumor necrosis factor (TNF)
(B) IL-4 and IL-5
(C) IL-10 and transforming growth factor beta (TGF-β)
(D) IL-12 and interferon gamma (IFN-γ)
(E) IFN-α and IFN-β

39 A person developed an extracellular bacterial infection, and IgM was made in response. What is the most important protective function of IgM in this infection?
(A) Antibody-dependent cell cytotoxicity
(B) Complement activation
(C) Direct lysis of bacterial cells
(D) Neutralization of bacterial toxins
(E) Opsonization

40 Neutrophils are attracted to the sites of extracellular bacterial infections by which two important chemotactic substances?
(A) Bacterial mannose and lipopolysaccharide
(B) Complement C5a and interleukin-8 (CXCL-8)
(C) Histamine and complement C3b
(D) Interleukin-7 and interleukin-16
(E) Leukotriene B4 and granulocyte colony-stimulating factor (G-CSF)

41 Plasma cells secreting IgA are especially abundant in which body site?

(A) Bone marrow
(B) Germinal centers of cervical lymph nodes
(C) Lamina propria of mucosa
(D) Thoracic duct
(E) White pulp of the spleen

42 Which immune system cells recognize body cells with reduced expression of MHC class I molecules?

(A) Cytotoxic T cells
(B) Dendritic cells
(C) Macrophages
(D) Natural killer cells
(E) Neutrophils

43 Activation of the complement system, directly results in which one of the following outcomes?

(A) Enhanced phagocytosis
(B) Expression of Toll-like receptors on phagocyte cell surface
(C) Enhancement of immune-mediated neutralization
(D) Proliferation of T cells
(E) Interaction of Fc receptors with antibodies bound to antigens on the pathogen cell surface

44 Which one of the following leukocytes is considered a "granulocyte"?

(A) Macrophage
(B) Neutrophil
(C) Dendritic cell
(D) Natural killer cell
(E) Natural killer T cell

45 A 45-year-old female presents with anorexia and some abdominal pain. Fecal smears reveal the presence of *Taenia* eggs, products of a parasitic tapeworm infection. Which one of the following cells would be most effective in defence against this parasite?

(A) Platelets
(B) Erythrocytes
(C) Neutrophils
(D) Eosinophils
(E) Monocytes

46 Antigen presenting cells (APCs) are required for T-cell recognition of specific antigen and activation. APCs accomplish this task by presenting antigen in the context of which of the following molecules?

(A) T-cell receptor (TCR)
(B) Toll-like receptor (TLR)
(C) Major histocompatibility complex (MHC)
(D) Killer inhibitory receptor (KIR)
(E) Fc receptor (FcR)

47 A 1-year-old female presented with symptoms of systemic autoimmunity (lupus, diabetes, and arthritis), and upon genetic analysis it was found that the patient had a mutation in the *Foxp3* gene locus. Which one of the following is an explanation for the clinical symptoms observed?

(A) Patient cannot produce antigen presenting cells
(B) Patient cannot generate regulatory CD4$^+$CD25$^+$ T cells
(C) Patient is unable to produce antibodies
(D) Patient cannot produce anti-inflammatory cytokines
(E) Patient NK cells have no inhibitory signal

48 Following an initial expansion of B cells in response to microbial peptides, a memory pool of B cells is generated and maintained in the individual in many cases throughout life. Recently, it was discovered that two memory cell types were generated in response to microbial challenge. Upon rechallenge with the microbe, the patient is protected from infection. Which one of the following explanations accounts for this observation?

(A) Circulating memory B cells are actively producing antibodies in the absence of antigen
(B) Circulating memory B cells will produce antibodies, however, only upon encounter with the microbial antigen
(C) Long-lived plasma cells are actively producing antibodies in the absence of antigen
(D) Long-lived plasma cells will produce antibodies, however, only upon encounter with the microbial antigen
(E) TLR signaling to the circulating memory B cells will induce rapid production of antibodies in response to antigen encounter

49 Which one of the following represents the mechanism by which immune complexes (ICs) are normally cleared from the circulation?

(A) ICs are solubilized by C3a
(B) ICs are solubilized by C5a
(C) Factor I releases complement-bound ICs to bind with complement receptors found on splenic/hepatic neutrophils
(D) Red blood cells capture ICs from blood via Fc receptors
(E) C3b solubilizes ICs and attaches to red blood cells via complement receptors

50 Which of the following is the site at which lymphocytes can leave the blood and gain entry into the lymph nodes and what lymphocyte cell surface protein mediates such access?

(A) Lymphoid follicle: CD4

(B) Germinal center: CD62L (L-selectin)

(C) Lymphoid follicle: CD62L (L-selectin)

(D) Periarterial lymphatic sheath (PALS): CCR7

(E) High endothelial venules (HEV): CD62L (L-selectin)

51 The difference between tolerance and immunity depends upon the maturation status of the antigen presenting dendritic cells. What is the T-cell outcome of an antigen presentation event by a mature dendritic cell?

(A) Anergy

(B) Apoptosis

(C) Activation

(D) Ignorance

(E) Suppression

ANSWERS

1 **The answer is C: Interleukin-7.** IL-1α and β (choice A) are inflammatory cytokines produced by phagocytes (and others) to promote inflammation. IL-4 (choice B) supports differentiation of Th2-type CD4+ T cells, while IL-12 and IL-18 (choices D and E) operate to differentiate Th1-type CD4+ T cells.

2 **The answer is E: Recurrent infections with extracellular bacteria.** Complement proteins function in innate immunity through enzymatic cleavage of C3 to liberate C3b which directly binds to pathogen surfaces. Following C3b insertion, enzyme cascade events result in lysis of the target cell by the membrane attack complex (complement protein scaffold C5–C9) and recruitment of phagocytes by C3a and C5a cleavage products. Chronic eczema (choice A), immune hemolytic anemia (choice B), incomplete recovery from viral infections (choice C), and poor response to vaccination (choice D) would not involve complement pathways and thus would be unaffected by a C3 deficiency.

3 **The answer is C: Neuralization.** Antibodies generated by the vaccination are produced by antigen-specific memory B cells which reside in the bone marrow. These antibodies (most likely IgG) can promote opsonization (choice A), Fc receptor-mediated phagocytosis, and complement activation (choice D) as well as ADCC (choice E). However, the infectious agent in most cases will have colonized tissues by the time these mechanisms act to limit growth. The most critical function of a vaccine-mediated humoral response is to generate antibodies which block attachment of infectious agents to host cell surfaces or neutralization. This blockade completely inhibits microbial colonization and ensures protection from the pathogen. Extravasation (choice B) refers to the process whereby immune cells can leave the circulation and enter tissues generally to migrate into areas of inflammation in order to destroy pathogens invading host tissues.

4 **The answer is E: T-cell receptor (TCR).** Immature T cells (double-positive or CD4+CD8+) interact with MHC class I and II-positive thymic epithelial cells and following this interaction, the T cells assume single positive status (either CD4 or CD8 expression) and express a functional TCR. CD28 (choice A) is a T-cell surface molecule involved in costimulation signals; however, it is not relevant for positive selection. While Fc receptors (choice B) and MHC class I (choice C) molecules are expressed by T cells, Fc receptors serve as a means to interact with antibodies and MHC to present antigens to T cells. There is, at present, some evidence that T cells can present antigens, albeit inefficiently, to other T cells, this interaction is included in the T–T interactions that have been described. T cells do not express MHC class II (choice D) molecules.

5 **The answer is A: Elimination of self-reactive T cells.** In fact, about 90% of all T cells that are produced are eliminated (apoptosis) during negative selection. Thymic medullary epithelial cells express the *Aire* gene (*autoimmune regulator* gene) and synthesize all self-antigens for presentation on MHC molecules to maturing thymocytes. Mature dendritic cells (DCs) also participate in the presentation of self-antigens to developing single positive T cells. Those T cells that respond too strongly or weakly undergo apoptosis (undetermined signals) while those responding intermediately are provided survival factors and complete maturation, and they migrate out of the thymus to seed the lymphoid organs in the body. While there may be some expansion of nonself-reactive T cells (choice B) due to provided survival/growth factors, this is not the major role of negative selection. DCs do mature but only serve to present self-antigens (choice C). TCR expression is completed following positive selection (choice D). Differentiation of CD4+ T cells (choice E) occurs after antigen exposure in the periphery (tissue, spleen, or lymph node).

6 **The answer is D: Negative selection.** Affinity maturation (choice A) refers to the process whereby immune receptors for specific antigen during a response are mutated to generate higher affinity, thereby allowing formation of memory B and T cells with the most reactive receptors to sense antigens upon re-encounter. Antigen processing (choice B) is the process of breaking down and loading antigen onto MHC molecules for surface recognition by responding T cells. Hematopoiesis (choice C) is the production of blood cellular components such as the many types of immune cells, and occurs in the bone marrow. Receptor editing (choice E) is a B cell process occurring in the bone marrow during development, and serves as a mode to reconfigure B-cell receptors that recognize self-antigen to identify foreign-antigens, otherwise, the self-reactive B cell will undergo apoptosis.

7 **The answer is A: IL-2.** IL-3 (choice B) is a differentiation factor for plasmacytoid dendritic cells. IL-4 and IL-5 (choices C and D) are factors involved in the differentiation and growth, respectively, of Th2 CD4+ T cells. IL-6 (choice E) is a proinflammatory cytokine that has been reported to suppress regulatory T cell activities and in conjunction with TGF-β can differentiate Th17 CD4+ T cells.

8 **The answer is D: CD80/86.** CD4 (choice A) and CD8 (choice B) are molecules which interact with antigen presenting cell MHC molecules to stabilize the MHC–peptide–TCR interaction. CD45 (choice C) is a cell surface protein found on hematopoietic cells. CD152 (choice E) or CTLA-4, cytotoxic T lymphocyte antigen-4, is expressed on activated T cells (CD4 and CD8) and interacts with B7 (CD80/86) molecules to suppress further T-cell activities (form of peripheral regulation). Only B7, expressed by antigen presenting cells, are used to engage CD28 to promote T-cell activation. CTLA-4 has a higher affinity for B7 than does CD28, thus providing a means of regulating T-cell activation status.

9 **The answer is B: Anergy.** Activation (choice A), differentiation (choice D), and proliferation (choice E) are T-cell outcomes following TCR interaction with peptide–MHC complexes in the presence of costimulatory signals (CD28-CD80/86 interactions). Apoptosis (choice C) is a signal generated in T cells through Fas–FasL (CD95–CD95L) and TNF–TNFR (tumor necrosis factor–TNF receptor) interactions. Anergy is a state of unresponsiveness, that is, upon re-exposure to the same antigen, even in the presence of appropriate costimulation, the T cells remain unable to proliferate although they do seem to be able to produce cytokines.

10 **The answer is E: CD152.** CD4 (choice A) and CD8 (choice B) are involved in MHC–TCR interactions. CD45 (choice C) is a cell surface marker for hematopoietic cells. CD28 (choice D) indeed binds to CD80/86 but the signal conveyed is stimulatory rather than inhibitory as for CD152 or CTLA-4.

11 **The answer is A: B cells.** Professional antigen presenting cells are those that express both MHC class I and II molecules. Basophils (choice B), eosinophils (choice C), mast cells (choice D), and neutrophils (choice D) all do not express MHC class II and thus cannot present antigens to CD4+ T cells. In addition, these cell types do not express the machinery for processing of exogenous antigens.

12 **The answer is D: Influenza virus.** MHC class I molecules express endogenous antigens, that is, antigens that were derived from the presenting cell interior. *A. lumbricoides* (choice A), a parasitic worm, *C. albicans* (choice B), a fungus, *H. influenzae* (choice C), and *S. pneumoniae* (choice E), extracellular bacteria, will generally only produce exogenous antigens due to their inability to invade cells. However, exogenous peptides from each of these pathogens can be presented on MHC class I molecules only by dendritic cells through a process termed crosspresentation. Macrophages do not have this capacity and thus could only present exogenous antigens on MHC class

II molecules. Influenza virus by nature is an intracellular parasite and thus endogenous antigens would be loaded onto MHC class I and presented to T cells.

13 **The answer is A: Interferon gamma (IFN-γ).** Upon antigen uptake, macrophages through toll-like receptor signaling, produce interleukin-12 which in turn promotes the differentiation of Th1 cells from naïve CD4+ T cell pools. These Th1 cells can then produce IFN-γ which is bound by macrophage IFN-γ receptors signaling to promote macrophage phagocytosis. GM-CSF (choice B) serves to differentiate granulocytes from stem cells. IL-1 (choice C) is produced by macrophages upon activation and stimulates inflammation. MCP (choice D) is a chemotaxis factor for both macrophages and T cells and at least at this point does not play a role in macrophage activation. TGF-β (choice E) is produced by many cells and serves to stimulate embryogenesis but functions to suppress activities of T cells.

14 **The answer is A: CD3.** CD4 (choice B) functions to stabilize interactions of TCR and MHC during T-cell activation. CD28 (choice C) is the costimulatory receptor for B7 molecules which promotes activation of T-cell responses. CD45 (choice D) is a cell surface marker of activation status but does not function in TCR signaling. CD152 or CTLA-4 (choice E) is a costimulatory receptor for B7 molecules which promotes suppression of T-cell responses.

15 **The answer is D: Fas (CD95).** B7 (choice A), expressed on antigen presenting cells, provides costimulatory signals for T-cell activation/suppression depending upon the interacting receptor. CD40 (choice B) is the receptor for CD40L. Signals generated by CD40L–CD40 interactions result in activation as in the case for B cells or maturation when occurring in dendritic cells. CTLA-4 (choice C) signaling mediated by binding with B7 from antigen presenting cells, suppresses T cell activation. FcR (choice E) are surface receptors that bind to Fc regions of antibodies and result in antibody-dependent cell cytotoxicity (ADCC) or opsonization. Only Fas–FasL interactions result in apoptosis caspase activation.

16 **The answer is B: Macrophages.** TNF-α, IL-1, and IL-12 are produced by activated macrophages to promote Th1 differentiation and inflammation. B cells (choice A) do not produce TNF-α or IL-12 but can produce IL-1. Mast cells (choice C) can produce only TNF-α and IL-1. Th1 (choice D) cells can produce TNF-α and IL-1 but not IL-12. However, activated CD8+ T cells (Tc1) can produce IL-12. Th2 (choice E) cells can only produce IL-1 of these three cytokines.

17 **The answer is E: Th2 cells.** B cells (choice A) can produce IL-4, IL-5, and IL-10. Macrophages (choice B) can produce IL-4 and IL-10. Mast cells (choice C) can produce IL-4. Th1 (choice D) cells do not produce any of these cytokines as these factors tend to suppress Th1 activation and differentiation. Interestingly, natural killer T cells can produce these cytokines as well upon initial activation in the presence of IL-4 production by macrophages, B cells, or mast cells.

18 **The answer is C: Macrophages.** All of the cells listed have the capacity to kill target cells. Cytotoxic T cells (choice A) or activated CD8$^+$ T cells kill primarily through Fas–FasL interactions or production of granzyme/perforin. Eosinophils, basophils, mast cells, macrophages, and neutrophils kill targets by secreting reactive oxygen species and enzymes. NK (choice D) and NKT (choice B) cells use killer activating receptor (recognize MHC class I-negative cells) signaling and produce granzyme/perforin. Th1 (choice E) cells can produce TNF-α and IFN-γ which has been shown to cause cell death.

19 **The answer is A: Cytotoxic T cells and natural killer cells/cell killing.** Perforin forms pores in the target cells and allows the passage of granzymes into the cytoplasm of the cells. Granzyme then initiates the process of apoptosis. Only cytotoxic T cells and NK cells produce perforin/granzyme while dendritic cells (choice B), eosinophils/basophils (choice C), macrophages/neutrophils (choice D), and mast cells (choice E) do not produce these molecules.

20 **The answer is E: Th1 cells.** Granulomas are the product of the immune system effort to control *Mycobacterium* replication. The two cells responsible for formation of the granuloma are macrophages and Th1 cells. There are relatively few cytotoxic T cells (choice A), dendritic cells (choice B), and natural killer cells (choice D) present in or near the granuloma. Eosinophils (choice C) do not appear to participate in the immune response against *Mycobacterium*.

21 **The answer is A: Interferon-γ.** In the formation of granulomas, two cell types predominate, Th1 cells and macrophages. Activated macrophages produce IL-12 which promotes Th1 differentiation. In turn, Th1 cells produce IFN-γ to further activate macrophages. IL-2 (choice B) is important in promoting early proliferation of Th1 cells but chronic infection (granuloma) with *Mycobacterium* would result in activation-induced cell cytotoxicity (AICC) driven by IL-2. IL-5 (choice C) and IL-10 (choice D) is produced by Th2 cells which do not play a role in *Mycobacterium* immunity. TNF-α (choice E) is produced by Th1 cells but in vivo studies suggests it only synergizes with IFN-γ in the containment of the bacterium.

22 **The answer is D: Hapten.** Allergens (choice A) are agents which stimulate an IgE response and subsequent re-exposure activates mast cells to degranulate. The allergens bind to IgE molecules captured by mast cell Fc receptors and these IgE-Fc receptor complexes are long-lived providing an opportunity to become re-exposed to the antigen. Cytokine (choice C) production is a result of hapten and allergen binding but does not define the role of urushiol (poison ivy oil). Immunogens (choice E) are chemicals which elicit an immune response. This response is correct but is a broad answer to the question posed. Carriers (choice B) are usually protein in nature and associate with haptens. These carriers do not necessarily induce an immune response. Haptens are small molecules which do induce an immune response only in the presence of a carrier.

23 **The answer is D: Type IV.** Type I (immediate hypersensitivity) (choice A) is an immune response mediated by IgE triggering of mast cell and basophil degranulation. Type II (choice B) are antibody-mediated responses in which antibodies against cellular or extracellular matrix antigens may deposit in any tissue expressing the target antigen. Thus, the disease is normally tissue-specific. An example of type II hypersensitivity is Goodpasture syndrome and myasthenia gravis. Type III (choice C) are immune-complex mediated events where antibodies to soluble antigens bind and form complexes which deposit in areas of high pressure such as blood vessel branches and the kidney glomeruli. An example of type III hypersensitivity is systemic lupus erythematosus. Poison ivy induces a delayed-type hypersensitivity in which CD4$^+$ T cells are activated and an inflammatory response develops.

24 **The answer is E: Th1 cells.** B cells (choice A) are associated with responses of type I, II, and III hypersensitivity. Cytotoxic T cells (choice B) can produce a type IV hypersensitive (cell-mediated) response by killing target cells expressing the antigen such as in rheumatoid arthritis. Eosinophils (choice C) can participate in type I as they express Fc receptors for IgE. Natural killer cells (choice D) are recruited participants in inflammatory responses but are not primarily responsible for hypersensitivity reactions. Delayed-type hypersensitivity reactions are primarily driven by Th1 cells producing IFN-γ.

25 **The answer is C: Mast cells.** Allergens such as dust, animal dander, and pollen bind to IgE expressed on the surface of mast cells. Such IgE is produced during the first exposure to the allergen and this IgE binds to high affinity Fc receptors on mast cells. This is known as sensitization. Secondary encounter with the allergen results in binding of the antigen to the IgE and activation of the mast cells (degranulation). Macrophages (choice B) play a role in type IV delayed-type hypersensitivity. B cells (choice A) produce the initial antibodies (IgE) to the allergen but do not release vasoactive amines as does mast cells. Th1 cells (choice D) are the mediators of type IV hypersensitivity and Th2 cells (choice E) do promote the IgE production but again are not responsible for the mediators.

26 **The answer is C: Histamine.** This is an allergic response to the yellow jacket venom involving mast cell degranulation. As a consequence of degranulation, histamine is released. Complement proteins (choice A) are a set of serum proteins which bind to microbial surfaces in order to promote opsonization and cell killing through formation of the membrane attack complex. IgG is an antibody isotype which can initiate complement activation and serve to promote opsonization of pathogens. TNF or tumor necrosis factor is a proinflammatory cytokine released by phagocytes and activated T cells, which elicits inflammatory activity. Norepinephrin is a hormone growth factor that plays a role during stress responses but is not responsible for allergic reaction.

27 **The answer is D: B cells utilize membrane immunoglobulin molecules to bind to antigen in its natural state.** CD4$^+$ and CD8$^+$ T cells can only respond to antigens once they have been processed and loaded onto major histocompatibility complexes (MHC) and displayed by antigen presenting cells. B cells recognize antigens directly. Upon initial B-cell encounter with antigen, B cells traffick to the paracortex of the lymph nodes to interact with helper T cells. This interaction involves CD40 ligand–CD40 which promote B-cell expansion as plasma cells (choice A). Once receiving the CD40 signal, the B cells traffick back into the lymphoid follicle and form a germinal center. Antigen is presented to the developing B cells by follicular dendritic cells, FDC (choice B). Only B cells expressing the highest affinity immunoglobulin receptors will remain bound to the FDC. All other B cells will undergo apoptosis. Helper T cells then produce the appropriate cytokines for isotype switching and cell survival signals are provided through CD40 ligand–CD40 interactions. Some of the B cells differentiate into antibody-producing plasma cells while others become memory B cells which leave the lymph node and traffick to the bone marrow where they remain as long-lived plasma cells. Receptor editing occurs in the bone marrow when B cells are undergoing central tolerance and involves rearrangement of Ig genes (choice C). Like all adaptive receptors each one is specific for only one antigen unlike innate

receptors which recognize conserved sequences on pathogens (choice E).

28 **The answer is E: IgM.** The first antibody isotype produced by B cells is IgM, that is, it is the first type of B cell antigen receptor. IgA (choice A) is the isotype of antibody synthesized and secreted primarily in the mucosa. IgD (choice B) is an isotype of antibody found in the blood in low levels and its exact function is unknown. IgE (choice C) is an isotype produced to mediate antibody-dependent cell cytotoxicity of parasites. It binds to Fc receptors on eosinophils, basophils, and mast cells and upon antigen binding results in granule release. IgG (choice D) is the highest concentration of antibody in the serum, mediates complement activation, opsonization, and can cross the placenta to protect fetus.

29 **The answer is A: IgA.** The antibody secreted in mucosal tissues is IgA, all other antibody isotypes, IgD (choice B), IgE (choice C), IgG (choice D), and IgM (choice E) are found predominantly in other fluids.

30 **The answer is D: IgG.** The predominant antibody isotype within the blood (site of viremia) is IgG. It functions to activate complement cascade, antibody-dependent cell cytotoxicity and opsonization. IgM (choice E) is also of high levels within the blood but not as significant as IgG. IgA (choice A) is found predominantly in the mucosal compartments. IgD (choice B) is found in low levels in the blood and its function is unknown. IgE (choice C) does not contribute to viral infection control.

31 **The answer is B: CD40 ligand and interferon-γ.** Interferon-γ promotes isotype switching from IgM to IgG, IL-4 (IL-13) induces switching to IgE; IL-2 and IL-7 do not influence isotype switching (choices A, C, D, and E). T helper cells and B cells interact through CD40 ligand–CD40 interactions whereas CTLA-4 and B7 are costimulatory signals, inhibitory and stimulatory, respectively. CD20 and antigen are not T helper cell-derived factors and cannot promote isotype switching.

32 **The answer is E: Secretory piece.** IgA is a structural dimer and is held together by the J chain (choice D). IgM can form pentamers also held together by the J chain. B cells produce IgA and the secretory piece permits translocation across mucosal epithelia, subsequent secretion and protection from proteolysis. The hinge region (choice C) is the flexible portion connecting the Fab (choice A) and Fc regions of an antibody. Fc receptors (FcR) (choice B) are receptors on cells which bind Fc regions of antibodies. These interactions result in cell signaling, activation, opsonization, and/or cytokine production.

33   **The answer is E: The variable beta portion of the T cell receptor.** Superantigens are molecules of microbial origin which can non-specifically activate T cells. Superantigens bind to certain domains on MHC Class II molecules and to certain domains on the variable region of the beta chain on the T cell receptor, forming a bridge between the two cells. A superantigen can bind to T-cell receptors (TCRs) from a number of different T cells, as long as the TCRs share similar amino acid sequences in a key region of the variable portion of the beta chain. None of the other molecules, although expressed on T cells, binds directly with superantigens.

34   **The answer is D: Cytokine secretion. Superantigen binding to T cells leads either to cell activation or anergy.** With regard to the pathogenesis of septic shock, TSST-1 acts as a polyclonal activator, stimulating a number of different T cells in a non-specific fashion and resulting in cytokine secretion. The hypersecretion of pro-inflammatory cytokines such as tumor necrosis factor-alpha can lead to septic shock as occurred in this patient. Anergic cells would not participate in the pathogenesis of this condition. The other choices are not typical responses of T cells to superantigen stimulation and would also not play a role in the pathogenesis of septic shock induced by TSST-1.

35   **The answer is E: Pattern recognition receptors.** Microbes express conserved amino acid and carbohydrate sequences on their cell (or viral capsid) surfaces called pathogen associated molecular patterns (PAMPs). These sequences are recognized by pattern recognition receptors (PRRs) on the surface of phagocytes. Antigen receptors (choice A) are adaptive immune response receptors structured to recognize specific antigens unique to pathogens. Complement receptors (choice B) are expressed on phagocytes and function to enhance phagocytosis of complement-coated (C3b, C4b) pathogens. Fc receptors (choice C) are expressed on numerous cell types and function to bind to immunoglobulin for opsonization and antibody-dependent cell cytotoxicity (NK cells and granulocytes such as mast cells). Membrane immunoglobulin (choice D) is expressed only on B cells and serves as the B cell antigen receptor.

36   **The answer is E: The variable portions of both receptor types are generated by random recombination of genes.** Innate receptors or pattern recognition receptors (PRRs) recognize conserved amino acid and carbohydrate sequences on the surface of pathogens.

This detection allows a rapid response in the form of phagocytosis and cytokine production to lead to adaptive immune activation. Antigen receptors on B and T cells are the product of gene segment rearrangement in order to devise receptors which can recognize various antigens from differing pathogens. Affinity maturation (choice A) is the process whereby activated B cells compete for binding with follicular dendritic cells in the germinal centers in order to generate the B cells synthesizing the highest affinity antibodies. T cells require interaction with MHC–peptide complexes in order to undergo activation, whereas B cells can recognize antigens in their natural state (choice B). The constant regions are not identical in nature, especially since soluble T-cell receptors do not bind to Fc receptors while B-cell receptors if solubilized will interact with Fc receptors (choice C). Specificity of both B- and T-cell antigen receptors is determined during development within the bone marrow and thymus, respectively, with those cells recognizing self-antigens undergoing apoptosis (choice D).

37   **The answer is B: Tolerogens.** Positive and negative selection processes make up the event termed central tolerance whose goal is to remove self-antigen-specific T cells. Allergens (choice A) are environmental antigens which are recognized by IgE molecules bound to Fc receptors on mast cells. Haptens (choice C) are chemicals which bind to carrier proteins and can then be immunogenic. Immunogens (choice D) are those antigens which promote immunity. The term antigens (choice E) refers to all chemical structures which can elicit immune responses, whether self- or foreign-derived in nature. Only tolerogens refers to self-antigens which are presented by thymic antigen presenting cells in order to facilitate negative selection.

38   **The answer is B: IL-4 and IL-5.** IL-1 and TNF (choice A) are cytokines produced by activated phagocytes and T cells promoting inflammation. IL-10 and TGF-β (choice C) are cytokines produced by Th2, macrophages, and regulatory T cells to suppress the immune response as a mechanism of regulating immunity. In addition, IL-10 can promote Th2 differentiation. TGF-β (combined with IL-6) can promote differentiation of Th17 cells involved in autoimmune diseases. TGF-β alone can promote differentiation of Th0 into regulatory T cells. IL-12 and IFN-γ (choice D) are cytokines which promote Th1 differentiation and activation of macrophages (enhance phagocytosis). Interferon alpha and beta (choice E) are cytokines induced by viral infections which result in establishment of the antiviral state. Since IgE bound to Fc receptor is critical for antibody-dependent cell cytotoxicity of helminths, the cytokines of importance are those which promote isotype switching from IgM to IgE, and production and chemotaxis of eosinophils that is, IL-4 and IL-5 respectively.

39 **The answer is B: Complement activation.** The most important defense against extracellular bacteria are opsonins and neutrophils. Complement activation generates the opsonin C3b and attracts neutrophils to the area via the action of C5a. IgM is the most efficient class of antibody at activating complement. IgM can function in neutralization of toxins; however, that is not the most effective protective function (choice D). IgM is not itself an opsonin (choice E), in contrast to IgG. No antibody class can induce bacterial cell lysis directly (i.e., without the assistance of complement) (choice C). IgM does not participate in antibody-dependent cell cytotoxicity (choice A), a function which is carried out against viral-infected cells, but not against extracellular bacteria. Lastly, natural killer cells are not important in defense against extracellular bacteria.

40 **The answer is B: Complement C5a and interleukin-8 (CXCL-8).** Bacterial mannose and lipopolysaccharide (LPS) (choice A) serve as ligands for pattern recognition receptors found on phagocytes. Histamine is a vasoactive amine released upon degranulation of mast cells, while C3b is an opsonin (choice C). IL-7 and IL-16 function in cell activation and survival but do not operate in chemotaxis (choice D). While leukotriene B4 is a pro-inflammatory product of mast cell activation, G-CSF is a growth stimulating factor for cells (choice E). Only the cleavage product C5a and IL-8 are both recruiting factors for neutrophils.

41 **The answer is C: Lamina propria of mucosa.** IgA is the isotype associated with mucosal immunity. While it can be produced in other anatomical regions, it is abundant in the mucosa. The bone marrow (choice A) contains long-lived plasma cells producing antibodies. Germinal centers (choice B) within the cervical nodes could also produce IgA, but B cells in the lamina propria produce significantly more IgA. The thoracic duct (choice D) is the lymph vessel responsible for returning cells and fluid from the lymph back into circulation. The white pulp of the spleen (choice E) contains areas of B cell differentiation into plasma cells and can produce IgA, but as IgA is an important neutralizing agent in the mucosa, it is localized in high levels within the mucosa.

42 **The answer is D: Natural killer cells.** Cytotoxic T cells (choice A) are CD8⁺ T cells which recognize antigens presented on MHC class I molecules, and act to kill targets expressing those antigens. Dendritic cells (choice B) are specialized antigen presenting cells.

Macrophages (choice C) and neutrophils (choice E) are phagocytes. Only natural killer cells recognize MHC class I expression on the surface of cells and kill those cells that have lost expression.

43 **The answer is A: Enhanced phagocytosis.** Activation of complement has three outcomes: promotion of inflammation through recruitment of phagocytes (C3a, C5a), opsonization to enhance phagocytosis by complement receptor-expressing phagocytes (C3b, C4b), and target cell killing (C5b–C9). Expression of Toll-like receptors is constitutive on phagocytes although this expression can be increased (choice B). Neutralization (choice C) is the process of blocking pathogen binding to host receptors (usually accomplished by antibodies), and is not a function of complement activation. Complement activation does not directly result in T-cell proliferation (choice D). Complement activation does not directly promote antibody binding to Fc receptors (choice E).

44 **The answer is B: Neutrophil.** Granulocytes are immune cells that contain granules in their cytoplasms. These granules are filled with enzymes and other inflammatory mediators which are released upon activation of the granulocytes. Neutrophils, easinophils and basophils are considered granulocytes. Although both NK cells and NKT cells have granules, they are referred to as large, granular lymphocytes, not granulocytes. Monocytic cells such as dendritic cells and macrophages (choices A and C) lack distinct cytoplasmic granules.

45 **The answer is D: Eosinophils.** Platelets and erythrocytes serve as blood components and do not generate immune responses against parasites (choices A and B). Neutrophils (choice C) are surveillance cells which may engage the parasite but the most effective response is generated by eosinophils which express Fc epsilon receptors. These receptors allow the eosinophils to bind to IgE directed against parasitic microbes. Such binding will result in antibody-dependent cell cytoxicity or ADCC. Monocytes (choice E) are bone marrow and circulating blood cells which can differentiate into macrophages and dendritic cells. However, these cells would not be as effective as the eosinophils in killing the parasite.

46 **The answer is C: Major histocompatibility complex (MHC).** APCs express TLR, FcR, and MHC. TLR (choice B) are innate pattern recognition receptors (PRR) which detect microbial antigens and initiate proinflammatory cytokine production by phagocytes (APCs as well). FcR (choice E) are important in the process of opsonization (FcR binding to antibody bound to the antigen on the pathogen surface and subsequent phagocytosis via this interaction). All nucleated somatic cells express MHC class I while only the professional APCs (B cells, macrophages, and dendritic cells) also express MHC class II. MHC displays antigens for recognition by T cell receptors (TCRs) (choice A).

47 **The answer is B: Patient cannot generate regulatory CD4⁺CD25⁺ T cells.** CD4⁺CD25⁺ T regulatory (Treg) cells or natural Treg cells function in peripheral tolerance to prevent self-antigen-specific T-cell activation. This is accomplished by still undefined cell-contact inhibitory mechanisms. What has been determined is that those inhibitory mechanisms are a product of the *Foxp3* gene; thus, cells with active gene expression of *Foxp3* (as determined by quantitative PCR) are regulatory T cells. *Foxp3* is a unique gene to Treg cells and not expressed in other cell types.

48 **The answer is C: Long-lived plasma cells are actively producing antibodies in the absence of antigen.** Following an initial B-cell proliferative event, cells termed plasmablasts differentiate into long-lived plasma cells which traffic to the bone marrow and reside there, actively producing antibodies to the specific antigen against which they were originally expanded (choice D). Circulatory memory B cells (choice A) also exist but do not actively secrete antibody and appear to serve as replacements for the long-lived plasma cells in the bone marrow over time (choice B). TLR signaling in memory B cells has not been described to impact antibody production as these circulating cells appear not to synthesize the antibodies (choice E).

49 **The answer is E: C3b solubilizes IC and attaches to red blood cells via complement receptors.** Defects in the complement pathway are associated with IC diseases due to the fact that complement is important for the removal of ICs that occur during normal B-cell immune responses to pathogens. ICs are created by soluble (or cell surface) antigen interaction with secreted antibodies. This normally results in opsonization and phagocytosis; however, another mechanism

of clearance is mediated in the spleen and liver by macrophages. C3 cleavage product, C3b, binds to the ICs and is attached to complement receptors on red blood cells. These cells then pass through the spleen and liver, and a tissue factor removes the ICs from the red blood cells and resident macrophages take up the ICs for degradation (choices A–D).

50 **The answer is E: High endothelial venules (HEV): CD62L (L-selectin).** Lymphocytes traffic between the blood and lymph circulation in order to maintain surveillance of the body for foreign invaders. Lymphoid and germinal center follicles (choices A–C) are areas in the lymph node where B cells and plasma cells, respectively, are found in high concentration. Periarterial lymphatic sheath (choice D) is the site in the spleen white pulp where T cells are heavily concentrated. In order for T cells to gain access to the lymph nodes from the circulation, specialized zones called high endothelial venules provide connections from the blood to the lymph node. The cells must arrest at the HEV via integrin binding, through CD62L found on naïve T cells, and then those arrested cells follow a chemokine (chemotactic) gradient extravasating through the endothelial cells of the HEV into the cortex of the lymph node.

51 **The answer is C: Activation.** Maturation indicates that the dendritic cell (DC) has been stimulated by Toll-like receptor binding to pathogen components. This in turn upregulates expression of B7 (costimulatory molecules) on the surface of the DC. Together with the MHC–peptide complex, the DC can now provide sufficient signaling to promote T-cell activation. Such interactions deficient in B7 result in anergy (choice A). Apoptosis (choice B) signals are the result of ligand–receptor interactions involving Fas–Fas ligand or TNF-related interactions. Ignorance (choice D) is the result of antigens being sequestered from access to T cells; thus, the T cells remain ignorant of the antigen presence (immune-privileged sites such as the sex organs utilize this mechanism). Suppression (choice E) is an active process mediated by cytokines or regulatory cells such as regulatory T cells.

Chapter 7

Clinical Immunology

1 A 67-year-old woman is hospitalized with a fever of unknown origin. An elevated C-reactive protein (CRP) and erythrocyte sedimentation rate (ESR) suggest an ongoing systemic inflammatory response. Which cytokine is especially important in inducing elevations in CRP and ESR?
(A) Interleukin-4
(B) Interleukin-6
(C) Interleukin-10
(D) Interleukin-12
(E) Interleukin-18

2 A 45-year-old woman presents to her primary care physician with complaints of fatigue, malaise, and pain and stiffness in the shoulders, hands, and knees for the past 6 weeks. Joint stiffness was particularly pronounced in the morning and improved within an hour. Physical exam reveals tenderness and warmth of affected joints with no deformations. Laboratory tests reveal a normocytic and normochromic anemia, and analysis of synovial fluid from the knee revealed a white blood cell count of 10,000 with a predominance of neutrophils. Which test would be most useful in establishing a diagnosis of her condition?
(A) Antinuclear antibody test
(B) Coombs test
(C) Erythrocyte sedimentation rate
(D) Radiographs
(E) Rheumatoid factor test

3 A 23-year-old female presents with fatigue, right eye pain, right leg weakness, and sensory loss. Her mother has multiple sclerosis (MS). Which lab test result, if found in this patient, supports a diagnosis of MS?
(A) Elevated erythrocyte sedimentation rate
(B) Elevated glucose in the cerebral spinal fluid (CSF)
(C) IgM to human herpesvirus type 6 in the serum
(D) Neutrophilic pleocytosis of CSF
(E) Oligoclonal bands of IgG in CSF

4 A 34-year-old inmate presented to the prison clinic with fever, cough, and night sweats. Tuberculosis was suspected and PPD (purified protein derivative) was injected intradermally. A skin reaction characterized by erythema and induration developed at the injection site within 2 days. Which cell type is primarily responsible for reacting to the PPD and releasing mediators that resulted in the skin manifestation?
(A) Endothelial cells
(B) Keratinocytes
(C) Langerhans cells
(D) Mast cells
(E) Th1 cells

5 A 66-year-old man with advanced pancreatic cancer develops cachexia. Which cytokine is primarily responsible for the cachexia seen in certain patients with cancer or debilitating infections?
(A) Interferon-α
(B) Interleukin-7
(C) Interleukin-17
(D) Transforming growth factor-β
(E) Tumor necrosis factor-α

6 A 24-year-old woman presents with airway obstruction secondary to laryngeal swelling. Her history is significant for episodes of recurrent facial swelling that began sometime in childhood. The swelling, which often involves the lips, begins suddenly without recognizable precipitating events and lasts for 2 to 3 days. Laboratory tests reveal a deficiency involving the complement system. Which component of the complement system is deficient in this woman?
(A) C1 inhibitor
(B) C3 convertase
(C) C5 convertase
(D) Mannose-binding lectin
(E) Membrane attack complex

The next two questions are linked.

7   An 8-month-old male has recurrent episodes of serious infections including otitis media, chronic sinusitis, and bacterial pneumonia. He is diagnosed with X-linked agammaglobulinemia after an immunologic workup. Which test result is consistent with this diagnosis?

(A) Absent CD16$^+$ and CD54$^+$ cells in peripheral blood

(B) Absent CD19$^+$ and CD20$^+$ cells in peripheral blood

(C) Absent serum IgG, very low levels of IgM

(D) Decreased CD3$^+$ cells in peripheral blood

(E) Lymphopenia

8   Which infectious agents are most likely causing the recurrent infections in the child in the above case?

(A) *Aspergillus flavus* and *Candida albicans*

(B) *Chlamydia pneumoniae* and *Legionella pneumophila*

(C) *Haemophilus influenzae* and *Streptococcus pneumoniae*

(D) *Mycobacterium tuberculosis* and *Mycobacterium avium* complex

(E) *Pneumocystis jeroveci* and *Cryptosporidium hominis*

The next two questions are linked.

9   A 10-month-old male with a history of recurrent, serious extracellular bacterial infections is hospitalized with pneumonia due to *Pneumocystis jeroveci*. An immunologic workup reveals neutropenia, normal numbers of T and B cells, normal complement levels and complement activity, elevated IgM and very low IgG and IgA. What is the molecular defect in this disease?

(A) Defective expression by lymphocytes of adenosine deaminase

(B) Lack of Bruton tyrosine kinase

(C) Mutation of the γ-chain of the IL-2 receptor

(D) Mutation of the NADPH oxidase enzyme

(E) Reduced expression of CD154 on T cells

10   What immunologic function is impaired in the child and best explains the infection in the above case?

(A) Antigen presentation by dendritic cells

(B) B-cell migration to follicles in secondary lymphoid tissue

(C) Differentiation of B and T cells from precursor cells

(D) Expression of functional antigen receptors on T cells

(E) T-cell activation of macrophages and class switching in B cells

11   What is the most common primary immune deficiency disorder?

(A) Bruton agammaglobulinemia

(B) Common variable immunodeficiency

(C) Leukocyte adhesion deficiency

(D) Selective IgA deficiency

(E) X-linked severe combined immunodeficiency

12   A 6-month-old male is hospitalized with disseminated *Mycobacterium avium* complex. His history is significant for recurrent episodes of otitis media which responded poorly to antibiotics and episodes of severe thrush and diaper rash. Based on this history, an immunologic workup was done and the child was diagnosed with an immune deficiency disorder. Deficiencies of which aspect of the immune response could best account for the child's medical history?

(A) B cells

(B) B and T cells

(C) Complement

(D) Macrophages

(E) Neutrophils

13   A drug in clinical trial for the treatment of multiple sclerosis inhibits matrix metalloprotease-9. If this drug leads to clinical improvement, how would it do so?

(A) Causing a shift in cytokine production in the CNS

(B) Degrading myelin antigens to prevent their presentation by oligodendrocytes

(C) Helping protect the blood–brain barrier and the myelin sheath from degradation

(D) Inducing apoptosis of activated CD8 cells

(E) Inhibiting the adherence of leukocytes to the endothelium of the blood–brain barrier

14   A 4-year-old male presents with a history of serious, recurrent bacterial infections including pneumonia, sepsis, and perianal abscesses. Physical exam reveals hepatosplenomegaly. An immune deficiency disease is suspected and his workup reveals WBC counts and serum IgG levels in the high normal range. The nitroblue tetrazolium (NBT) test indicated that the patient's neutrophils did not reduce NBT dye. Which of the following best explains these results?

(A) Deficiency in NADH or NADPH oxidase

(B) Presence of endotoxin in the blood

(C) Human immunodeficiency virus reactivation

(D) Deficiency in the common γ-chain (CD132)

(E) Deficiency in adenosine deaminase

15 A 1-year-old male born to term apparently healthy has for the last 5 months suffered from numerous bacterial, viral, and fungal infections. Upon examination, tonsils and lymph nodes are nearly undetectable and total leukocyte counts as well as serum immunoglobulin levels are abnormally low. Which of the following deficiencies is primarily responsible for the leukopenia in this patient?

(A) Adenosine deaminase
(B) IL-2 receptor γ-chain (CD25)
(C) IL-7 receptor α-chain (CD127)
(D) Janus tyrosine kinase 3 (JAK 3)
(E) T box-1 (TBX1)

The next two questions are linked.

16 A male infant developed tonic convulsions a few days after birth and was found to be hypocalcemic. Of note, he was born with a cleft palate, widely spaced eyes, and ears residing lower than normal. Cardiac defects also became apparent in the neonatal period. A lateral view chest radiograph revealed a diminished thymic shadow. What genetic defect could account for the problems seen in this child?

(A) A deletion in chromosome 22q11.2
(B) A mutation in adenosine deaminase
(C) Defect in recombination-activating genes (RAG)
(D) Janus tyrosine kinase 3 (JAK 3) deficiency
(E) Toll-like receptor signaling defect

17 A 45-year-old AIDS patient was enrolled in a drug development study. As part of the study, he underwent anergy skin testing. He was inoculated intradermally with candidal and mumps virus antigens. No reaction was demonstrable after 48 h. What is the most likely explanation for this?

(A) Antiretroviral drugs are known to interfere with this type of test
(B) He has neutropenia and cannot control the growth of *Candida*
(C) He lacks antibodies to both *Candida* and mumps virus
(D) His CD8 cells are not being activated due to decreased CD4 cell numbers
(E) His Th1 cells are unable to carry out a delayed type hypersensitivity reaction

18 A 3-week-old female child presents with omphalitis (swelling and redness surrounding the remains of the umbilical cord), a fever, and persistent diaper rash. History revealed that a few years earlier her brother had presented in a similar fashion and died at the age of 18 months due to bacterial pneumonia. Physical examination and radiology do not shown any abnormalities. A white blood cell count reveals leukocytosis; however, a Rebuck skin window test (abrade skin with scalpel, repeat placing cover slip over area) was negative for leukocytes. Which of the following is a likely explanation for this result?

(A) Defect in production of nucleotide oligomerization (NOD) proteins
(B) Defect in tumor necrosis factor (TNF) production
(C) Deficiency in expression of CD18
(D) Deficiency in expression of toll-like receptor 4 (TLR4)
(E) Deficiency in NADH or NADPH oxidase

19 A 25-year-old male is brought by ambulance to the emergency department after collapsing at a restaurant. His history is significant for peanut allergy. Physical exam reveals a blood pressure of 50/30 mm Hg, cold, clammy skin, diffuse urticaria, dyspnea, and wheezing. What drug is best to rapidly reverse the man's symptoms?

(A) Inhaled β-agonist
(B) Intravenous β-blocker
(C) Intravenous methylprednisolone
(D) Oral diphenhydramine
(E) Parenteral epinephrine

20 A 21-year-old female presented to the college infirmary in January with sore throat, cough, and fever. Auscultation reveals rhonchi, rale, and wheezing and she is treated for mild pneumonia as an outpatient. Following completion of a course of antibiotics, her initial symptoms resolved but she now complains of persistent fatigue and occasional pain in the extremities, particularly while walking between buildings on campus. In addition, she reports occasional bluish discoloration of her finger tips when her hands are cold. Physical exam reveals pallor and tachycardia. Her hematocrit, hemoglobin level, and red cell count reveal anemia. Which of the following is the most appropriate test to order at this point?

(A) Chest X-ray
(B) Direct and indirect Coombs test
(C) Glucose tolerance test
(D) Monospot test
(E) Screen for lupus by detection of anti-SR protein antibodies

21 An 18-month-old male child has a history of recurrent viral and fungal infections including respiratory syncytial virus and *Candida*. Examination revealed a marked reduction in T lymphocyte absolute numbers but a normal level of B cells. Furthermore, a chest radiograph reveals that the patient's thymus is hypoplastic. Assuming past infections were not severe, which of the following is the most appropriate therapeutic modality?

(A) No treatment
(B) Pharmacological intervention for future infections
(C) Bone marrow transplant
(D) Fetal thymic transplantation
(E) Intravenous interleukin-2 (IL-2)

The next three questions are linked.

22 A 20-year-old male was hospitalized with fever, hemoptysis, and respiratory distress. He had a 2-week history of fever, chills, cough, and shortness of breath that was unresponsive to a course of azithromycin. His cough had recently become tinged with blood. Urinalysis also showed hematuria. Blood, urine samples, and bronchoalveolar lavage samples were taken for culture and he was placed on empiric, broad spectrum antibiotics. He quickly deteriorated, developing pulmonary hemorrhage and azotemia. Direct immunofluorescent staining of a renal biopsy is shown in the photograph. What is the diagnosis?

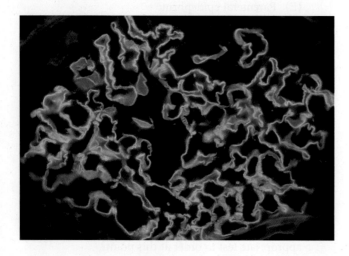

(A) Goodpasture syndrome
(B) IgA nephropathy
(C) Postinfectious glomerulonephritis
(D) Systemic lupus erythematosus
(E) Wegener granulomatosis

23 What antigen is targeted by the immune system in the above case?

(A) Desmoglein-3
(B) Neutrophil cytoplasmic antigens
(C) Nuclear antigens
(D) Pathogen antigens
(E) Type IV collagen

24 How should the patient in the above case be initially treated?

(A) Azathioprine
(B) Corticosteroids
(C) Diuretics
(D) Plasmaphoresis
(E) Transfusion

25 A 43-year-old woman has a diagnosis of relapsing and remitting multiple sclerosis. Which cytokines predominate in the CNS during periods of remission and what is their effect?

(A) CC-chemokines/recruit Th1 cells into CNS
(B) γ-Interferon and tumor necrosis factor-α (TNF-α)/support proliferation of oligodendrocytes
(C) IL-2, IL-5, TNF-α/activate microglia and astrocytes to secrete matrix metalloproteases
(D) IL-4, IL-10, TGF-β/downregulate Th1 cells
(E) IL-17 and TNF-α/activate endothelial cells and memory T cells

26 A 25-year-old male complains of a persistent (6 months) cough, severe pain in the left lower back, and blood in his urine. He is afebrile, a nonsmoker, and has not recently traveled. The chest radiograph reveals bilateral hilar lymphadenopathy while blood analysis indicates increased levels of calcium in the serum. A CT scan demonstrates the presence of many granulomatouslike lesions in the lungs in addition to the hilar lymphadenopathy. Which of the following would be the most appropriate test to order?

(A) Mantoux test
(B) Pulmonary function test
(C) Lung biopsy
(D) Determination of angiotensin-converting enzyme (ACE)
(E) Bone scan

27 A 10-year-old male child has seasonal episodes of runny nose, sneezing, nasal congestion, and itchy, watery eyes. His symptoms are most severe in the spring and interfere with school performance and outside activities. His symptoms have not been well controlled with over-the-counter antihistamines and his physician prescribes a medication that inhibits the cysteinyl leukotriene receptor. Which of the following drugs was he given?
(A) Beclomethasone
(B) Diphenhydramine
(C) Loratadine
(D) Montelukast
(E) Pseudoephedrine

The next two questions are linked.

28 A 56-year-old male with end stage renal disease receives a kidney transplant. He is treated post-transplant with an immune suppressive regimen including an antilymphocyte antibody, a calcineurin inhibitor, and an anti-proliferative drug in addition to corticosteroids. Which drugs, in addition to corticosteroids, is he given?
(A) Anti-CD3, cyclosporine, and mycophenolate, respectively
(B) Anti-CD4, cyclophosphamide, and tacrolimus, respectively
(C) Anti-CD8, mycophenolate, and sirolimus, respectively
(D) Anti-CD19, azathioprine, and mycophenolate, respectively
(E) Anti-CD20, tacrolimus, and cyclosporine, respectively

29 Despite the immunosuppressive regimen given to the patient in the above question, within a month posttransplant, signs of rejection began to appear as evidenced by rising creatinine levels. Acute rejection was diagnosed by biopsy. What is the immunopathologic basis for the rejection of this transplanted kidney?
(A) Delayed type hypersensitivity reaction of host T cells leading to atherosclerotic vascular damage in the grafted kidney
(B) Dendritic cells in the transplanted kidney presenting recipient antigens to and activating recipient cytotoxic T cells
(C) Presence in the recipient of preformed antibodies to the donor ABO blood group antigens
(D) Polyclonal activation of T cells that cross-react with allogeneic MHC molecules on the transplanted kidney
(E) T-cell response to reactivated cytomegalovirus causing damage to renal tubular epithelial cells

The next three questions are linked.

30 A 1-year-old male child who has experienced recurrent serious infections with staphylococcal and streptococcal bacteria is evaluated for immune deficiency during a time when he has no ongoing infection. His white blood cell count is within the normal range; however, flow cytometry analysis reveals an absence of $CD19^+$ lymphocytes and normal numbers of CD4 and $CD8^+$ lymphocytes. Nephelometry reveals very low levels of IgG and no measurable IgM or IgA. What is the most likely diagnosis?
(A) Acquired immunodeficiency syndrome (AIDS)
(B) Adenosine deaminase deficiency
(C) DiGeorge syndrome
(D) Systemic lupus erythematosus (SLE)
(E) X-linked agammaglobulinemia

31 Regarding the above case, which molecule is defective in this disease?
(A) Bruton tyrosine kinase (btk)
(B) CD40
(C) CD80/86
(D) Fas ligand
(E) Rag

32 What is the pathogenesis of this condition?
(A) An inability of B cells to differentiate into plasma cells
(B) An inability of B cells to undergo cognate binding with T helper cells
(C) An inability of B cells to undergo VDJ gene recombination
(D) An inability of plasma cells to secrete IgM
(E) An inability of pro-B cells to differentiate into B cells

33 A 14-year-old male child with extensive third-degree burns from a house fire receives a skin graft. Skin grafted from which donor has the lowest risk of immunologic rejection?
(A) The patient
(B) The patient's father
(C) The patient's fraternal twin brother
(D) The patient's fraternal twin sister
(E) The patient's mother

The next two questions are linked.

34 A 36-year-old female is diagnosed with myasthenia gravis. What were her most likely clinical manifestations?

(A) Abdominal pain, weight loss, and bloody diarrhea

(B) Ascending weakness and paresthesia

(C) Drooping of her eyelids and muscle weakness that improves with rest

(D) Fatigue, pallor, and mild jaundice

(E) Goiter, palpitations, and proptosis of the eyes

35 What is the immunopathogenesis of the disease in the above case?

(A) Antibody-mediated hemolysis of red blood cells

(B) Antibody-mediated interference with neuromuscular transmission

(C) Antibody-mediated stimulation of the thyroid gland

(D) Immunologic attack of peripheral nerve myelin sheath

(E) Inflammation of colonic mucosa

36 Tumor editing is one of the most difficult clinically relevant problems to overcome in the course of tumor therapy. Which one of the following accounts for the mechanism of tumor editing?

(A) Survival of tumors with moderate expression of class II MHC molecules

(B) Survival of tumors with low expression of class I MHC molecules

(C) Survival of tumors with low expression of class II MHC molecules

(D) Survival of tumors with high expression of class II MHC molecules

(E) Survival of tumors with moderate expression of class I MHC molecules

37 Which one of the following represents a mechanism of tumor evasion from the immune response?

(A) Deviation of helper T cells to type-1 or Th1 cells

(B) Production of interferon-γ (IFNγ) by the tumor

(C) Cross-presentation of tumor antigen by dendritic cells to activate CD8⁺ T cells

(D) Decreased expression of class I MHC on tumor cells

(E) Tumor inhibition of angiogenesis

38 A 4-month-old girl child is hospitalized with a serious staphylococcal skin infection without pus formation. Her history is significant for delayed separation of the umbilical cord, recurrent infections, gingivitis, and poor wound healing. Her CBC and differential shows marked leukocytosis; however, flow cytometry studies showed a lack of expression of β_2-integrins on leukocytes. What immunologic problem would this lead to?

(A) Failure of lymphopoiesis

(B) Reduced antigen processing by dendritic cells

(C) Reduced diapedesis of neutrophils

(D) Reduced expression of tolllike receptors

(E) Reduced angiogenesis

39 A 57-year-old woman with chronic joint pain receives a diagnosis of rheumatoid arthritis (RA). What pathologic process, ongoing in the synovial membranes of her affected joints, is the most important contributor to joint damage?

(A) B-cell autoantibody production and immune complex deposition

(B) Complement-mediated lysis of synovial membranes

(C) Cytokine activation of synoviocytes, chrondocytes, and osteoclasts

(D) Cytotoxic T cell-mediated destruction of cartilage

(E) Mast cell degranulation and infiltration of neutrophils

40 A 2-month-old infant presents with severe pyoderma over much of her body. Her history is significant for other infections including pneumonia and for bruising very easily. Both parents are healthy with no significant medical history. Physical exam reveals an ill infant with large areas of hypopigmentation of the skin, silvery hair, and very pale eyes. Gingival inflammation and bleeding of the gums and generalized lymphadenopathy are noted. A white blood cell count reveals moderate leukopenia and thrombocytopenia. Definitive diagnosis is made by examination of a peripheral blood smear which showed unusually large granules within neutrophils and eosinophils. What is the most likely diagnosis?

(A) Bare lymphocyte syndrome

(B) Chediak–Higashi syndrome

(C) Thrombocytopenia purpura

(D) Wegener granulomatosis

(E) Wiskott–Aldrich syndrome

41 A 25-year-old female presents with marked bilateral weakness in her legs and arms. She has difficulty standing and lifting. The condition began 3 days ago with altered sensations in both feet and legs. The weakness in her legs was noted with difficulty getting up from a chair. Within 24 hours, she experienced difficulty raising her arms and now feels short of breath. She has no significant medical history except for a diarrheal illness 2 weeks ago following consumption of undercooked chicken. Physical exam reveals normal muscular development, impaired proprioception, and absent deep tendon reflexes. Cerebral spinal fluid analysis reveals elevated protein with no pleocytosis. Results of nerve conduction studies are consistent with demyelination of peripheral nerves. What is the most likely diagnosis?

(A) Botulism
(B) Guillain–Barre syndrome
(C) Multiple sclerosis
(D) Polymyositis
(E) Systemic lupus erythematosus

The next two questions are linked.

42 A 22-year-old female presents with an erythematous malar rash as seen in the accompanying photograph after spending spring break on the beach. Prior to this incident, she had been feeling increasingly fatigued and noticed painful swelling in her hands and wrists. Which of the following test results would yield a definitive diagnosis of her condition?

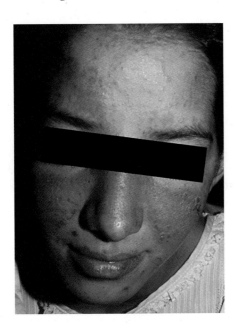

(A) Antibodies to double-stranded DNA
(B) Decreased serum complement levels
(C) Elevated antinuclear antibody levels
(D) Elevated C-reactive protein
(E) Positive Coombs test

43 The patient in the above case is prescribed a drug that reduces inflammation without causing generalized immune suppression. What drug is she given?
(A) Azathioprine
(B) Cyclophosphamide
(C) Hydroxychloroquine
(D) Methotrexate
(E) Methylprednisolone

44 The 56-year-old woman in the accompanying photograph has been under the care of an endocrinologist and receiving radioactive iodine for a hyperthyroid condition in which thyroid-stimulating immunoglobulins are present in the serum. What is the diagnosis?

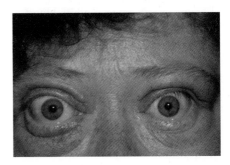

(A) Graves disease
(B) Goodpasture syndrome
(C) Hashimoto thyroiditis
(D) Myasthenia gravis
(E) Sjogren syndrome

45 A 15-year-old girl is being evaluated for Addison disease. Her history is significant for hypoparathyroidism diagnosed at age 10 and recurrent bouts of mucocutaneous candidiasis since early childhood. She is diagnosed eventually with polyglandular autoimmune syndrome type-1. Which gene is associated with this condition?
(A) AIRE
(B) Complement C1q
(C) CTLA-4
(D) FoxP3
(E) HLA-DR4

46 A 60-year-old man presents with fatigue, weight loss of several months duration, and tingling sensations in his feet for the past few weeks. Physical exam reveals pallor and tachycardia. A complete blood count reveals anemia with increased mean corpuscular volume, as well as mild leukopenia and thrombocytopenia. The peripheral smear shows large red cells with abnormal shapes along with hypersegmented neutrophils. Having ruled out nutritional causes, the physician decides to look for autoantibodies in the patient's serum. For which antibodies will she test?
(A) ABO antibodies
(B) Antinuclear antibodies
(C) Antiparietal cell antibodies
(D) Antired cell antibodies
(E) Rh antibodies

47 A 21-month-old male child is being evaluated for recurrent otitis media that returns rapidly following completion of an antibiotic regimen. His history is significant for pneumonia at 14 months of age. Physical exam reveals eczema and a petechial rash. His mother reports he is prone to nose bleeds. A complete blood count reveals normal white blood cell number and distribution, thrombocytopenia, and decreased mean platelet volume. Immunoglobulin levels show decreased IgM and IgG, but elevated IgA and IgE. Isohemagglutinins were not detected even though the child's blood type was O. What is the cellular defect characteristic of this condition?

(A) Defective expression of chemokine receptors
(B) Defective expression of costimulatory molecules on T cells
(C) Defective expression of signal transduction molecules
(D) Defective maturation of stem cells into white blood cells
(E) Defective polymerization and depolymerization of actin

48 A 36-year-old male has been treated for 10 years for the scaly, plaquelike lesions shown in the accompanying photograph. The plaques are widespread on his body and have been resistant to several different therapies. His physician prescribes cyclosporine that leads to a rapid reduction in lesions. Which cell is implicated in the pathogenesis of this disease as demonstrated by the response to this drug?

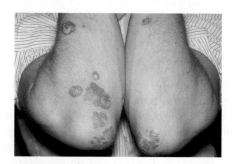

(A) B cells
(B) Dendritic cells
(C) Eosinophils
(D) Neutrophils
(E) T cells

49 A 68-year-old man presents with low back pain. Physical exam reveals a pale white male with petechiae on the mucous membranes of the mouth. Tenderness of L4 was elicited by palpation. Blood tests reveal mild anemia, leucopenia, thrombocytopenia, an elevated erythrocyte sedimentation rate, and increased blood calcium. Radiographs reveal lytic bone lesions, and an MRI of the spine reveals a destructive lesion in L4 with extrusion of a mass and compression of the spinal cord. Serum electrophoresis reveals a spike in the γ-globulin region. What would most likely be found in the urine?

(A) Bence–Jones proteins
(B) Glucose
(C) Leukocyte esterase
(D) Red cell casts
(E) White cell casts

The next two questions are linked.

50 A 33-year-old woman is pregnant with her second child. Her blood type is B, Rh-negative, and her husband's is AB, Rh-positive. Her first child has type B blood and expresses the D antigen in his red blood cells. What test can be used to determine if her fetus is at risk for hemolytic disease of the newborn?

(A) ABO blood typing of the fetus prior to birth
(B) Bilirubin level in umbilical cord blood
(C) Direct Coombs test on the mother's red cells
(D) Indirect antiglobulin test on the mother's serum
(E) Ultrasound

51 How is hemolytic disease of the newborn prevented?

(A) Administration of anti-Rh antibodies to Rh-negative women after the birth of each Rh-positive child
(B) Infusion of intravenous immune globulin to Rh-negative women during each pregnancy
(C) Periodic plasmaphoresis of Rh-negative women during pregnancy
(D) Transfusion of Rh-negative women with Rh-positive blood after delivery of each child
(E) Transfusion of Rh-negative women with Rh-positive blood prior to each pregnancy

The next two questions are linked.

52 A 55-year-old Jewish man presented to his dentist with a few painful oral lesions which appeared as irregularly shaped erosions on the gingiva. The dentist suspected aphthous ulcers and suggested an over-the-counter topical preparation. Within weeks, the number of lesions increased appearing on the palate, tongue, uvula, and buccal surface. In addition, a small ulcerative sore appeared on his face and enlarged to form a fluid-filled bulla before he was able to see his physician. By this time, the man is noticeably hoarse and unable to eat or drink without pain. His physician took a biopsy of the skin lesion and surrounding normal skin and sent it to a laboratory which performed a direct fluorescent antibody test. The test result showed intercellular fluorescence as shown in the accompanying photograph. What is the diagnosis?

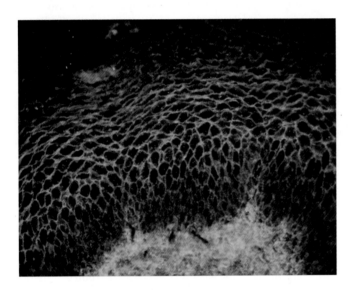

(A) Contact dermatitis
(B) Discoid lupus
(C) Herpes simplex type 1 infection
(D) Pemphigus vulgaris
(E) Psoriasis

53 What is the pathogenesis of the disease in the above question?
(A) Antidesmoglein antibodies causing acantholysis
(B) Antigen–antibody complex mediated inflammation of the epidermis
(C) Complement-mediated lysis of keratinocytes
(D) Neutrophil infiltration and necrosis of the dermis
(E) Underlying immune suppression allowing uncontrolled viral-mediated cell lysis

54 A 42-year-old male presents with fever, fatigue, malaise, and cough occasionally productive of bloody sputum. His history is significant for sinusitis for the past several months. Physical exam reveals tenderness over the maxillary sinus, a serosanguineous discharge from the nose, and chest dullness to percussion. Auscultation reveals crackles and decreased breath sounds. A urinalysis reveals increased protein and microscopic hematuria. Chest radiographs reveal bilateral nodules. Antineutrophil cytoplasmic antibodies (ANCA) were detected in his serum. What is the diagnosis?
(A) Chronic granulomatous disease
(B) Goodpasture syndrome
(C) Sarcoidosis
(D) Systemic lupus erythematosus
(E) Wegener granulomatosis

55 A 6-year-old boy is diagnosed with asthma after repeated episodes of wheezing and chest tightness. Frequent use of a bronchodilator does little to reduce the frequency of his symptoms. His visits to the emergency department decline after being placed on inhaled corticosteroids. What is the most important explanation for the clinical improvement seen with inhaled corticosteroids?
(A) Decreased histamine production by mast cells
(B) Decreased inflammatory cell infiltrates into bronchial wall
(C) Decreased number of allergen-reactive B cells
(D) Inhibition of Th17 cell function
(E) Switch from Th2 cell activity to Th1 cell activity

56 The repression of which transcription factor explains on a molecular level the anti-inflammatory effect of corticosteroids?
(A) FoxP3
(B) ITAM
(C) MAP kinase
(D) NF-κB
(E) Protein kinase C

ANSWERS

1　**The answer is B: Interleukin-6.**　When the body experiences a significant inflammatory reaction, many physiological responses are generated. Interleukin-6, released into the circulation from activated macrophages and other cells, stimulates hepatocytes to release acute phase reactants. These proteins include components of the complement system, clotting system, and variety of others that play a role in promoting inflammation, or serving as opsonins. Some even down-regulate inflammation. Fibrinogen is a protein of the clotting system and causes an elevated ESR. In this test, a tube of heparinized blood is allowed to stand on end while the red blood cells settle to the bottom of the tube. When the red cells settle, they stack on top of one another. The more fibrinogen in the blood, the faster the red cells settle. Thus, the more inflammation, the more IL-6 is released and this in turn causes a greater release of acute phase reactants including fibrinogen. Another acute phase reactant is CRP, which functions as an opsonin. Both IL-1 and tumor necrosis factor (TNF)-α can also cause the release of acute phase reactants.

2　**The answer is E: Rheumatoid factor test.**　The case describes early rheumatoid arthritis. Early in this disease, patients present with bilateral, polyarticular joint pain, and tenderness. Joint deformity is generally a late-stage process indicative of severe joint pathology. Recognition of rheumatoid arthritis at an early stage is essential as pharmacologic intervention can delay the onset of joint deformity. The rheumatoid factor test is positive in about 70% of patients with rheumatoid arthritis; however, it may be negative early in the disease. The test detects the presence of autoantibodies (called rheumatoid factors), which bind to the Fc region of IgG. These autoantibodies are most commonly of the IgM isotype; however, IgG rheumatoid factors can also be found. While the presence of rheumatoid factor in a patient's serum is an aid to the diagnosis of rheumatoid arthritis, it is not used to make a definitive diagnosis. Rheumatoid factor can also be detected in patients with other types of connective tissue diseases as well as in normal individuals. The antinuclear antibody test is most commonly used as an aid to the diagnosis of systemic lupus erythematosus. This test may also be positive in some patients with rheumatoid arthritis, as well as several other connective tissue diseases. The Coombs test is used to make a diagnosis of immune hemolytic anemia. Anemia, common in patients with rheumatoid arthritis, is characterized as normocytic and normochromic, and is not diagnosed with the Coombs test. The erythrocyte sedimentation rate is elevated in chronic inflammatory states and is not diagnostic for any particular disease. Radiographs would not be expected to be diagnostic during the early stage of the disease, prior to joint deformity.

3　**The answer is E: Oligoclonal bands of IgG in CSF.** Multiple sclerosis is an autoimmune disease with demonstrated genetic predisposition. In monozygotic twins, the concordance rate for the disease is about 30%. Individuals with second and third degree relatives with MS are also at increased risk of developing the disease when compared to the general population. Clinical diagnosis of MS is difficult because the disease is quite heterogeneous in its presentation. Neurological manifestations depend upon the location of demyelinating lesions within the central nervous system. Laboratory and imaging tests are essential in establishing a diagnosis of MS. Oligoclonal bands of IgG in CSF are found in about 85% of patients and are one of the most important diagnostic findings. The term oligoclonal indicates that the IgG was produced by a few different clones of B cells. This term is in contrast to "monoclonal," meaning from a single clone, and "polyclonal," meaning from a large number of clones of B cells. An oligoclonal response is consistent with a response of B or T cells to a pathogen. Several clones of T or B cells would have specificity for the dominant antigens of the pathogen and would become activated. The finding of oligoclonal bands of IgG in the CSF supports the idea that MS is an antigen-driven response, perhaps even a pathogen-driven response. The oligoclonal IgG present in the CSF appears to have been synthesized in the CNS, rather than in the periphery and crossing the blood–brain barrier. The variable regions of the oligoclonal IgG of patients with MS have been studied, but do not point to a single nervous system antigen or to a particular pathogen as the stimulus for the antigen-driven response. In fact, there appears to be person-to-person variability in the nature of these antibodies. Certain viral pathogens have been suggested to play a role in the pathogenesis of MS, including herpesvirus type 6; however, none has a proven association, and the finding of antiviral IgM is not useful in making a diagnosis of MS. Glucose levels are usually normal in the CSF of MS patients, and although pleocytosis may occur, it is frequently mononuclear. An elevated erythrocyte sedimentation rate is a nonspecific indicator of systemic inflammation and is not diagnostic for MS or any other disease.

4　**The answer is E: Th1 cells.**　The reaction to PPD in a tuberculosis patient is the result of *Mycobacterium tuberculosis*-specific memory T helper 1 (Th1 cells that encounter the antigen presented by skin dendritic cells (Langerhans cells). Following antigen interaction, the

Th1 cell releases cytokines and chemokines, which recruit and activate mononuclear cells from the blood. The inflammatory response that develops, with its vasodilation and cellular infiltrate, accounts for the erythema and induration seen at the site of antigen injection. If any of the other cells were primarily involved in this reaction, even uninfected individuals would respond by mounting an inflammatory response following antigen injection. The skin test is used to detect memory cells elicited following primary exposure to *M. tuberculosis*.

5 **The answer is E: Tumor necrosis factor-α.** Cachexia is a loss of body mass irreversible by nutrition. Tumor necrosis factor (TNF)-α is the main cytokine involved in cachexia. High levels of TNF-α in the blood lead to several metabolic changes in conjunction with increased energy utilization by the growing tumor. TNF-α induces mobilization of fatty acids and protein catabolism leading to a breakdown of adipose tissue and skeletal muscle wasting. The other cytokines listed are not responsible for causing cachexia.

6 **The answer is A: C1 inhibitor.** This case is descriptive of hereditary angioedema, a condition attributed to a decrease in or dysfunction of C1 inhibitor (C1-INH). This protein is a multifunction serine protease normally found in large amounts in serum. It binds to and inactivates C1r and C1s. It also inactivates proteins of the clotting and kinin systems. Decreased amounts of this protein result in subcutaneous and/or submucosal edema through compromised inactivation of the complement and/or the kinin system. Hereditary angioedema is an autosomal dominant trait. Deficiencies in the other complement components listed do not lead to hereditary angioedema.

7 **The answer is B: Absent CD19⁺ and CD20⁺ cells in peripheral blood.** X-linked agammaglobulinemia (XLA), also called Bruton agammaglobulinemia, is a congenital immune deficiency disease characterized by a lack of B-cell production by the bone marrow. B cells express CD19 and CD20, and these two markers are exploited in flow cytometry studies to enumerate B cells in the peripheral blood. The lack of these cells in peripheral blood of a male infant is diagnostic for XLA. Natural killer cells express CD16⁺ and CD54⁺ and are not affected in this disease. Absent serum IgG, very low levels of IgM is inconsistent with XLA since without B cells no IgM could be produced. Infants with this disease have maternal IgG in their serum which declines at about 5 to 6 months of age, leaving them at increased risk for infections such as those seen in this patient. Infants with XLA have normal to elevated levels of CD3⁺ T cells. Lymphopenia is not seen, as the majority of circulating lymphocytes are T cells.

8 **The answer is C: *Haemophilus influenzae* and *Streptococcus pneumoniae*.** The absence of B cells and thus antibody makes an individual susceptible to those organisms controlled by humoral immune responses. The most important defenses against extracellular bacteria are opsonins (including IgG, in addition to complement C3b) and neutrophils. The ability of neutrophils to phagocytize microorganisms is markedly enhanced when they are opsonized with both complement and IgG. Thus, a lack of IgG renders phagocytosis much less efficient and increases the risk for infection with extracellular bacteria. *H. influenzae* and *S. pneumoniae* are two of the most important bacterial causes of otitis media, sinusitis, and pneumonia, and both are extracellular organisms. *Aspergillus flavus* and *Candida albicans* are both opportunistic fungi which cause infections in patients with profound neutropenia. Patients with T-cell deficiencies also suffer serious infections with these organisms. *Chlamydia pneumoniae*, *Legionella pneumophila*, and *Mycobacterium* sp. are intracellular bacteria. Legionnaires disease is seen most often in T-cell immune compromised patients, such as the elderly, transplant patients, or cancer patients. Patients with disseminated *Mycobacterium avium* are profoundly T-cell immune suppressed. On the other hand, both *C. pneumoniae* and *Mycobacterium tuberculosis* are able to infect immune competent individuals. *Pneumocystis jeroveci* and *Cryptosporidium hominis* are pathogens that cause serious disease in the profoundly T-cell immune suppressed, including AIDS patients. *P. jeroveci* is a fungus, whereas *C. hominis* is a sporozoan parasite.

9 **The answer is E: Reduced expression of CD154 on T cells.** This case is descriptive of hyper-IgM syndrome, a disease whose molecular defect is caused by mutations in the gene for CD40 ligand otherwise known as CD154. See next question for further explanation of this disease.

10 **The answer is E: T-cell activation of macrophages and class switching in B cells.** The case describes a child with T-cell dysfunction, as demonstrated by his infection with *Pneumocystis jeroveci* a fungal organism thought to be part of the normal oropharyngeal flora and that causes disease in patients with compromised T-cell–mediated immunity. As the T cells are normal in number, their activation must be impaired, and his current infection supports this idea. The fact that the patient has elevated IgM and very low levels of IgG and IgA, suggests that the T cells cannot interact adequately with B cells to induce class switching. In addition to cytokine stimuli, the interaction of CD40 on the B cell with CD40 ligand (also known as CD154) on the T cell is essential to stimulate class switching in B cells. This molecule is also essential for contact-mediated activation of macrophages by Th1 cells, and activated macrophages are important for the control of *P. jeroveci*. The other immunologic processes listed are not affected in this disease.

11   **The answer is D: Selective IgA deficiency.**   Estimates of the frequency of this disease range from 1 in 700 to 1 in 3,000 live births. The other diseases listed have a much lower incidence. The frequency of Bruton agammaglobulinemia has been estimated to be 1 in 250,000 to 1 in 379,000 live births. Common variable immunodeficiency in contrast to its name is not common, occurring in about 1 in 10,000 to 1 in 50,000. Leukocyte adhesion deficiency is extremely rare, having been reported in only a few hundred infants in the United States. X-linked severe combined immunodeficiency is one of several diseases under the umbrella term of severe combined immunodeficiency diseases. The frequency of this group of diseases is estimated to be between 1 in 50,000 and 75,000 live births.

12   **The answer is B: B and T cells.**   Control of intracellular pathogens is primarily dependent on intact cell-mediated immunity and control of extracellular pathogens is primarily dependent on intact humoral immunity. The pathogens causing disease in this child include both intracellular and extracellular organisms. Disseminated *M. avium* complex infections occur in patients with compromised cell-mediated immunity. Organisms causing otitis media requiring antibiotics are extracellular bacteria such as *Streptococcus pneumoniae*, *Haemophilus inlfuenzae*, or *Moraxella catarrhalis*. The agent that causes thrush and diaper rash, *Candida albicans*, is controlled by phagocytes. Uncontrolled growth of *C. albicans* occurs in patients with neutrophil dysfunctions or in patients whose T cells are unable to activate phagocytic macrophages.

13   **The answer is C: Helping protect the blood–brain barrier and the myelin sheath from degradation.**   MMPs are tissue degrading enzymes released from activated glial cells in the CNS as well as by infiltrating lymphocytes and monocyte-derived macrophages. These enzymes play an important role in the pathogenic process in MS and other immune-mediated diseases. Some studies have shown that β-interferon, a drug used in the treatment of MS, acts in part by down-regulating the production of MMPs. Metalloproteases are not involved in any of the other activities listed in the question, thus interfering with the function of MMPs would not lead to any of the other effects listed.

14   **The answer is A: Deficiency in NADH or NADPH oxidase.**   This case describes a child with chronic granulomatous disease. The key clinical clue to this diagnosis is the recurrent serious bacterial infections. The key

lab result is the NBT test which assesses the capacity of phagocytes to produce superoxides by NADPH oxidase. These superoxides can then be converted to hydrogen peroxide and hydroxyl radicals. A lack of NBT reduction (i.e., a negative test result) indicates a deficiency in the enzyme. While endotoxin (choice B) can increase WBC counts and IgG levels, the NBT test will be positive in this case. Accordingly, HIV reactivation (choice C), CD132 (choice D), or ADA (choice E) deficiencies will result in lowered WBC counts and serum IgG levels (CD132 and ADA). Consequently, CD132 or ADA deficiencies are indicative of severe combined immunodeficiency.

15   **The answer is A: Adenosine deaminase.**   Susceptibility to bacterial infections implicate B-cell defects (lack of tonsil and lymph node tissue), while increased viral and fungal infections characterize a defect in the T-cell compartment. All of the answers result in severe combined immunodeficiency; however, only adenosine deaminase deficiencies will present with marked decreases in both T- and B-cell numbers. Mutations in CD25, JAK 3, CD127, and TBX1 result in reduced T-cell numbers, while B-cell counts remain in the normal range or may be slightly increased. In all cases, serum immunoglobulin levels are reduced.

16   **The answer is A: A deletion in chromosome 22q11.2.**   This child has congenital thymic aplasia or DiGeorge syndrome, which is associated with a deletion in chromosome 22q11.2. Other syndromes associated with this deletion include velocardiofacial syndrome and conotruncal anomaly face syndrome. All these syndromes share characteristic facial features, cardiac abnormalities and recurrent infections. These syndromes represent a developmental defect involving the pharyngeal arches and pouches. Embryologic development of these areas, which include the thymus, parathyroids, heart, and face, is dependent on the migration of neural crest cells to the region of the pharyngeal pouches. Defects in RAG, adenosine deaminase, JAK3 molecules, which result in severe combined immunodeficiency and tolllike receptor signaling, are not associated with the distinctive physical features of this patient.

17   **The answer is E: His Th1 cells are unable to carry out a delayed type hypersensitivity reaction.**   Intradermal inoculation of candidal or mumps antigens in immune competent individuals results in an infiltration of mononuclear cells at the inoculation after 48 hours. This reaction is due to the activation of memory Th1 cells by antigen presenting macrophages and dendritic cells in the skin. Activated memory Th1 cells release cytokines that recruit mononuclear cells to the area. This reaction requires about 48 hours to develop and results in the induration and erythema characteristic of a positive delayed type hypersensitivity (DTH) reaction. The inability to carry out a DTH reaction to commonly encountered antigens such as *Candida* and mumps virus indicates a dysfunction of Th1 cells. Antiretroviral drugs do not interfere with this type of test. Neutropenia can lead to uncontrolled candidal infections but it does not result in skin test anergy. Antibodies and CD8 cells do not play a role in the DTH reaction.

18 **The answer is C: Deficiency in expression of CD18.** Recurrent skin infections and delayed umbilical cord separation suggest a defect in leukocyte migration. The Rebuck skin window test supports this notion as no leukocytes appeared over the course of observation (typically up to 8 hours). TNF, NADH/NADPH oxidase, TLR4, and NOD proteins are molecules involved in cell signaling and/or effector functions but not cell migration. CD18, however, is the common chain of β_2-integrins, namely, LFA-1 and Mac-1. These molecules are found on phagocytes and lymphocytes and guide those cells to sites of infection. In normal individuals, neutrophils appear in the first cover slip and about 4 hours later; monocytes would be predominant at 8 hours. A lack of CD18 prevents such migration patterns.

19 **The answer is E: Parenteral epinephrine.** The patient in this case is experiencing shock. A number of clinical syndromes can be responsible for these symptoms including trauma, septic shock, dehydration, and heart damage. This patient, however, experienced these conditions suddenly upon consumption of food. Thus, this is a case of systemic anaphylaxis, possible due to exposure to peanut antigens in the food he ingested. Clues to this diagnosis include the extremely low blood pressure and other physical signs. Cold and clammy skin is the classic sign of impending shock. It suggests that the patient is not delivering sufficient blood to the peripheral tissues. The low blood pressure is a result of increased vascular permeability and vasodilation secondary to wide-spread mast cell and basophil degranulation. Mediators from these cells are responsible for the development of urticaria and bronchoconstriction leading to dyspnea and wheezing. Since total respiratory collapse could occur in minutes, urgent therapeutic intervention is required. Epinephrine, given either subcutaneously or intramuscularly, is the drug of choice for rapid reversal of hypotension, wheezing, and dyspnea in anaphylaxis. An inhaled β-agonist is also effective for bronchospasm, but would not have an effect on hypotension. β-blockers are used to treat hypertension, and may interfere with the actions of epinephrine in patients taking these drugs. Corticosteroids are used to treat anaphylaxis; however, their protective effects are slow to develop, and they are not used to reverse hypotension. Likewise, antihistamines such as diphenhydramine are used in anaphylaxis, primarily to reverse urticaria and other cutaneous manifestations.

20 **The answer is B: Direct and indirect Coombs test.** The case description should raise the suspicion of cold agglutinin disease. This diagnosis is suggested by the postinfection onset of anemia, discoloration of the fingers, and extremity pain associated with exposure to the cold. A second possibility is drug-induced hemolytic anemia; however, her symptom association with the cold more strongly suggests cold agglutinin disease. In this disease, IgM antired cell antibodies transiently attach to red cells when the temperature is less than 37°C, as the blood passes through the extremities. Although dissociation of these antibodies occurs as the blood enters the central circulation, the initial attachment of the red cell-specific antibodies results in clumping and hemolysis of the cells. Transient ischemia can result in pain in the extremities and discoloration of the digits. The diagnosis of cold agglutinin disease is confirmed by the results of the direct and indirect Coombs tests. A direct Coombs test using reagents that include only monoclonal anti-IgG is usually negative, as the red cells are coated with IgM antibodies. However, as IgM activates the complement cascade, the red cells are also coated with C3 break down products, which can be detected using reagents containing antibodies to C3b and C3d. Indirect Coombs test run at 37°C is negative in this disease, as the antibody does not bind to red cells at this temperature. When run at 4°C, however, the indirect test is positive. By contrast, if the patient had drug-induced hemolytic anemia, the direct test would be reactive using antibodies to IgG and the indirect test would be negative at both 4°C and 37°C. Thus, the direct and indirect Coombs tests would be the most useful to distinguish between cold agglutinin disease and drug-induced hemolytic anemia. Because the patient's respiratory symptoms have resolved, a chest radiograph is not indicted. The other tests listed would not be useful at this point, although both mononucleosis and SLE might be included in a broad differential.

21 **The answer is B: Pharmacological intervention for future infections.** Recurrent viral and fungal infections suggest a defect in the T-cell compartment. This suggestion is confirmed by lab results indicating normal levels of B cells but reduced numbers of T cells. Radiograph reveals that an abnormal development of thymic tissue and suggest a diagnosis of DiGeorge syndrome. Since the patient has had no severe complications from past infections and responds well but slowly with pharmacological intervention, continuing this treatment strategy should be sufficient therapy as T-cell function often improves by the age of 5 years in these patients. Acquisition of such T-cell improvement is probably due to as yet unidentified maturation site for the T cells. If past infections had been severe to life threatening, bone marrow or fetal thymic transplantation would be an appropriate mode of action. Intravenous IL-2 will be ineffective in expanding T-cell numbers as the T cells in the patient are immature and do not express the receptor to respond to this cytokine. In addition, the small percentage of T cells that express the IL-2 receptor constitutively are regulatory cells and activation with this cytokine may dampen any response to infectious challenge resulting in more severe disease. Due to the lack of T cells required for clearance of viral and fungal challenges, no treatment would result in prolonged and perhaps increased severity of all future infections.

22 **The answer is A: Goodpasture syndrome.** The patient in this case was suffering from a form of pulmonary-renal syndrome, characterized by the simultaneous occurrence of pulmonary hemorrhage and glomerulonephritis. Differential diagnosis of pulmonary-renal syndrome includes Goodpasture syndrome, systemic lupus erythematosus (SLE), and Wegener granulomatosis. The smooth, uniform pattern of fluorescence seen on the biopsy is typical for Goodpasture syndrome. A more heterogenous fluorescence, often called "lumpy bumpy," is typical for immune complex mediated glomerulonephritis as occurs in SLE. Postinfectious glomerulonephritis is also due to immune complex deposition and would appear similarly; this disease is not part of the pulmonary-renal syndrome. Kidney biopsies from patients with IgA nephropathy show IgA deposition in the mesangium, while kidney biopsies from Wegener granulomatosus show little or no deposition of IgG or complement, and thus weak or no fluorescence.

23 **The answer is E: Type IV collagen.** This type of collagen is found in the basement membranes of the lung and kidney. Type IV collagen fibers are made up of a triple helix containing mixtures of one of the six different α-chains. The collagen epitope targeted in Goodpasture syndrome is at the carboxyl terminal of the noncollagenous domain of the α3-chain. Desmoglein-3 is a protein component of desmosomes found between keratinocytes. It is targeted by autoantibody in the disease pemphigus vulgaris. Neutrophil cytoplasmic antigens are targeted in Wegener granulomatosus. Nuclear antigens are targeted in systemic lupus erythematosus. Pathogen antigens would be found in immune complexes deposited in the kidneys in postinfectious glomerulonephritis.

24 **The answer is D: Plasmaphoresis.** It is essential to remove the offending autoantibodies as rapidly as possible. Once plasmaphoresis has been initiated and the autoantibody levels have declined, medications to prevent further production of these antibodies can begin. This usually consists of cyclophosphamide and corticosteroids. The other therapies listed are not used in this situation.

25 **The answer is D: IL-4, IL-10, TGF-β/downregulate Th1 cells.** Human and animal studies suggest that these cytokines are present in the brain during times of disease remission and act to regulate Th1 cells. The other cytokines listed are not associated with MS remission, and many (CC-chemokines, γ-interferon, TNF-α, IL-12, and IL-17) are associated with disease progression. The recruitment of Th1 cells into the CNS would accelerate the disease. Proliferation of oligodendrocytes is not promoted by γ-IFN or TNF-α. T cells secrete matrix metalloproteases in patients with MS. Activation of endothelial cells and memory T cells is not consistent with disease remission.

26 **The answer is A: Mantoux test.** Interestingly, in this case both lungs and kidneys are affected. Some autoimmune immunoglobulin depositions can give similar symptoms; however, these conditions do not account for the granulomatouslike lesions found in the lungs. Elevated calcium levels may be due to multiple causes including diet, bone metabolism, renal secretion abnormalities, and hormonal problems (parathyroid hormone). However, there is no link with the elevated calcium and the granulomatouslike lesions suggesting the altered calcium levels are due to an effect upon the kidneys as opposed to a bone disease. Therefore, a bone scan (choice E) would not be the next course of action but could be used to confirm that no such bone disease exists. Granulomatouslike lesions are present in tuberculosis patients in addition to the persistent cough. For this reason, the most appropriate test to order is the Mantoux test (choice A) to rule out tuberculosis. If the test is positive, then the patient is diagnosed with tuberculosis. If the test is negative, sarcoidosis is a potential alternate diagnosis as this multisystem disease of unknown etiology produces granulomatouslike lesions in the lungs and also promotes the hilar lymphadenopathy observed in this patient. While there is no gold standard test for diagnosis, one must use the process of elimination to make a diagnosis. Pulmonary function test (choice B), lung biopsy (choice C), and determination of ACE concentrations (choice D) would be supportive tests for a sarcoidosis diagnosis. One additional test would be the Kveim test which operates in the same way as the Mantoux test with the exception that spleen homogenate from a sarcoidosis patient is injected intradermally into the test subject rather than tuberculin protein. Given the symptoms and the lower flank pain suggestive of kidney stone formation (due to increased calcium levels), a presumptive diagnosis of sarcoidosis could be proposed.

27   **The answer is D: Montelukast.**   The child in this case suffers from allergic rhinitis. Similar in pathogenesis to asthma, allergic rhinitis has an immediate phase and a late phase response. In the immediate phase, antigens bind to IgE on mast cells in the nasal mucosa, inducing their activation and degranulation. Degranulation leads to histamine release and histamine is an important contributor to the increase in nasal secretions (runny nose). Arachidonic acid metabolism also occurs upon mast cell activation and this leads to the release of leukotrienes and other metabolites. The cysteinyl leukotrienes (CysLTs) play a very important role in the immediate phase of allergy by increasing vascular permeability and inducing vasodilation. This leads to rhinitis and nasal congestion. In addition, CysLTs cause upregulation of adhesion molecules on endothelial cells and promote the recruitment and survival of eosinophils, thus participating in the late phase response. Eosinophilic infiltration and release of toxic granule components lead to further mast cell degranulation and perpetuation of the allergic response. Montelukast is a leukotriene receptor antagonist that blocks type 1 CysLT receptors found on leukocytes, smooth muscle cells, and endothelial cells of the respiratory mucosa, leading to clinical improvement in patients with allergic rhinitis. It was first used in patients with allergic asthma and more recently in patients with allergic rhinitis. Other pharmacologic approaches to allergic rhinitis include the use of antihistamines and inhaled corticosteroids. Antihistamines, including diphenhydramine (first generation antihistamine) and loratadine (second generation antihistamine) act only on the immediate phase of the response while inhaled corticosteroids such as beclomethasone target the late phase by reducing inflammation in the nasal mucosa.

28   **The answer is A: Anti-CD3, cyclosporine, and mycophenolate, respectively.**   Induction of immune suppression following renal transplantation usually involves a regimen of four drugs in the indicated catagories, thus this choice could be used. The antilymphocyte antibody should target all T cells, as both CD4 and CD8 cells play a crucial role in graft rejection. Thus, anti-CD3 antibodies are used since all T cells express this molecule as part of the antigen receptor complex. Only helper T cells express CD4 and only cytotoxic T cells express CD8, thus antibodies to either of these molecules would only lead to a decline in the respective population of cells. B cells express CD19 and CD20

and, although antibodies can play a role in graft rejection, their reduction would not prevent acute graft rejection. Calcineurin inhibitors include cyclosporine and tacrolimus. Both of these agents block the production of cytokines by effector T cells. The antiproliferative agents used to prevent transplant rejection are azathioprine, cyclophosphamide, and mycophenolate. Azathioprine is a purine analog that inhibits DNA replication. Mycophenolic acid inhibits *de novo* synthesis of purines. Compared to most other cells, lymphocytes are particularly sensitive to inhibition of purine synthesis as they are less able to generate this nucleotide by the purine salvage pathway. Cyclophosphamide is an alkylating agent that interferes with DNA replication. Sirolimus is a rapamycin that binds to the same intracellular protein as the calcineurin inhibitors (the FK506-binding protein).

29   **The answer is D: Polyclonal activation of T cells that cross-react with allogeneic MHC molecules on the transplanted kidney.**   Acute transplantation rejection is mediated by T cells and represents an alloreactive response against MHC antigens expressed by the donated tissues. Prior to transplantation, MHC molecules of the host are matched with MHC molecules of a potential donor. Rejection reactions are made less likely the more MHC molecules the two have in common. However, finding a perfect match, except between identical twins, is highly unlikely. This is because of the tremendous heterogeneity of MHC molecule expression in the human population. Even if a single MHC molecule is mismatched between the donor and the recipient, immunologic reactivity of the recipient will occur and could lead to an acute rejection reaction. Multiple T-cell clones are activated in response to a single unrelated MHC molecule because each allogeneic MHC molecule offers several distinct epitopes for T cells of the recipient to react against. Thus, the polyclonal nature of the immune reaction against transplanted tissues makes the response far stronger than the immune response against pathogens. Other forms of rejection of transplanted tissue can occur. Chronic rejection, occurring about 6 months posttransplantation, is characterized by a delayed type hypersensitivity reaction of host T cells against donor endothelial cells leading to atherosclerotic vascular damage in a grafted organ. Other nonimmunologic factors, including the use of nephrotoxic immune suppressants and reactivation of cytomegalovirus (though not necessarily the host's immune response to the virus) can also play a role in chronic rejection. The presence in the recipient of preformed antibodies to the donor ABO blood group antigens would lead to hyperacute rejection beginning within hours of transplantation. This type of rejection can be avoided by using donors and recipients with the same blood type. While donor dendritic cells are present in the grafted tissue and can interact with recipient T cells in all activation, they do not play a role in acute rejection through presentation of the recipient own proteins.

30 **The answer is E: X-linked agammaglobulinemia.** The major clinical clues to this diagnosis include the sex of the patient and the history of serious recurrent bacterial infections. X-linked agammaglobulinemia is also known as Bruton agammaglobulinemia. The laboratory test results that support this diagnosis are the lack of CD19+ cells. The molecule CD19 is part of the B-cell coreceptor complex involved in B-cell activation. Typically, in Bruton agammaglobulinemia, T-cell numbers are normal to slightly elevated and neutrophils and monocyte numbers are normal. Immunoglobulin levels are low to absent in Bruton's as a result of the lack of B cells. Laboratory findings in acquired immunodeficiency syndrome (AIDS), adenosine deaminase (ADA) deficiency, and DiGeorge syndrome would show reduced numbers of T cells. ADA deficiency is one of the most common forms of severe combined immunodeficiency (SCID). This condition is due to a deficiency in expression of the ADA enzyme which functions in the salvage pathway of purines. Since developing lymphocytes are particularly sensitive to ADA deficiency (inefficient in degrading dATP into 2'-deoxyadenosine), B- and T-cell numbers are impacted. DiGeorge syndrome is characterized by low to absent T-cell numbers depending on the extent of the disease. T cells can be found in patients with partial DiGeorge syndrome. AIDS is a disease resulting from an infection with human immunodeficiency virus or HIV. Generally, CD4+ T-cell numbers are significantly reduced over time and the CD4:CD8 ratio is altered. B-cell number and function are affected as these cells depend on T helper cells for responses to protein antigens. SLE is an autoimmune disease, not an immune deficiency disease.

31 **The answer is A: Bruton tyrosine kinase (btk).** See answer 32 for the role of this molecule in B-cell development.

32 **The answer is E: An inability of pro-B cells to differentiate into B cells.** B-cell differentiation in the bone marrow begins with the first committed cell in B-cell development, the pro-B cell. This cell expresses the B-cell marker, CD19. Rearrangement of the variable genes of the heavy chain occurs at this stage, and the cell is considered a pre-B-cell when it expresses the first version of its antigen receptor, called the pre-B cell receptor. Further development of the B cell from this stage relies on signals generated by the receptor and delivered to the nucleus by a signal transduction molecule known as Bruton tyrosine kinase. Bruton

agammaglobulinemia or X-linked agammaglobulinemia (XLA) is associated with a defect in the gene for btk. The *BTK* gene is required for the proliferation and differentiation of B lymphocytes. Therefore, mutations in *BTK* results in deficient B-cell development and subsequent lack of antibody production in response to antigens.

33 **The answer is A: The patient.** Autografts are transplants of tissues from one part of the body to another in the same individual. These transplants are often performed on patients with burns or those with disfiguring injuries. Graft failure does occur in autologous skin grafts; however, it is not due to immunologic rejection reactions. All of the other choices are allografts and are thus prone to immunologic rejection reactions.

34 **The answer is C: Drooping of her eyelids and muscle weakness that improves with rest.** See answer 35 for explanation.

35 **The answer is B: Antibody-mediated interference with neuromuscular transmission.** Myasthenia gravis results from antibody directed against the acetylcholine receptor. Receptors bound by antibody are not stimulated by acetylcholine, and the neurotransmitter is then degraded by acetylcholine esterase. Use of the affected muscles results in progressive weakness as more and more acetylcholine is degraded. Improvement of muscle weakness with rest is attributed to regeneration of acetylcholine stores. Acetylcholine esterase inhibitors are used in therapy of this disease. Abdominal pain, weight loss, and bloody diarrhea have a number of causes including inflammation of colonic mucosa in inflammatory bowel disease. Ascending weakness and paresthesia suggest Guillian Barre syndrome, which is due to an immunologic attack on the peripheral nerve myelin sheath. Fatigue, pallor, and mild jaundice suggest a form of anemia such as autoimmune hemolytic anemia mediated by antired blood cell antibodies. Goiter, palpitations, and proptosis of the eyes are consistent with Graves disease caused by antibody-mediated stimulation of the thyroid gland.

36 **The answer is B: Survival of tumors with low expression of class I MHC molecules.** Tumors have numerous mechanisms to escape immune responses. The most important antitumor immune response is the activation of tumor-specific CD8+ T cells. It is the CTL which eradicates the tumor from the patient and the focus of much cellular immunotherapies (infusion of modified CTL into tumor patients). Since CTL are responsible for eradication of tumors and these cells require antigen recognition for targeting their cytotoxic machinery, these cells would need to interact with tumors expressing class I MHC (choices A, C, and D). Only tumors expressing low levels of class I MHC are capable of escaping CTL-mediated killing. Even moderately class I MHC-expressing tumors are susceptible to CTL lysis.

37 **The answer is D: Decreased expression of class I MHC on tumor cells.** Tumor immunity requires inflammatory responses, namely, Th1 cells and IFNg-producing CTL (choices A and B). Tumor evasion tactics function to eliminate this immune response. In order to maximally activate those CTL, a specialized antigen presenting cell, the dendritic cell, can internalize exogenous tumor antigens, reroute those antigens to the class I MHC pathway, and present effectively to CD8$^+$ T cells to generate tumor-specific CTL (choice C). This process of rerouting exogenous antigens to the class I MHC pathway is called cross-presentation and the dendritic cell is the only cell capable of this function. In order for a tumor to grow in size, it requires a large supply of nutrients obtained by the construction of new blood vessels to service the tumor directly (angiogenesis) (choice E). In addition, these new blood vessels can limit the accessibility of tumor-specific cells into the tumor. A number of antiangiogenesis drugs are in clinical trials to block this mechanism of tumor escape. One of the primary mechanisms of tumor escape from CTL responses is to down-regulate gene or surface expression of class I MHC. This tends to render the tumors susceptible to lysis by NK cells; however, the recruitment of Th2 and regulatory T cells (by tumor products) to the tumor site has been implicated to impede NK cell activities.

38 **The answer is C: Reduced diapedesis of neutrophils.** This case is descriptive of leukocyte adhesion deficiency, a diagnosis strongly suggested by the lack of pus formation in the current infection and confirmed by the lack of β_2-integrins on leukocytes. β_2-integrins are membrane-associated protein heterodimers consisting of CD18 and one of the families of CD11 glycoproteins. Leukocyte function antigen-1 (LFA-1) is comprised of CD18 and CD11a, and is found on leukocytes; whereas the expression of CD11b/CD18 and CD11c/CD18 is restricted to myeloid cells. These molecules interact with ligands on endothelial cells during inflammation, and a lack of expression prohibits the migration of leukocytes into areas of infection. Pus formation is evidence of an acute inflammatory response. The lack of pus formation in this child indicates an inability of the neutrophils to bind to endothelium and migrate into tissues in response to infection. β_2-integrins are also important in other cell-to-cell interactions including the interaction of T cells with antigen-presenting cells. CD18 forms a part of the complement receptor on phagocytes, thus its deficiency impairs

phagocytosis. The association of deficient β_2-integrin expression, delayed umbilical cord separation, and poor wound healing is poorly understood. The other immunologic processes listed are not affected in this disease.

39 **The answer is C: Cytokine activation of synoviocytes, chrondocytes, and osteoclasts.** RA is considered to be a T helper cell-driven autoimmune disease. Many of the pathological processes are mediated by T cell-derived cytokines which activate joint-associated cells for further cytokine secretion as well as proliferation and enhanced function. Under the influence of cytokines, the synovial membrane thickens to form a granulation tissue called pannus. Pannus consists of proliferating fibroblastlike synoviocytes, as well as infiltrating mononuclear cells. Cytokines and other mediators activate osteoclasts and chrondrocytes. Activated osteoclasts lead to bone resorption and degradation of bone. Activation of chrondrocytes leads to increased secretion of matrix metalloproteases which cause tissue degradation. Neovascularization occurs within pannus and is also stimulated by cytokines (chemokines). B-cell production of autoantibodies and immune complex deposition also occurs in RA and makes an important contribution to joint pathology; however, its role is not as great as that of cytokines. Complement activation is ongoing, particularly in synovial fluid where decreased complement levels indicate activation of complement; however, complement-mediated lysis of synovial membranes is not part of the pathologic process of RA. Mast cells may play a role in joint inflammation in RA; however, their role is not as important as that of cytokines. Cytotoxic T cells do not cause cartilage damage in RA.

40 **The answer is B: Chediak–Higashi syndrome.** This autosomal recessive genetic disease is characterized by partial hypopigmentation of the skin, hair, and eyes, as well as immune deficiency and abnormal bleeding. This child manifested all these problems. Nonneoplastic lymphoid cell infiltration into various organs also occurs in most patients. The disease results from mutations in the gene for a protein involved in organelle protein trafficking called lysosomal-trafficking regulator protein or LYST. Any cell whose function depends on storage or secretory granules is adversely affected. Thus, melanocytes are unable to secrete melanin, leading to hypopigmentation. Neutrophils are unable to fuse lysosomes with the phagosome, resulting in defective microbicidal activity and increased infection. The function of platelets and natural killer cells, which rely on substances within granules, is impaired. Even the maturation of granule-containing cells is affected leading to the moderate decrease in neutrophils and platelets seen in this patient. Bare lymphocyte syndrome is a form of severe combined immune deficiency syndrome, manifesting as defects in T and B cells. Hypopigmentation and defects in neutrophil and platelet functions are not seen in this disease. Thrombocytopenia purpura manifests with bleeding disorders. Wegener granulomatosis is an immunopathologic disease involving the small- and medium-sized vessels of the respiratory tract and kidney whose manifestations include chronic sinusitis, hemoptosis, and hematuria. Wiskott–Aldrich syndrome is an X-linked recessive immune deficiency disease affecting the function of platelets, T cells, and B cells. Infants present with recurrent infections, bleeding disorders, and eczema.

41 **The answer is B: Guillain–Barre syndrome.** The most important clues to this diagnosis are the acute onset and rapid progression of ascending muscular weakness and demyelination of peripheral nerves. Guillain–Barre syndrome (GBS) develops rapidly, involving muscles of the extremities, trunk, head, and face. Patients may require mechanical ventilation during the peak of its severity. GBS is frequently postinfectious, and *Campylobacter jejuni*, an infection associated with the consumption of undercooked chicken, is the most common infection linked with this condition. Antigens within the carbohydrate structure of lipooligosaccharide of *C. jejuni* are similar to the GM1 ganglioside of the myelin sheath of peripheral nerves. The demyelination in GBS results from an immune attack against the myelin by antibody stimulated during the antecedent bacterial infection. Immune-based treatments include plasmaphoresis to remove offending antibodies, and intravenous immune globulin (IVIG). The mechanism of action of IVIG is uncertain but may involve blocking of Fc receptors on macrophages and other cells involved in antibody-dependent cell cytotoxicity against the myelin sheath, and feedback inhibition of antibody production and other mechanisms. Most patients with GBS recover fully within 6 to 12 months. Although the other disease entities listed can present with muscular weakness, the clinical manifestations are different from those described in the case, and demyelination of peripheral nerves is not involved.

42 **The answer is A: Antibodies to double-stranded DNA.** This case is descriptive of a new onset of systemic lupus erythematosus (SLE). Patients with SLE make a variety of autoantibodies, particularly antinuclear antibodies. These autoantibodies are also found in other immune disorders of connective tissue, thus, the finding of antinuclear antibodies is suggestive of, but not diagnostic of SLE. It is considered a screening test for SLE. Antibodies to double-stranded DNA are unique to SLE, and are found in about 60% of patients

with this disease. Anti-Sm antibodies are even more specific for SLE. All the other test results listed could be positive in a patient with SLE, but do not confirm the diagnosis. Decreased serum complement levels are seen in diseases marked by complement activation, such as occurs in the Type III hypersensitivity reactions that are at the heart of the pathology of SLE. Elevated C-reactive protein is a nonspecific marker of systemic inflammation, similar to elevated erythrocyte sedimentation rates. Hemolytic anemia, indicated by a positive Coombs test, and other immune-mediated cytopenias can be seen in patients with SLE who develop antibodies to blood cells.

43 **The answer is C: Hydroxychloroquine.** This drug is an antimalarial used in the initial therapy of SLE. Its mechanism of action is primarily aimed at neutrophil and monocyte/macrophage chemotaxis and phagocytosis. It has been shown to inhibit the release of lysosomal contents by stabilizing the membranes of these organelles. In addition, it blocks arachidonic acid metabolism thereby preventing the release of prostaglandins. Azathioprine, cyclophosphamide, and methotrexate are immune suppressant, cytotoxic drugs, and methylprednisolone is a corticosteroid. All of these drugs increase the risk of infection and neoplasia in patients.

44 **The answer is A: Graves disease.** The photograph shows a woman with ophthalmopathy secondary to the hyperthyroidism of Graves disease. Graves disease is due to the formation of antibodies to the thyroid stimulating hormone receptor. These antibodies constantly stimulate the thyroid to secrete thyroid hormones in the absence of normal physiological feedback mechanisms that control hormone secretion. None of the other conditions listed are associated with hyperthyroidism. Goodpasture syndrome is an autoimmune disease affecting the lung and kigney. Hashimoto thyroiditis is mediated by T-cell infiltration into the thyroid, resulting in hypothyroidism. Myasthenia gravis is an immune-mediated condition resulting in profound muscle weakness. Sjogren syndrome is an inflammatory connective tissue disease leading to dry eyes, dry mouth, and enlarged parotid glands.

45 **The answer is A: AIRE.** The AIRE (autoimmune regulator gene) codes for a transcription factor that regulates the expression of many genes. It is particularly active in the thymus where it is thought to allow the expression of genes encoding proteins found outside of the thymus. Thus, it enables thymic epithelial cells and dendritic cells to present extrathymic antigens in the process of central tolerance induction. A mutation in this gene would interfere with normal negative selection against self-reactive thymocytes, thereby allowing autoreactive T cells to enter the peripheral circulation. Numerous studies have associated mutations in AIRE with the development of polyglandular autoimmune syndrome Type-1. Genes of the complement system including C1 and C4 have been associated with systemic lupus erythematosus. A number of animal models and human genetic studies have linked polymorphisms of CTLA-4 with various autoimmune diseases including allergic encephalomyelitis, SLE, and Type-1 diabetes. This molecule is important in the maintenance of peripheral tolerance by down-regulating T-cell activation. FoxP3 is a transcription factor expressed by regulatory T cells. Deficiencies of FoxP3-expressing regulatory T cells have been associated with a variety of autoimmune diseases in animal models. The association of major histocompatability genes and autoimmune diseases is a strong one, and the relative risk of developing rheumatoid arthritis, Type-1 diabetes, or pamphigus vulgaris is increased in individuals expressing HLA-DR4. Surprisingly, there is no strong association of any MHC gene and the development of polyglandular autoimmune syndrome Type-1.

46 **The answer is C: Antiparietal cell antibodies.** This case is descriptive of pernicious anemia, which has a variety of etiologies including autoimmunity. Clues to the diagnosis of pernicious anemia are the man's clinical manifestations (pallor, fatigue, weight loss, and tingling sensations) as well as the hematology results showing megaloblastic anemia, leucopenia, and thrombocytopenia. This disease results from a decrease in the body's intake of vitamin B_{12}, which is essential for coenzymes involved in cell proliferation. The absorption of B_{12} in the body is dependent on the secretion of a glycoprotein called intrinsic factor from parietal cells in the stomach. Release of B_{12} from ingested food occurs in the intestine, where it binds to intrinsic factor and the complex then binds to receptors on cells of the ilium and is absorbed. Manifestations of the lack of B_{12} include pancytopenia, megaloblastic anemia, and neurological disorders. In the autoimmune form of the disease, antibodies to parietal cells and to intrinsic factor are found in the patient's serum. The manifestations of the patient in this case are not consistent with antibodies that would attack red blood cells (antired cell antibodies or anti-Rh-antibodies). He does not present with symptoms of connective tissue disease in which antinuclear antibodies would be found. Finally, ABO antibodies are detected during blood typing.

47 **The answer is E: Defective polymerization and depolymerization of actin.** This case is descriptive of Wiscott–Aldrich syndrome (WAS). This disease classically presents with increased susceptibility to infection, eczema, and thrombocytopenia. The finding of unusually small platelets, as indicated by the decreased mean platelet volume, is particularly helpful in making a diagnosis of this condition. In addition, low IgM and IgG are characteristic of this disease, as is the lack of isohemagglutinins. Elevations in IgA and IgE are often found. WAS is an X-linked recessive disease due to a mutation in the WAS protein or WASP. This protein, found in leukocytes and megakaryocytes, binds to actin and is involved in its reorganization. Actin polymerization and depolymerization are essential for the normal functioning of cells. In T lymphocytes for instance, actin reorganization follows engagement of the T-cell receptor to antigen presented on MHC molecules and results in the clustering of relevant receptors and their ligands to one pole of the cell. This clustering of receptors and ligands holds the two cells together to form the immunologic synapse across which cytokines can be exchanged between the T cell and the antigen-presenting cell. Actin reorganization is also essential for the movement of thymocytes as they mature within the thymus, the migration of mature lymphocytes into lymph nodes and sites of infection, as well as in cell division. Mitogen stimulation of lymphocytes often reveals decreased responsiveness. Although lymphocyte numbers are relatively normal early in life, patients with WAS develop lymphopenia with time. Bone marrow stem cell transplantation is the treatment of choice for this condition.

48 **The answer is E: T cells.** This case is descriptive of psoriasis, an inflammatory skin disease characterized by excessive proliferation of keratinocytes. Several different forms of the disease exist. This individual has plaque psoriasis. In addition to skin lesions, individuals frequently have arthritis and nail problems. The pathogenesis of psoriasis is uncertain; however, recent evidence supports a role for T cells. It is believed that dendritic cells present a skin antigen to T cells which than migrate as effector cells into the skin where they secrete cytokines which stimulate keratinocyte proliferation. One key cytokine involved in psoriasis is tumor necrosis factor. In fact, inhibitors of tumor necrosis factor have been used with success in this disease. Cyclosporine is a drug used to prevent transplant rejection. It works by blocking the calcineurin-mediated activation of a transcription factor necessary for the expression of IL-2 and other cytokines by T cells. Thus, T-cell activation is inhibited. The efficacy of cyclosporine in reducing psoriasis lesions was one of the first pieces of evidence suggesting that T cells play a role in the pathogenesis of this disease. There are many different pharmacologic approaches to the treatment of this disease, but none of them lead to complete resolution of symptoms.

49 **The answer is A: Bence–Jones proteins.** This case is descriptive of multiple myeloma, a neoplasia of plasma cells. Bone pain is often the presenting symptom for patients who develop this cancer. The neoplastic plasma cells are produced in the bone marrow where they crowd out other hematopoietic cell lines leading to pancytopenia. This explains the anemia and petechiae. Interleukin-6 produced by the neoplastic plasma cells induces osteoclast activity leading to lytic bone lesions and also stimulates the liver to release acute phase proteins, resulting in elevated erythrocyte sedimentation rates. The malignant plasma cells are from a single clone and therefore secrete a monoclonal immunoglobulin. The isotype of the myeloma immunoglobulin is most commonly IgG or IgA. Excess light chains called Bence–Jones proteins are found in the urine and help confirm the diagnosis of multiple myeloma. The other items listed are found in the urine during certain types of kidney disease.

50 **The answer is D: Indirect antiglobulin test on the mother's serum.** Hemolytic disease of the newborn results from Rh incompatibility between the mother and the fetus. It can occur when an Rh-negative mother is carrying an Rh-positve fetus. Fetal blood mixes with maternal blood during gestation or during the birth process. The mother becomes sensitized to the Rh antigens and makes anti-Rh antibodies. In a subsequent pregnancy with an Rh-positive fetus, these IgG anti-Rh antibodies can cross the placenta and cause hemolysis of the fetal red blood cells. Sensitization of the mother to fetal Rh antigens can be detected by the indirect antiglobulin test, also called the indirect Coombs test. In this test, the mother's serum is mixed with Rh-positive red blood cells. If anti-Rh antibodies are present in maternal serum, they will bind to the Rh-positive red blood cells. Rabbit antihuman globulin, made by injecting rabbits with the γ-globulin fraction of human serum, is added to the mixture, and the anti-Rh antibody-coated red cells agglutinate, giving a positive reaction. This test should be done at the first prenatal visit. A direct Coombs test done on the mother's red cells would indicate, if positive, that her cells were attacked by antired cell antibodies. ABO incompatibility between the mother and fetus does not lead to hydrops fetalis, or hemolytic disease of the newborn. Testing for fetal bilirubin levels and ultrasound studies are methods of assessing the severity of hemolysis in an affected fetus.

51 **The answer is A: Administration of anti-Rh antibodies to Rh-negative women after the birth of each Rh-positive child.** Rhogam is a preparation of anti-Rh antibodies used to prevent sensitization of an Rh-negative mother by Rh-positive fetal red blood cells. These antibodies cause hemolysis of fetal cells that enter the maternal circulation, destroying the cells before the Rh antigens have a chance to be presented to the mother's immune system and stimulate antibody production. An Rh-negative mother should receive this preparation after the birth of each Rh-positive child. Intravenous immune globulin can be given to affected infants after birth to help prevent destruction of red cells by maternal anti-Rh antibodies that crossed the placenta during gestation. Plasmaphoresis is not used in the prevention or management of this disease. Transfusion of the mother with Rh-positive blood before pregnancy or after delivery will stimulate her immune system to make anti-Rh antibodies, thereby promoting, not preventing, hemolytic disease in any Rh-positive fetuses that she carries.

52 **The answer is D: Pemphigus vulgaris.** This autoimmune disease causes erosive lesions on mucous membranes and fluid-filled bullae on the skin. It is most prevalent in individuals of Ashkenazi Jewish ancestry. Oral lesions usually appear first and can spread to the larynx to cause hoarseness. The disease is diagnosed by the finding of IgG deposits between keratinocytes by direct immunofluorescent staining of biopsy material. None of the other conditions listed present as described in this case. Contact dermatitis very rarely involves the mucous membranes. Lesions of discoid lupus are dry, erythematosus, scaly and crusty in appearance. Herpes simplex infection can cause oral vesicular lesions, but this type of presentation is seen in children with primary infection. Cold sores are the typical manifestation of recurrent HSV-1. Psoriasis can present in a number of ways; however, oral erosions and fluid-filled bullae are not found in any variant of this disease.

53 **The answer is A: Antidesmoglein antibodies causing acantholysis.** The autoantibodies formed in this disease are directed against the desmosomal antigen desmoglein-3. This antibody is predominantly of the IgG4 subclass which does not activate complement. Instead, the binding of the autoantibody causes disruption of adhesion between keratinocytes, with subsequent weakening of the dermal layer with erosions and/or bullae formation. The pathogenesis is a form of Type II immune hypersensitivity. Type III hypersensitivity is mediated by antigen–antibody complex formation, and is not a part of this pathogenesis. Neutrophils do not cause the erosions or bullae to form, although they are involved should these lesions become infected. Pemphigus vulgaris is not an immune deficiency disease.

54 **The answer is E: Wegener granulomatosis.** This case is descriptive of the vasculitic disease Wegener granulomatosis, which typically affects the respiratory system and kidney. Patients often present with sinusitis that is unresponsive to antibiotics. Antineutrophil cytoplasmic antibodies can be demonstrated in most patients with this disease. None of the other diseases listed present in the manner described in this case. Chronic granulomatous disease is an immune deficiency disease manifesting in young children and due to an inability of neutrophils to make oxygen-reactive products. It presents as recurrent bacterial infections. Goodpasture syndrome is a rapidly progressing autoimmune disease affecting the lungs and kidney and presenting with hemoptosis and frank hematuria. It is due to the formation of antibodies to type IV collagen found in the basement membranes of those organs. Sarcoidosis is an immune system disorder in which granulomas develop in a variety of organs and tissues. ANCA are not produced in this disease. Systemic lupus erythematosus can present in a number of ways, depending on the organ system involvement. Autoantibodies associated with this disease are primarily directed against nuclear constituents of cells and ANCA are not associated with this disease.

55 **The answer is B: Decreased inflammatory cell infiltrates into bronchial wall.** Corticosteroids are used in a variety of inflammatory diseases because they block the transcription of multiple genes involved in the inflammatory process. Inflammation is crucial to the pathogenesis of asthma, and is far more important than the early effects of mast cell degranulation leading to initial bronchoconstriction. Inflammation of the airways occurs in the "late response" of allergic asthma, leading to an infiltration of eosinophils and mononuclear cells that promote continued asthma symptoms. The most effective therapies for asthma are aimed at reducing allergic inflammation, and affected genes include those encoding proinflammatory cytokines and chemokines as well as genes for adhesion molecules. In addition, corticosteroids block the metabolisms of arachidonic acid, decreasing the production of leukotrienes and prostaglandins that play important role in inflammatory diseases such as asthma. A reduction in inflammatory cells occurs in bronchial walls of patients successfully treated with inhaled corticosteroids. The other choices listed are not activities attributed to corticosteroids or their role in asthma therapy.

56 **The answer is D: NF-κ B.** This transcription factor, along with AP-1 and NFAT (nuclear factor of activated T cells), promotes activation of genes for proinflammatory cytokines and proteins necessary for cell activation and proliferation. They are inhibited by corticosteroids. FoxP3 is a transcription factor found in regulatory T cells. The other molecules listed are not transcription factors, but are instead involved with signal transduction following antigen binding to T-cell receptors.

Figure Credits

Chapter 1

Q1-1: From Winn WC. Koneman's Color Atlas and Textbook of Diagnostic Microbiology. 6th Ed. Baltimore: Lippincott Williams & Wilkins, 2006, Color plates 10-1C and 10-1A.

Q1-6: Photograph courtesy of Lauritz Jensen, DA.

Q1-7: Photograph courtesy of Lauritz Jensen, DA.

Q1-9: Photograph courtesy of Lauritz Jensen, DA.

Q1-10: Photograph courtesy of Lauritz Jensen, DA.

Q1-14: Photograph courtesy of Lauritz Jensen, DA.

Q1-23: Photograph courtesy of Lauritz Jensen, DA.

Q1-27: Photograph courtesy of Lauritz Jensen, DA.

Q1-32: Photograph courtesy of Lauritz Jensen, DA.

Q1-43: Photograph courtesy of CDC/M. Rein, VD. Public Health Image Library #6803.

Q1-44: Photograph courtesy of Lauretz Jensen, DA.

Q1-48: Photograph courtesy of Lauritz Jensen, DA.

Q1-50: Photograph courtesy of Lauritz Jensen, DA.

Q1-51: Diagram courtesy of Lauritz Jensen, DA.

Q1-52: Photograph courtesy of Lauritz Jensen, DA.

Q1-58: Photograph courtesy of Lauritz Jensen, DA.

Q1-70: Photograph from Public Health Image Library # 6704

Q1-75: From Engleberg NC. Schaechter's Mechanisms of Microbial Disease. 4th Ed. Baltimore: Lippincott Williams & Wilkins, 2006, p. 218, Figure 18-2.

Q1-95: From Harvey RA. Lippincott's Illustrated Reviews: Microbiology. 2nd Ed. Baltimore: Lippincott Williams & Wilkins, 2006, p. 94, Figure 10-5.

Q1-101: Image courtesy of CDC/Dr. Brodsky. Public Health Image Library #6423.

Q1-105: From Winn WC. Koneman's Color Atlas and Textbook of Diagnostic Microbiology. 6th Ed. Baltimore: Lippincott Williams & Wilkins, 2006, Color plates 13-1 E and 13-1 B.

Q1-107: Photograph courtesy of Lauritz Jensen, DA.

Q1-110: Photograph courtesy of CDC/Dr. Mike Miller. Public Health Image Library # 2896.

Chapter 2

Q2-12: Photograph courtesy of CDC/Dr. Hermann. Public Health Image Library #5434.

Q2-18: From Goodheart HP. Goodheart's Photoguide of Common Skin Disorders. 2nd Ed. Philadelphia: Lippincott Williams & Wilkins, 2003, Figure 6-33.

Q2-42: From Sloane PD. Essentials of Family Medicine. 5th Ed. Baltimore: Lippincott Williams & Wilkins, 2007, Figure 40-3.

Q2-71: From Tasman W, Jaeger E. The Wills Eye Hospital Atlas of Clinical Ophthalmology. 2nd Ed. Baltimore: Lippincott Williams & Wilkins, 2001, Figure 8-24B.

Q2-75: From Hall JC. Sauer's Manual of Skin. 8th Ed. Philadelphia: Lippincott Williams & Wilkins, 2000, p. 197, Figure 22-6.

Q2-92: Photograph courtesy of CDC. Public Health Image Library # 4284.

Q2-97: Photographs courtesy of Bonnie A. Buxton, PhD.

Chapter 3

Q3-1: Photograph courtesy of Christine Saraceni, DO.

Q3-2: Photograph courtesy of Christine Saraceni, DO.

Q3-3: Photograph courtesy of Lauritz Jensen, DA.

Q3-4: Photographs courtesy of Lauritz Jenson, DA.

Q3-6: Photograph courtesy of Lauritz Jensen, DA.

Q3-7: Photograph courtesy of Lauritz Jensen, DA.

Q3-9: Photograph courtesy of Lauritz Jensen, DA.

Q3-11: Photograph courtesy of Lauritz Jensen, DA.

Q3-12: Photograph courtesy of Christine Saraceni, DO.

Q3-13: Photograph courtesy of Lauritz Jenson, DA.

Q3-18: From Engleberg NC. Schaechter's Mechanisms of Microbial Disease. 4th Ed. Baltimore: Lippincott Williams & Wilkins, 2006, p. 466, Figure 48-3.

Q3-27: Photograph courtesy of Lauritz Jensen, DA.

Q3-28: Photographs courtesy of Lauritz Jensen, DA.

Q3-29: Photograph courtesy of Lauritz Jensen, DA.

Q3-30: Photograph courtesy of Lauritz Jensen, DA.

Q3-32: Photograph courtesy of Lauritz Jensen, DA.

Q3-34: Photograph courtesy of Lauritz Jensen, DA.

Q3-35: Photograph courtesy of Christine Saraceni, DO.

Q3-37: Photograph courtesy of Christine Saraceni, DO.

Q3-38: Photograph courtesy of CDC/Edwin Ewing, Jr., M.D. M.D.Public Health Library Image #960.

Chapter 4

Q4-3: Photograph courtesy of Lauritz Jensen, DA.

Q4-4: Photograph courtesy of Lauritz Jensen, DA.

Q4-5: Photograph courtesy of Lauritz Jensen, DA.

Q4-6 & A4-6: Photograph courtesy of Lauritz Jensen, DA.

Q4-7: Photographs courtesy of Lauritz Jensen, DA.

Q4-10: Photographs courtesy of Lauritz Jensen, DA.

Q4-11: Photograph courtesy of Lauritz Jensen, DA.

Q4-14: Photograph courtesy of Lauritz Jensen, DA.

Q4-16: Photographs courtesy of Lauritz Jensen, DA.

Q4-17: Photograph courtesy of Lauritz Jensen, DA.

Q4-19: Copyright Lippincott Williams & Wilkins

Q4-20: Photograph courtesy of Lauritz Jensen, DA.

Q4-21: Photograph courtesy of Lauritz Jensen, DA.

Q4-22: Photograph courtesy of Lauritz Jensen, DA.

Q4-24: Photograph courtesy of Lauritz Jensen, DA.

Q4-25: Photograph courtesy of Lauritz Jensen, DA.

Q4-26: Photograph courtesy of Lauritz Jensen, DA.

Q4-27: Photograph courtesy of Lauritz Jensen, DA.

Q4-28: Photographs courtesy of Lauritz Jensen, DA.

Q4-29: Photograph courtesy of Lauritz Jensen, DA.

Q4-30: Photograph courtesy of Lauritz Jensen, DA.

Q4-31: Photographs courtesy of Lauritz Jensen, DA.

Q4-32: Photograph courtesy of Lauritz Jensen, DA.

Q4-33: Photograph courtesy of Lauritz Jensen, DA.

Q4-34: Photograph courtesy of Lauritz Jensen, DA.

Q4-35: Photographs courtesy of Lauritz Jensen, DA.

Q4-36: Photographs courtesy of Lauritz Jensen, DA.

Q4-37: Photograph courtesy of Lauritz Jensen, DA.

Q4-38: Photograph courtesy of Lauritz Jensen, DA.

Q4-39: Photograph courtesy of Lauritz Jensen, DA.

Q4-43: Photograph courtesy of Lauritz Jensen, DA.

Q4-46: Photograph courtesy of Lauritz Jensen, DA.

Q4-47: Photographs courtesy of Lauritz Jensen, DA.

Q4-48: Photograph courtesy of Lauritz Jensen, DA.

Q4-52: Photograph courtesy of Lauritz Jensen, DA.

Q4-58: Photograph courtesy of CDC/Dr. Mae Melvin. Public Health Image Library #899.

Q4-60: Photograph courtesy of Lauritz Jensen, DA.

Q4-62: Photograph courtesy of Lauritz Jensen, DA.

Q4-63: Photograph courtesy of Lauritz Jensen, DA.

Q4-64: Photograph courtesy of Lauritz Jensen, DA.

Q4-65: Photograph courtesy of Lauritz Jensen, DA.

Q4-66: Photograph courtesy of Lauritz Jensen, DA.

Q4-67: Photograph courtesy of Lauritz Jensen, DA.

Q4-68: Photograph courtesy of Lauritz Jensen, DA.

Q4-69: Photograph courtesy of Lauritz Jensen, DA.

Q4-70: Photographs courtesy of Lauritz Jensen, DA.

Q4-71: Photographs courtesy of Lauritz Jensen, DA.

Q4-72: Photograph courtesy of Lauritz Jensen, DA.

Chapter 5

Q5-5: Photograph courtesy of CDC/Dr. Libero Ajello. Public Health Image Library #4219.

Q5-8: Photographs courtesy of the CDC. Public Health Image Library #5177 and #3798.

Q5-29: Photograph courtesy of CDC/Dr. George P. Kubica. Public Health Image Library #5789.

Q5-30: Photograph courtesy of Lauritz Jensen, DA.

Q5-35: Photograph courtesy of CDC/Dr. Lucille K. Georg. Public Health Image Library #4232.
Q5-39: Photographs courtesy of Lauritz Jensen, DA.
Q5-47: Photograph courtesy of Lauritz Jensen, DA.
Q5-50: Photograph courtesy of Lauritz Jensen, DA.
Q5-57: From Engleberg NC. Schaechter's Mechanisms of Microbial Disease. 4th Ed. Baltimore: Lippincott Williams & Wilkins, 2006, p. 456, Figure 47-1.
Q5-58: Photograph courtesy of Bonnie A. Buxton, PhD.
Q5-61: Photograph courtesy of Lauritz Jensen, DA.
Q5-63: Photograph courtesy of CDC/ Gilda Jones. Public Health Image Library # 10775.
Q5-72: Photograph courtesy of CDC/ Teresa Hammett. Public Health Image Library #10131.
Q5-83: Photograph courtesy of CDC/Dr. Edwin P. Ewing, Jr. Public Health Image Library # 846.
Q5-93: Photograph courtesy of Bonnie A. Buxton, PhD.

Chapter 7

Q7-22: From Fenderson BA, Rubin R. Lippincott's Review of Pathology. Baltimore: Lippincott Williams & Wilkins, 2007, p. 161, Figure 16-28.
Q7-42: From Goodheart HP. Goodheart's Photoguide of Common Skin Disorders. 2nd Ed. Philadelphia: Lippincott Williams & Wilkins, 2003, Figure 25-24.
Q7-44: From Goodheart HP. Goodheart's Photoguide of Common Skin Disorders. 2nd Ed. Philadelphia: Lippincott Williams & Wilkins, 2003, Figure 25-9.
Q7-48: From Goodheart HP. Goodheart's Photoguide of Common Skin Disorders. 2nd Ed. Philadelphia: Lippincott Williams & Wilkins, 2003, Figure 3-2.
Q7-52: From Fenderson BA, Rubin R. Lippincott's Review of Pathology. Baltimore: Lippincott Williams & Wilkins, 2007, p. 247, Figure 24-10.

Index

A

Acne, *Propionibacterium acne,* 111, 126
Actinomyces israelii, 4, 21
Acute phase response, 155, 164
Acute pulmonary histoplasmosis, 67, 74
Acute rheumatic fever (ARF), 124, 140
Acyclovir, mechanism of action, 42, 55
Adenosine deaminase deficiency, 157, 166
Adenovirus
    conjunctivitis, 42, 54
    respiratory illness, 40, 53
African sleeping sickness, 96, 107
AIDS
    B cell lymphoma, 120, 136
    case definition, 119, 134
    delayed type hypersensitivity (DTH), Th1 cells, 157, 166–167
    efavirenz, 123, 139
    cryptococcal meningitis, 70, 76, 114, 129
    cytomegalovirus retinitis, 44, 58
    Epstein–Barr virus, 120, 136
    invasive cervical carcinoma, 44, 57, 119, 134
    Pneumocystis jiroveci, 71, 77, 111, 125, 126
    Progressive multifocal leukoencephalopathy, 46, 59
    toxoplasmosis, 112, 128
    treatment of, 123, 139–140
    tuberculosis, 113, 128
Amantadine, 36, 50
Amphotericin B, mechanism of action, 68, 75
Anaphylaxis, 143, 150, 157, 167
Anisakis, 84, 101
Antacids, 10, 26
Antibiotic sensitivity test, 9, 25
Antigen presentation, 142, 145, 148, 152, 153
Antigen-presenting cells, 142, 148
Antigen receptors, 144, 151
Antiparietal cell antibodies, 161, 173
Antistreptolysin O antibodies, 18, 32–33
Antitumor immune response, CD8+ T cells, 160, 170–171
Apoptosis, 142, 148
Appendicitis, 110, 125
Ascaris lumbricoides, 92, 105
    ascarid eggs, 92, 105
    biliary involvement, 94, 106
    transmission, 94, 106
Aspergillus fumigatus
    Angioinvasive disease, 71, 76–77, 124, 140

Aspergillomas, 63, 72
    Otitis externa, 70–71, 76
    Pneumonia, 114, 130
Atherosclerosis, 121, 138
Atopic asthma, 163, 175
Atopic dermatitis, 143, 149–150
Atopic rhinitis, 159, 169
Autoimmune regulator gene (AIRE), 161, 172–173
Autoimmunity, and T reg cells, 145, 153
Azidothymidine, 50
Azithromycin, 109, 125
Azoles, mechanism of action, 68, 75
Aztreonam, 14, 30

B

B cells
    antigen presentation, 142, 148
    antigen recognition, 143, 150
    isotype switching, 144, 150
    lymphoma, 129
    memory, 145, 153
Babesia microti, 94, 106
Bacillary dysentery, 5, 22–23
Bacillus anthracis, 2, 20
Bacillus cereus, 123, 138–139
Bacterial vaginosis, 9, 25
Bacteroides fragilis, 14, 29
Balantidium coli, 80, 99
Bartonella henselae, 14, 29
Bordetella pertussis, 12, 28, 117, 132
Borrelia burgdorferi, 5, 23
Borrelia hermsii, 8, 24
Bacterial vaginosis, 9, 25
Bence–Jones proteins, 162, 174
Biofilm production, 15, 31
Botulism, 7, 24
Bronchiolitis, 119, 134
Bruton agammaglobulinemia, see
        X-linked agammaglobulinemia
Bruton tyrosine kinase (btk), 159, 170
Burkholderia cepacia, 21
Burkitt lymphoma, 113–114, 129

C

C1 inhibitor (C1-INH), 155, 165
Cachexia, 155, 165
Calicivirus, 35, 49
Campylobacter jejuni
    diarrhea, 10, 13, 15, 26, 28, 31, 111, 126
    Guillain–Barre syndrome, 160–161, 172
Candida spp.
    candidiasis, HIV infection, 64, 72
    esophagitis, 67, 74, 120, 135
    pneumonia, 66, 73

    thrush, nystatin, 64, 72
    vaginal yeast infection, 69, 76, 120, 136
Catalase test, 3, 21
Cat scratch fever, 14, 29
Caspofungin, 67, 74
Cellulitis, 14, 30
CD3, 142, 148
CD4+CD25+ T regulatory (Treg), 145, 153
CD18 expression deficiency, 157, 167
CD40L, 144, 150
CD80/86, 141–142, 147–148
CD152, 142, 148
CD154, 156, 165–166
CD62L (L-selectin), 146, 153
Cellulitis, 123, 139
Cephalexin, 15, 30
Cervical cancer, 45, 58
    in AIDS, 44, 57, 119, 134
Chagas' disease, 94–95, 106, 121, 136
Chediak–Higashi syndrome, 160, 171–172
Chlamydia trachomatis, 11, 27, 121, 136
Chlamydophila pneumoniae, 14, 29, 122, 138
Cholera, 13, 29
Chromoblastomycosis, 68, 75
Chronic granulomatous disease, 156, 166
Ciprofloxacin, 110, 126
Clindamycin, 16, 32, 111, 117, 126, 132
Clonorchis sinensis
    cholangiocarcinoma, 85, 92, 102, 105
    transmission, 102
Clostridium botulinum, 7, 24
Clostridium difficile, 111, 127, 128
Clostridium perfringens
    gas gangrene, 2, 20–21
    lecithinase, 2, 20
Clotrimazole, 120, 136
Coccidioides immitis
    coccidioidomycosis, 68, 75
    osteomyelitis, 70, 76
Cold agglutinin disease, 157, 167
Colorado tick fever, 46, 59
Common cold, 137–138
Complement activation, 145, 152
Complement proteins
    C1 inhibitor, 155, 165
    C3 deficiency, 141, 147
    C5a, 144, 152
Condyloma acuminatum, 45, 58
Congenital rubella syndrome, 47, 60–61
Congenital thymic aplasia, see also
        DiGeorge syndrome, 157, 166
Conidia
    arthroconidia, 69, 76
    inhalation, 71, 76
    macroconidia (Fusarium), 66, 73

Conjunctivitis, 121, 136
Contact hypersensitivity, 143, 149
Coombs test, 157, 162, 167, 174
Corticosteroids, mechanism of, 163, 175
Corynebacterium diphtheriae, 15, 31
Co-stimulation, 141–142, 147–148
Coxsackieviruses
    Hand, foot and mouth disease, 48, 62
    myocarditis, 44, 57, 118, 133
    vesicular lesions, 48, 62
Croup, 39, 53, 110, 126
Cryptococcus neoformans
    cryptococcosis, 63, 68, 72, 74–75
    cryptococcal meningitis, 63, 70, 72,
        76, 114, 129
    cutaneous lesions, 63, 72
    transmission, 76
Cryptosporidium parvum, 98, 108
Cutaneous larva migrans, 84, 101
Cyclospora, 93, 105
Cystic fibrosis (CF), 3, 21
Cytomegalovirus (CMV)
    diagnosis, 47, 61
    incidence of congenital infection, 43, 56
    mental retardation and deafness, 43, 56
    retinitis, 44, 58
    treatment, 47, 61
    in utero infection, 117, 132–133

D

Delayed type hypersensitivity, 157,
    166–167
Dendritic cells
    maturation, 146, 153
    T cell activation 141, 147–148
Dengue virus, 47, 60
Dermatophyte, 64–65, 72
    tinea capitis, 68, 75
    tinea corporis, 65, 69, 72–73, 76
Dextran production, 17, 32
Diarrhea,
    antibiotic associated, 111, 127
    bloody, 15, 31
    Camplyobacter, 10, 26, 13, 15, 28, 31,
        111, 126
    Calicivirus, 35, 49
    Cyclospora, 93, 105
    Escherichia coli, EHEC, bloody
        diarrhea and HUS, 4–5, 7, 10,
        16, 22, 24, 26, 31
    Giardia lamblia, 88–89, 98, 103, 107,
        118–119, 133
    Hymenolepis nana, 80–81, 100
    Norovirus, 123, 138
    Rotavirus, 119, 134
    Shigella sonnei, 113, 128–129
    watery, 16, 32, 113, 128
        pathogenesis of, 12, 28
DiGeorge syndrome
    chromosome 22q11.2 deletion, 157, 166
    partial, 158, 167–168

Dimorphic fungi, 67, 73, 74
Diphtheria, 15, 31
Diphyllobothrium latum
    anemia, 82–83, 100–101
    transmission, 93, 105
Doxycycline
    Lyme disease, 5, 23
    Rocky Mountain spotted fever
        (RMSF), 7, 24
Dysentery
    Ameobic, 89, 103
    Enteroinvasive *E. coli*, 7, 24
    Shigella dysentery, 5, 22–23

E

Eastern equine encephalitis virus,
    42, 56
Ebola virus, 46, 59–60
Echinococcosis, 81, 92, 100, 105
Echinococcus granulosus, 82, 100
Ehrlichiosis, 116, 131
Elephantiasis, 87, 103
Encephalitis
    acyclovir, 123, 139
    cytomegalovirus, 132, 136
    herpes simplex virus, 136–137
    progressive multifocal
        leukoencephalopathy, 46, 59
    toxoplasmosis, 112, 128
    West Nile virus, 46, 60
Endocarditis
    Enterococcus faecalis, 11, 27
    HACEK group, 119, 133–134
    Subacute, 117, 132
    Viridans group streptococci, 17, 32,
        117, 132
Endotoxic shock, 16, 32
Entamoeba histolytica
    amebiasis, 89, 103
    cytotoxins, 93, 106
    liver abscess, 95, 107
Enterobius vermicularis, 80, 90, 99,
    103–104
Enterococcus faecalis, 18, 33–34
    vancomycin resistance, 11, 27
Enterococcus faecium, 112, 128
Eosinophils, 144, 145, 151, 152
Epidemic typhus, 96, 107
Epiglottitis, 119, 134
Epstein–Barr virus
    B cell lymphoma, 120, 136
    Burkitt lymphoma, 113–114, 129
    CNS lymphoma, 120, 136
    mononucleosis, 39–40, 53
Ergosterol, 65, 67, 68, 73–75
Escherichia coli
    EHEC, bloody diarrhea and HUS,
        4–5, 7, 10, 16, 22, 24, 26, 31,
    EIEC, 7, 24
    meningitis, 7, 24
    urinary tract infection, 6, 23

Esophagitis, 67, 74, 120, 135
Eumycotic mycetoma, 68–69, 75–76

F

Fas, Fas ligand, 142, 148
Fimbriae, 6, 23
Flow cytometry, 35, 49
Flucytosine, 68, 74–75
Fluoroquinolone, mechanism of action,
    14, 29
Food poisoning, 138–139
Foscarnet, 50, 52
FoxP3 gene, 145, 153
Francisella tularensis, 115, 130
Fusarium, 66, 73

G

Ganciclovir, 50, 51, 58, 61
Gardnerella vaginalis, 123, 139
Gas gangrene, 20–21
Gastroenteritis, norovirus, 122, 138
Genital herpes, 41, 55
Gentamicin toxicity, 112, 128
Giardia lamblia, 88–89, 98, 103, 107,
    118–119, 133
Gonorrhea, *Neisseria gonorrhoeae*
    disseminated infection, 110, 125–126
    genital discharge, 136
    symptoms, 137
    treatment, 9, 25
    urethral exudate, 9, 25
Goodpasture syndrome, 158, 168
Granulocytes, 145, 152
Graves disease, 161, 172
Group A streptococci, see *Streptococcus
    pyogenes*
Group B streptococci, see *Streptococcus
    agalactiae*
Guillain–Barre syndrome, 160–161, 172

H

HACEK group endocarditis, 118–119,
    133–134
Haemophilus influenzae b, 2, 20
    epiglottitis, 119, 134
    meningitis, 11, 27
    vaccine, 2, 20, 11, 27
Hand, foot and mouth disease, 48, 62
Hantavirus pulmonary syndrome, 122,
    138
Haptens, 143, 149
Helicobacter pylori, 7, 24, 112, 127
    gastric adenocarcinoma, 7, 24
    virulence factors, 7, 12–13, 24, 28
Helminth infections, immunity to, 144,
    145, 151–152, 153
Hemolytic uremic syndrome (HUS), 4–5,
    7, 22, 24
Hemolytic disease of the newborn, 162,
    174

Hepatitis A virus, 121, 137
  diagnosis, 40, 54
  vaccination, 41, 54
Hepatitis B virus infection
  α-interferon, 38, 52
  acute infection, 38, 52
  chronic infection, 39, 52
  lamivudine, 38, 52
  perinatal infection, 38, 51–52
  transmission mode, 38, 52
  vaccination, 41, 55
Hepatitis C virus infection
  genotype testing, 41, 54
  RT-PCR, 41, 54
  transmission, 42–43, 56
  treatment, 41, 43, 54, 56
  window period, 40, 53
Hereditary angioedema, 155, 165
Herpes simplex virus, 44, 57
  cold sores, 36, 50
  neonatal disease, 121, 136–137
  primary infection, Type-1, 42, 55
  primary infection, Type-2, 42, 55
  recurrences and immune response, 42, 55–56
  replication, 44, 57
High endothelial venules (HEV), 146, 153
Histamine, 143, 150
Histoplasma capsulatum, 67, 74, 109, 110, 117, 125, 133
Hookworm
  microcytic anemia, 93, 105–106
  parasite eggs, 96, 107
Hortaea wernickii, 67, 74
Human herpes virus type 6, 38, 52
Human herpes virus type 8, 45, 58
Human immunodeficiency virus (HIV)
  acute retroviral syndrome, 43, 57
  co-receptors, 42, 56
  cytotoxic T lymphocytes and, 37, 50
  enfuvirtide, 41, 54
  epidemiology, 43, 56–57
  flow cytometry, 35, 49
  group-specific antigen, 46, 60
  HIV Vpr, 37–38, 51
  invasive cervical cancer and, 44, 57
  macrophages, 36, 50
  pol gene, 45, 58
  protease inhibitors, 124, 139
  reverse transcriptase inhibitors, 124, 139
  transcription factors and polymerases, 36, 50
  tuberculosis in HIV patients, 113, 128
  virus replication, 36, 44, 50, 57
  VZV and CD4 cells, 41, 54
  western blot and test sensitivity, 39, 52–53
Human parvovirus B-19, 35, 45–46, 49, 59
Humoral immune response, See B cells, Complement proteins, Immunoglobulins

Hydrops fetalis, 35, 49
Hymenolepis nana, 80–81, 100
Hyper-IgM syndrome, 156, 165–166

I

Imiquimode, 45, 58
Immune complex (IC) clearance, 145, 153
Immune hypersensitivity, 143, 149
Immunoglobulins
  IgA, 143, 144, 145, 150–151, 152
  IgE, 144, 151
  IgG, 143–144, 150
  IgM 143, 144, 150, 152
Impetigo 9–10, 15, 26, 30
Inactivated polio vaccine (IPV), 47–48, 61–62
Inflammatory response
  asthma, 163, 175
  interleukin-6, 155, 164
  tumor immunity, 160, 171
Infectious mononucleosis, 39–40, 53, 117, 132
Influenza virus, 37, 50–51, 39, 52
  antigenic changes, 47, 61
  vaccine, 47, 61
Interferon, antiviral effect, 37, 51
Interferon gamma (IFN-γ)
  isotype switching, 144, 150
  macrophage activation, 142, 148
  Mycobacterium tuberculosis, 143, 149
Interleukin-2, 141, 147
Interleukin-4, 144, 151–152
Interleukin-5, 144, 151–152
Interleukin 6, 155, 164
Interleukin-7, 141, 147
Interleukin-8, 144, 152
Isotype switching, 144, 150
Itraconazole, 66, 73, 118, 133

J

J chain, 150
JC virus, 46, 59

K

Kaposi sarcoma, 45, 58
Klebsiella pneumoniae, 6–7, 23–24

L

Legionella pneumophila
  intracellular growth, 2, 20
  pneumonia, 1, 14, 20, 30
Leishmaniasis, 97, 107
Leptospira interrogans, 13, 29, 116, 131
Leukocyte adhesion deficiency, 157, 167
  neutrophil diapedesis, 160, 171
Leukopenia, 157, 166
Linezolid, 112, 128
Listeria monocytogenes, 19, 34

Lyme disease, 5, 23
Lymphocyte migration, 146, 153
Lymphocytes, see B cells, Natural Killer cells, T cells

M

M antigens, 11, 27
M protein, 18, 33
MacConkey agar, 16, 31
Macrophages,
  activation of, 142, 148
  cytokine secretion, 142, 148
  intracellular killing mechanism, 142, 149
Major histocompatibility molecules, see also Antigen presentation, 145, 152
Malaria, 90–91, 104
Mantoux test, 158, 168–169
Mast cells, 143, 149–150
Measles virus, 40, 53–54
Measles, mumps, rubella (MMR) vaccine, 39, 53
Meningitis
  Cryptococcus neoformans, 63, 70, 72, 76, 114, 129
  CSF findings, 130, 131
  diagnosis, 124, 140
  Escherichia coli, 7, 24
  Haemophilus influenzae b, 11, 27
  mumps virus, 112, 127–128
  Naegleria fowleri, 98, 107–108
  Neisseria meningitidis, 1–2, 11, 16, 20, 26, 32, 110, 126
  signs and symptoms, 114, 129–130
  Streptococcus agalactiae, 111, 126
  tuberculosis meningitis, 115, 130
  viral, 115, 130–131
Metagonimus yokogawai, 86, 102
Methicillin-resistant *Staphylococcus aureus,* 3, 21
Metronidazole, 14, 30, 111,127
Microsporum canis, 64–65, 72
Molluscum contagiosum, 44, 58
Montelukast, 159, 169
Moraxella catarrhalis, 18, 34
Multiple myeloma, 162, 174
Multiple sclerosis (MS)
  matrix metalloproteases in, 156, 166
  oligoclonal IgG bands, CSF, 155, 164
  remission, 158, 168
Mumps virus, 39, 53, 112, 127–128
Myasthenia gravis, 159–160, 170
Mycetoma, 4, 21
Mycobacterium avium complex, 19, 34
Mycobacterium tuberculosis
  BCG vaccine, 18, 33
  miliary tuberculosis, 115, 130
  tuberculosis, 17, 32
    hemoptysis, 123, 140
    isoniazid, 124, 140
    meningitis, 114, 129

PPD test, 155, 164–165
  signs and symptoms, 111, 127
  treatment, 112, 127
  virulence, 112, 127
  transmission, 119, 135
Mycology
Myocarditis
  Coxsackievirus B, 44, 57, 118, 133
  diphtheria toxin interaction, 15, 31
  Trypanosoma cruzi, 121, 136
Mycoplasma pneumoniae, 14, 29

N

Naegleria fowleri, 98, 107–108
Natural killer (NK) cells, 35, 49, 142,
    145, 149, 152
Negative selection, 141, 144, 147, 151
Neisseria gonorrhoeae
  antigenic variation, 14, 30
  genital discharge, 136
  manifestations, 110, 125
  symptoms, 137
  urethral exudate, 9, 25
Neisseria meningitidis
  ciprofloxacin, 110, 126
  latex agglutination, 123, 140
  lipooligosaccharides, 1–2, 20
  meningitis, 16, 32
  prophylaxis, 110, 126
  treatment, 16, 32
  septic arthritis, 11, 26
  vaccination, 16, 32, 109, 125
Neurocysticercosis, 92, 105
Neutralizing antibody, 147
Neutrophils, 144, 145, 152, 153
Nitroblue tetrazolium (NBT) test,
    156, 166
Nocardia asteroides, 114, 129
Norovirus, 123, 138
Northern blot, 35, 49
Nosocomial pneumonia, 116, 131
Nucleoside analogs, 38, 51
Nystatin, 64, 72

O

Ocular larval migrans, 85, 102
Oligoclonal IgG bands, CSF, 155, 164
Oncocerca volvulus, 8, 103
Onychomycosis, 65, 73
Opsonization, 152
Oral polio vaccine (OPV), 47–48, 61–62
Oral rehydration therapy, 119, 134
Orientia tsutsugamushi, 4, 22
Oseltamivir, 37, 50–51
Osteomyelitis, 70, 76

P

Papillomavirus, 45, 46, 58, 59
  vaccine, 46, 59
Paragonimus westermani, 85, 102
Parainfluenza virus
  croup, 39, 53, 110, 126

Poxvirus, 44, 58
Parenteral epinephrine, 157, 167
Parvovirus B-19, 35, 45–46, 49, 59
Pasteurella multocida, 13, 28–29
Pattern recognition receptors, 144, 151
Pediculosis capitis, 85, 96, 101–102, 107
Pelvic inflammatory disease, 14, 29
Pemphigus vulgaris, 163, 174
Penciclovir, 36, 50
Penicillin-binding proteins, 18, 33
Peptic ulcer disease, 7, 24, 112, 127
Perforin, 142, 149
Permethrin, 115, 130
Pernicious anemia, 161, 173
Pertussis, 12, 28, 117, 132
Pharyngitis, 110, 116, 126, 131
Phthirus pubis, 84, 101
Plague, 13, 29
Plasmaphoresis, 158, 168
Plasmodium falciparum, 90, 104
Plasmodium vivax, 90–91, 104
Pneumocystis jiroveci, 71, 77
Pneumonia
  Adenovirus, 40, 53
  Aspergillus, 114, 130
  Candida albicans, 66, 73
  Chlamydophila pneumoniae, 14, 29
  Klebsiella pneumoniae, 6–7, 23–24
  Legionella 1, 14, 20, 30
  Nocardia 114, 129
  Nosocomial, 116, 131
  Pneumocystis jiroveci, 71, 77
  Psuedomonas aeruginosa, 117, 131
  Respiratory syncytial virus, 40, 54
  Treatment, 15, 30, 109, 125
Pneumocystis jiroveci, 71, 77, 111, 126
Poison ivy rash, Th1 cells, 143, 149
Poliomyelitis
  eradication program, 123, 139
  OPV and IPV, 47–48, 61–62
  transmission, 120, 135
Polyglandular autoimmune syndrome
    Type-1, AIRE, 161, 171–172
Positive selection, 141, 147
Postherpetic neuralgia (PHN), 37, 51,
    118, 133
Post-streptococcal glomerulonephritis,
    9–10, 26, 121, 137
Poxvirus, 44, 58
Praziquantel
  intestinal tapeworm infection, 81–82,
    100
  Schistosoma mansoni, 87, 102
Primary amebic meningoencephalitis, 98,
    107–108
Prion diseases, 135
Progressive multifocal
    leukoencephalopathy, 46, 59
Propionibacterium acne, 111, 126
Protease inhibitors,
  mechanism of action, 124, 139
  toxicity, 124, 139–140
Proteus mirabilis, 6, 23

Pseudomonas aeruginosa
  burn infection, 13, 29
  cystic fibrosis (CF), 3, 21
  malignant otitis externa, 116, 131
  pneumonia, 117, 131
  treatment, 113, 128
  wound infection, 113, 128
Psoriasis, 162, 173
Pulmonary-renal syndrome, *(see)*
    Goodpasture syndrome;
    Wegener granulomatosis
Pyoderma, 121, 137
Pyrazinamide toxicity, 120, 134–135

R

Rabies virus, 36, 50
Ramsey Hunt syndrome, 118, 133
Rebuck skin window test, 157, 167
Renal transplantation
  immune suppression, 159, 169
  T-cell polyclonal activation, 159,
    169–170
Respiratory syncytial virus
  bronchiolitis, 119, 134
  fusion protein and palivizumab, 41,
    54–55
  pneumonia, 40, 54
Rh factor incompatibility, 162, 174
Rheumatic fever, 11, 17–18, 27, 32–33,
    119, 124, 133, 140
Rheumatoid arthritis (RA), 160, 171
Rheumatoid factor test, 155, 164
Rhinocerebral mucormycosis, 71, 77
Rhinocerebral zygomycosis, 64, 72
Rhinovirus, 122, 137–138
Ribavirin, mechanism of action, 43, 56
Rickettsia rickettsii, 4, 21–22, 7, 24
River blindness, 88, 103
Rocky Mountain spotted fever, 4, 7,
    21–22, 24, 115, 130
Roseola, 38, 52
Rotavirus, 119, 134
  rotavirus vaccine, 45, 59, 120, 134
Rubella virus
  congenital rubella syndrome, 47, 60–61

S

Sabouraud dextrose agar, fungal culture,
    65, 72–73
Salmonella, 10, 26
Salmonella typhi, 12, 28, 111, 126–127
Sarcoptes scabiei, 92, 94, 104–105, 106,
    114, 130
Schistosoma haematobium, 86, 102
Schistosoma mansoni, 86–87, 102
schistosomiasis
  endemicity, 86, 102
  transmission, 87, 102–103
Scrapie, 120, 135
Scrub typhus, 4, 22
Secretory piece, IgA, 144, 150
Selective IgA deficiency, 156, 166

Serratia marcescens, 10–11, 26
Severe acute respiratory syndrome
(SARS), 46, 60
Severe combined immunodeficiency, 157,
166
Shigella dysenteriae, 5, 22–23
Shigella flexneri, 10, 26
Shigella sonnei, 16, 32, 113, 128–129
Shingles, see also Varicella-zoster virus,
37, 41, 51, 54, 118, 133
Smallpox virus, 46, 59, 122, 138
Sporothrix schenckii, 66, 73, 75
Staphylococcus aureus
catalase test, 3, 21
cephalexin, 30
clindamycin for treatment, 16, 32
coagulase test, 8, 25
food contamination, 18, 33
MRSA, 3, 21
vancomycin resistance, 34
Staphylococcus epidermidis, 15, 31
biofilm production, 15, 31
Streptococci
Group A, see *Streptococcus pyogenes*
Group B, see *Streptococcus agalactiae*
Streptococcus agalactiae, 111, 123, 126,
138
Streptococcus pneumoniae
penicillin resistance, 18, 33
pneumoniae, 18, 33
Streptococcus pyogenes, 118, 133
cellulitis, 14, 30
gomerulonephritis, 9–10, 26
impetigo, 9–10, 26
pharyngitis, 11, 27, 116, 131
rheumatic fever, 11, 17–18, 27, 32–33
Stevens–Johnson syndrome, 28, 109, 125
Streptokinase, 14, 30
Strongyloides stercoralis, 93, 106
Struvite stones, 6, 23
Superantigens, 144, 151
Systemic lupus erythematosus (SLE)
antinuclear antibody test, 164
double-stranded DNA, antibodies,
161, 172
hydroxychloroquine, 161, 172
Syphillis, 8, 13, 25, 29

T

T cells
activation, 141–142, 146, 147–148,
153
anergy, 142, 148
CD154 expression, 156, 165
cytotoxic T cells, 142, 149
differentiation in thymus, 141, 147
down-regulation, 142, 148
Fas (CD95), 142, 148
Pneumocystis jeroveci infection and,
156, 165–166
polyclonal activation, 159, 169–170

proliferation, IL–2, 141, 147
psoriasis, 162, 173
regulatory, 145, 152
Th1 cells
delayed type hypersensitivity
(DTH), 143, 149, 157, 166–167
downregulation, 168
tuberculosis, 143, 149, 155,
164–165
Th2 cells, 142, 149
viral and fungal infections and, 158,
167–168
Taenia saginata, 82, 100
Taenia solium
cysticercosis, 83, 92, 101, 105
gastrointestinal disease, 80, 99
meningoencephalitis, 98, 107–108
Terbinafine, 65, 73
Tetanus toxoid vaccine, 8, 25
Thrush, 64, 72
Tickborne encephalitis, 46, 59
Tickborne relapsing fever, 8, 24
Tinea capitis, 68, 75
Tinea corporis, 65, 72–73
Tolerance mechanism, 141, 142, 144, 147,
148, 151
Tolerogens, 144, 151
Toxocara canis, 85, 102
Toxoplasma gondii, 112, 128
Trachoma, 11, 27
Transplantation, 159, 169–170
Treponema pallidum, 8, 13, 25, 29
Triatoma infestans, 95, 106
Trichina nativa, 79, 99
Trichinella spiralis, 79, 99
Trichomonas vaginalis, 95, 107
Trichuris trichiura
albendazole, 89, 103
pseudoappendicitis, 88, 103
rectal prolapse, 93, 105
Trypanosoma brucei, 96, 107
Trypanosome cruzi 94–95, 106, 121, 136
Tuberculosis, see also *Mycobacterium
tuberculosis,* 17, 32
and HIV, 113, 128
hemoptysis, 123, 140
isoniazid, 124, 140
Mantoux skin test, 158, 168
meningitis, 115, 130
miliary tuberculosis, 115, 130
signs and symptoms, 111, 127
treatment, 112, 127
virulence, 112, 127
transmission, 119, 135
Tularemia, 115, 130
Tumor necrosis factor-alpha, 155, 165
Tumors, immunity to, 160, 170–171
Type I interferons, 37, 51
Type I hypersensitivity, 143, 149–150
Type IV hypersensitivity, 143, 149
Typhoid fever, *Salmonella typhi,* 12, 28,
111, 126–127

U

Uncoating process
influenza virus, 36, 50
Urea breath test, 112, 127
Urinary tract infection
Enterococcus faecalis, 18, 33–34
Escherichia coli, 6, 16, 23, 31
Proteus mirabilis, 6, 23
Serratia marcescens, 10–11, 26
treatment, 12, 27–28, 109, 125

V

Vaccinia virus vaccine, 46, 59,
122, 138
Vaccination, see also individual
organisms and diseases,
141, 147
Vaginal discharge, 121, 175
Vaginitis
bacterial, 123, 139
candidal, 69, 76, 120, 136
Trichomonas vaginalis, 95, 107
Varicella-zoster virus, 37, 51, 118, 133
Variant Creutzfeldt-Jacob Disease, 120,
135
Vibrio cholerae, 13, 29
Vibrio vulnificus, 19, 34
Viridans group streptococci
endocarditis, 17, 32
Virus replication cycle, 35, 49
Voriconazole, 71, 76, 124, 140

W

Wegener granulomatosis, 163, 174–175
Weil disease, *Leptospira interrogans,* 13,
29, 115, 131
West Nile virus (WNV), 46, 60
Whipworm
albendazole, 89, 103
pseudoappendicitis, 88, 103
rectal prolapse, 93, 105
Wiscott–Aldrich syndrome (WAS), 162,
173
Wuchereria bancrofti, 88, 103

X

X-linked agammaglobulinemia 156, 159,
165, 170

Y

Yeasts, 67, 73
Yellow fever virus, 45, 58
Yersinia pestis, 13, 29
Yersinia enterocolitica, 19, 34

Z

Zanamivir, 39, 52